Mast Cells

METHODS IN MOLECULAR BIOLOGY™

John M. Walker, SERIES EDITOR

METHODS IN MOLECULAR BIOLOGY™

Mast Cells

Methods and Protocols

Edited by

Guha Krishnaswamy
David S. Chi

Quillen College of Medicine,
James H. Quillen Veterans Affairs Medical Center,
East Tennessee State University, Johnson City, TN

HUMANA PRESS ✳ TOTOWA, NEW JERSEY

© 2006 Humana Press Inc.
999 Riverview Drive, Suite 208
Totowa, New Jersey 07512

www.humanapress.com

This publication is printed on acid-free paper. ∞
ANSI Z39.48-1984 (American Standards Institute)

Permanence of Paper for Printed Library Materials.

Production Editor: Jennifer Hackworth

Cover design by Patricia F. Cleary

Cover illustration: Scanning electron microscopic photograph of mast cells taken by Fred E. Hossler, PhD, using cells generated in Guha Krishnaswamy's laboratory. Artwork provided by Guha Krishnaswamy.

For additional copies, pricing for bulk purchases, and/or information about other Humana titles, contact Humana at the above address or at any of the following numbers: Tel.: 973-256-1699; Fax: 973-256-8341; E-mail: orders@humanapr.com; or visit our Website: www.humanapress.com

Printed in the United States of America. 10 9 8 7 6 5 4 3 2 1
1-59259-967-2 (e-book)
ISSN 1064-3745

Library of Congress Cataloging-in-Publication Data

Mast cells : methods and protocols / edited by Guha Krishnaswamy, David S. Chi.
    p. ; cm. – (Methods in molecular biology ; 315)
  Includes bibliographical references and index.
  ISBN 1-58829-374-2 (alk. paper)
 1. Mast cells–Laboratory manuals.
 [DNLM: 1. Mast Cells. 2. Cell Communication. 3. Cell Culture
Techniques. 4. Gene Expression. 5. Immunity. 6. Inflammation. QS
532.5.C7 M4238 2005] I. Krishnaswamy, Guha. II. Chi, David S. III. Series:
Methods in molecular biology (Clifton, N.J.) ; v. 315.
  QR185.8.M35M373 2005
  612.1'12–dc22
                                                                    2005006271

Dedication

I would like to dedicate this book to my father, Dr. Narayanaswamy Krishnaswamy, MBBS, an immunologist and clinician extraordinaire, who encouraged me to enter academic medicine, and who continues to inspire me with his clinical acumen, wide-armed compassion, and his practical yet gentle wisdom.

Guha Krishnaswamy

Preface

Mast cells are multifunctional, tissue-dwelling cells consisting of two well-described subsets, MC_T and MC_{TC} cells. They are distinguished on the basis of their tissue location, T-lymphocyte dependence, and ability to synthesize granule contents such as tryptase and chymase. Following activation, these cells express mediators, such as histamine, leukotrienes, and prostanoids, proteases, and various cytokines and chemokines, all of which are pivotal to the genesis of an inflammatory response. By their interaction with endothelium, macrophages, fibroblasts, and B and T cells, mast cells further amplify the inflammatory cascade. Mast cells directly interact with bacteria and appear to play a vital role in host defense against pathogens. Additionally, recent data suggests that mast cells may play an active role in such diverse diseases as asthma, pulmonary fibrosis, atherosclerosis, malignancy, and arthritis. As research in mast cells has expanded exponentially, a technical procedure manual for working with these cells is timely. Thus, the aim of *Mast Cells: Methods and Protocols* is to present selected molecular and cellular techniques used in studying various aspects of this fascinating, multifunctional cell.

Mast Cells: Methods and Protocols follows the objective of the *Methods in Molecular Biology* series to present step-by-step protocols that can be easily applied in the laboratory. Although it is impossible to present all mast cell research protocols, this book attempts to cover a range of procedures that provides a sound base of methodology for mast cell research. *Mast Cells: Methods and Protocols* has been divided into nine parts. Part I consists of three chapters presenting a review and the history of mast cells. Part II reviews techniques used frequently in the identification of mast cells. Part III provides protocols for the development of mast cells in vitro. Part IV offers methods for studying mast cell signaling and gene expression. Part V reviews various techniques of measuring mast cell expression of inflammatory mediators. Part VI suggests methods for studying mast cell interactions with other cell types. Part VII introduces novel aspects of mast cell activation and regulation, and Part VIII analyzes various methodologies used to study roles of mast cells in host defense. Part IX reviews techniques that have been utilized to study mast cell apoptosis.

We hope that this collection of mast cell protocols will provide researchers with basic techniques for their own mast cell studies. We would like to take this opportunity to thank the series editor, John Walker, and the staff at Humana Press for their invitation and assistance in pursuing the publication of this book. We also want to express our sincere appreciation and gratitude to the contributing authors for taking time off their busy schedules to provide these excellent chapters. Finally, we wish to acknowledge the superb secretarial assistance of Dolores Moore.

Guha Krishnaswamy
David S. Chi

Contents

Contributors

SOMAN N. ABRAHAM • *Departments of Pathology, Molecular Genetics and Microbiology, and Immunology, Duke University Medical Center, Durham, NC*

OMAR AJITAWI • *Department of Internal Medicine, Quillen College of Medicine, East Tennessee State University, Johnson City, TN*

STEPHEN C. ARMSTRONG • *Cardiovascular Research Institute, University of South Dakota School of Medicine, Sioux Falls, SD*

IDO BACHELET • *Department of Pharmacology, School of Pharmacy, Faculty of Medicine, The Hebrew University of Jerusalem, Jerusalem, Israel*

ANN L. BALDWIN • *Department of Physiology, University of Arizona, Tucson, AZ*

STEPHAN C. BISCHOFF • *Chair of Clinical Nutrition and Immunology, University of Hohenheim, Stuttgart, Germany*

JEAN-YVES BONNEFOY • *Transgene, Strasbourg, France*

KEVIN F. BREUEL • *Department of OB/GYN, Quillen College of Medicine, East Tennessee State University, Johnson City, TN*

MELISSA A. BROWN • *Department of Microbiology and Immunology, Northwestern University School of Medicine, Chicago, IL*

DAVID S. CHI • *Department of Internal Medicine, Quillen College of Medicine, East Tennessee State University, Johnson City, TN*

ISABELLE COGNET • *Département de Pharmacologie, Université de Montréal, Montreal, Canada*

W. KEITH DE PONTI • *Department of OB/GYN, Quillen College of Medicine, East Tennessee State University, Johnson City, TN*

KOTTARAPPAT N. DILEEPAN • *Department of Internal Medicine, University of Kansas Medical Center, Kansas City, KS*

GREG C. ELSON • *Hybridoma Technologies Section, NovImmune SA, Geneva, Switzerland*

MARK L. ENTMAN • *Section of Cardiovascular Sciences, Department of Medicine, Baylor College of Medicine, Houston, TX*

S. MATTHEW FITZGERALD • *Department of Internal Medicine, Quillen College of Medicine, East Tennessee State University, Johnson City, TN*

STEFAN FLORIAN • *Department of Internal Medicine I, Division of Hematology and Hemostaseology, University of Vienna, Vienna, Austria*

NIKOLAOS G. FRANGOGIANNIS • *Section of Cardiovascular Sciences, Department of Medicine, Baylor College of Medicine, Houston, TX*

JEAN-FRANÇOIS GAUCHAT • *Département de Pharmacologie, Université de Montréal, Montreal, Canada*

ALEXANDER GERBAULET • *Department of Dermatology, University of Cologne, Cologne, Germany*

GREGORY D. GREGORY • *Graduate Program in Immunology and Molecular Pathogenesis, Emory University School of Medicine, Atlanta, GA*

ANGÉLIQUE GUAY-GIROUX • *Département de Pharmacologie, Université de Montréal, Montreal, Canada*

PAUL GUGLIELMI • *Institut National de la Santé et de la Recherche Médicale, Unite 454, Centre Hospitalier Universitaire Arnauld de Villeneuve, Montpellier, France*

FLORENCE GUILHOT • *Département de Pharmacologie, Université de Montréal, Montreal, Canada*

TUANZHU HA • *Department of Surgery, Quillen College of Medicine, East Tennessee State University, Johnson City, TN*

KARIN HARTMANN • *Department of Dermatology, University of Cologne, Cologne, Germany*

ALEXANDER W. HAUSWIRTH • *Department of Internal Medicine I, Division of Hematology and Hemostaseology, Medical University of Vienna, Vienna, Austria*

GREGORY HEMONTOLOR • *Department of Internal Medicine, Quillen College of Medicine, East Tennessee State University, Johnson City, TN*

FRED E. HOSSLER • *Department of Anatomy and Cell Biology, Quillen College of Medicine, East Tennessee State University, Johnson City, TN*

SHAU-KU HUANG • *Asthma and Allergy Center, Johns Hopkins University School of Medicine, Baltimore, MD*

DAVID A. JOHNSON • *Department of Biochemistry and Molecular Biology, Quillen College of Medicine, East Tennessee State University, Johnson City, TN*

TOSHIAKI KAWAKAMI • *Division of Cell Biology, La Jolla Institute for Allergy and Immunology, San Diego, CA*

YUKO KAWAKAMI • *Division of Cell Biology, La Jolla Institute for Allergy and Immunology, San Diego, CA*

JIM KELLEY • *Department of Internal Medicine, Quillen College of Medicine, East Tennessee State University, Johnson City, TN*

ARNOLD S. KIRSHENBAUM • *Laboratory of Allergic Diseases, Mast Cell Biology Section, NIH/NIAID, Bethesda, MD*

JIRO KITAURA • *Division of Cellular Therapy, Advanced Clinical Research Center, Institute of Medical Science, University of Tokyo, Tokyo, Japan*

MARIA-THERESA KRAUTH • *Department of Internal Medicine I, Division of Hematology and Hemostaseology, Medical University of Vienna, Vienna, Austria*

GUHA KRISHNASWAMY • *Division of Allergy and Immunology, Department of Internal Medicine, James H. Quillen VAMC and the Quillen College of Medicine, East Tennessee State University, Johnson City, TN*

JACQUELINE M. LANGDON • *The Johns Hopkins Asthma and Allergy Center, Department of Medicine, Johns Hopkins University School of Medicine, Baltimore, MD*

FRANCESCA LEVI-SCHAFFER • *Department of Pharmacology, School of Pharmacy, Faculty of Medicine, The Hebrew University of Jerusalem, Jerusalem, Israel*

CHUANFU LI • *Department of Surgery, Quillen College of Medicine, East Tennessee State University, Johnson City, TN*

SUSAN M. MACDONALD • *The Johns Hopkins Asthma and Allergy Center, Department of Medicine, Johns Hopkins University School of Medicine, Baltimore, MD*

JAMES B. MCLACHLAN • *Department of Pathology, Duke University, Durham, NC*

YOSEPH A. MEKORI • *Department of Medicine B, Meir General Hospital, Sackler School of Medicine, Tel-Aviv University, Kfar-Saba, Israel*

DEAN D. METCALFE • *Laboratory of Allergic Diseases, Mast Cell Biology Section, NIH/NIAID, Bethesda, MD*

DENISE M. MILHORN • *Department of Internal Medicine, Quillen College of Medicine, East Tennessee State University, Johnson City, TN*

LOU ELLEN MILLER • *Department of Pathology, Quillen College of Medicine, East Tennessee State University, Johnson City, TN*

ARIEL MUNITZ • *Department of Pharmacology, School of Pharmacy, Faculty of Medicine, The Hebrew University of Jerusalem, Jerusalem, Israel*

JÉRÔME PÈNE • *Institut National de la Santé et de la Recherche Médicale, Unite 454, Centre Hospitalier Universitaire Arnauld de Villeneuve, Montpellier, France*

ZHENHONG QU • *Department of Pathology and Laboratory Medicine, University of Texas Health Science Center in Houston, Houston, TX*

MIN QUI • *Department of Pediatrics, Quillen College of Medicine, East Tennessee State University, Johnson City, TN*

HIROHISA SAITO • *Department of Allergy and Immunology, National Research Institute for Child Health and Development, Okura, Setagaya-ku, Tokyo, Japan*

GERIT-HOLGER SCHERNTHANER • *Department of Internal Medicine II, Division of Angiology, Medical University of Vienna, Vienna, Austria*

EDGAR SCHMITT • *Institute for Immunology, Johannes Gutenberg-University, Mainz, Germany*

LAWRENCE B. SCHWARTZ • *Department of Internal Medicine, Virginia Commonwealth University, Richmond, VA*

GERNOT SELLGE • *Department of Cell Biology and Infection, Institute Pasteur, Paris, France*

CHRISTOPHER P. SHELBURNE • *Department of Pathology, Duke University, Durham, NC*

SHRUTI A. SHUKLA • *Department of Pathology, Quillen College of Medicine, East Tennessee State University, Johnson City, TN*

KAROLINE SONNECK • *Department of Internal Medicine I, Division of Hematology and Hemostaseology, Medical University of Vienna, Vienna, Austria*

WOLFGANG R. SPERR • *Department of Internal Medicine I, Division of Hematology and Hemostaseology, Medical University of Vienna, Vienna, Austria*

MICHAEL STASSEN • *Institute for Immunology, Johannes Gutenberg-University, Mainz, Germany*

DANIEL J. STECHSCHULTE • *Department of Internal Medicine, University of Kansas Medical Center, Kansas City, KS*

WILLIAM L. STONE • *Department of Pediatrics, Quillen College of Medicine, East Tennessee State University, Johnson City, TN*

CHARLES A. STUART • *Department of Internal Medicine, Quillen College of Medicine, East Tennessee State University, Johnson City, TN*

TSUNG-HSIEN TSAI • *Division of Allergy and Clinical Immunology, Johns Hopkins University School of Medicine, Baltimore, MD*

PETER VALENT • *Department of Internal Medicine I, Division of Hematology and Hemostaseology, Medical University of Vienna, Vienna, Austria*

ANGELA VALEVA • *Institute of Medical Microbiology and Hygiene, Johannes Gutenberg-University, Mainz, Germany*

RANJITHA VEERAPPAN • *Department of Pathology, Quillen College of Medicine, East Tennessee State University, Johnson City, TN*

HARSHA VYAS • *Department of Internal Medicine, Quillen College of Medicine, East Tennessee State University, Johnson City, TN*

IWAN WALEV • *Institute of Medical Microbiology and Hygiene, Johannes Gutenberg-University, Mainz, Germany*

ELAINE S. WALKER • *James H. Quillen VAMC, and Department of Internal Medicine, Quillen College of Medicine, East Tennessee State University, Johnson City, TN*

JUDY S. WHITTIMORE • *Department of Pathology, Quillen College of Medicine, East Tennessee State University, Johnson City, TN*

HONGSONG YANG • *Department of Pediatrics, Quillen College of Medicine, East Tennessee State University, Johnson City, TN*

DELING YIN • *Department of Internal Medicine, Quillen College of Medicine, East Tennessee State University, Johnson City, TN*

GEORGE A. YOUNGBERG • *James H. Quillen VAMC, and Department of Pathology, Quillen College of Medicine, East Tennessee State University, Johnson City, TN*

WALID YOUNIS • *Department of Internal Medicine, Quillen College of Medicine, East Tennessee State University, Johnson City, TN*

HANS YSSEL • *Institut National de la Santé et de la Recherche Medicale, Unite 454, Centre Hospitalier Universitaire Arnauld de Villeneuve, Montpellier, France*

I

OVERVIEW OF MAST CELL BIOLOGY

1

Paul Ehrlich's "Mastzellen"— From Aniline Dyes to DNA Chip Arrays

A Historical Review of Developments in Mast Cell Research

Harsha Vyas and Guha Krishnaswamy

Summary

It has been more than a century since the discovery of the mast cell by the genius and tenacity of Paul Ehrlich, who described this cell when he was a medical student. One cannot deny that this discovery also coincides with the golden age of immunology. The discovery of this important cell type in immunological history was no serendipity: it was a result of Ehrlich's prodigious laboratory talent and his ability to combine intuition and deduction despite the limited resources of his times. Since then, we have learned much more about the immune response, immunoglobulin E, and the development and function of mast cells in various pathological states. What follows is a review of Paul Ehrlich's discovery of the mast cell (mästzellen) and a chronological review of subsequent developments in mast cell research, including the recent use of proteomics and genomics to understand mast cell biology.

Key Words: Mast cells; immunoglobulin E; cytokine; gene expression; host defense; inflammation; history.

1. Ehrlich's "Mastzellen"

Paul Ehrlich (**Fig. 1**) is credited with the initial discovery of mast cells (**Fig. 2**) as we know them today. He was born near Breslau, now known as Wroclaw, Poland, in 1854. He studied to become a medical doctor at the university in Breslau, followed by training in Strasbourg, Freiburg, and Leipzig *(1)*. Ehrlich was greatly influenced by his cousin, Karl Weigert, an eminent histopathologist who pioneered the use of aniline dyes for staining bacteria and tissue sections *(1)*. Weigert had a strong and positive influence throughout Ehrlich's life *(1a)*. As a result, even as a medical student, Ehrlich had a precocious knowledge of structural organic chemistry and a fascination with dyes as probes of

From: *Methods in Molecular Biology, vol. 315: Mast Cells: Methods and Protocols*
Edited by: G. Krishnaswamy and D. S. Chi © Humana Press Inc., Totowa, NJ

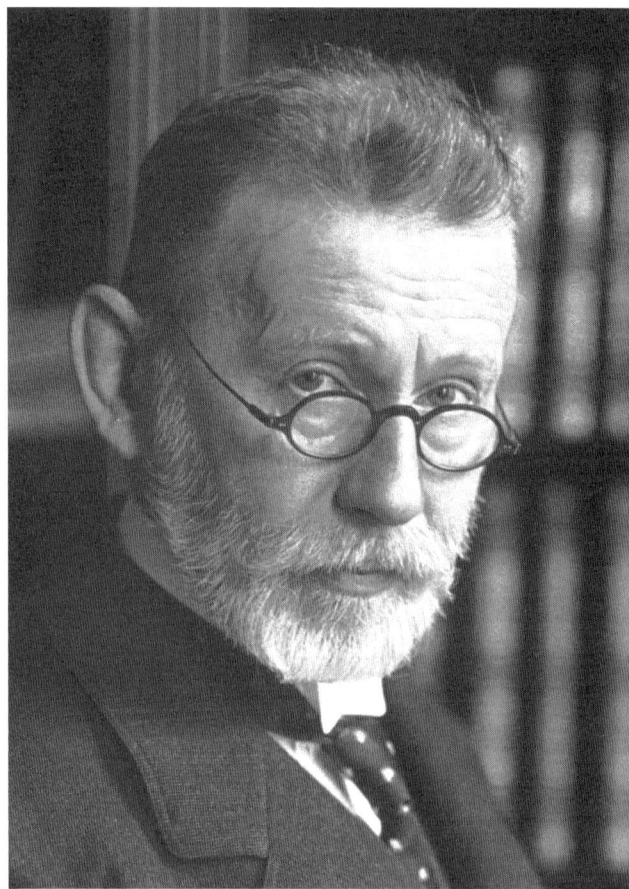

EHRLICH, Paul
Nobel Laureate PHYSIOLOGY OR MEDICINE 1908
© Nobelstiftelsen

Fig. 1. Picture of Paul Ehrlich (courtesy of © The Nobel Foundation).

cellular activity *(1a)*. He already was exposed to the idea that organic chemicals can have differential and specific reactions with various tissues and bacteria.

On June 17, 1878, Ehrlich's date with history was set. On that day, the 24-yr-old medical student presented his doctoral thesis, "Contributions to the theory and practice of histological staining," to the Medical Faculty of Leipzig. The medical student divided his thesis into two halves. In the first part, he talked about the chemical basis of many important histological reactions. In the second part, he gave a detailed discussion about aniline dyes *(1)*. The first description of the mast cell comes in the portion of the thesis dedicated to the

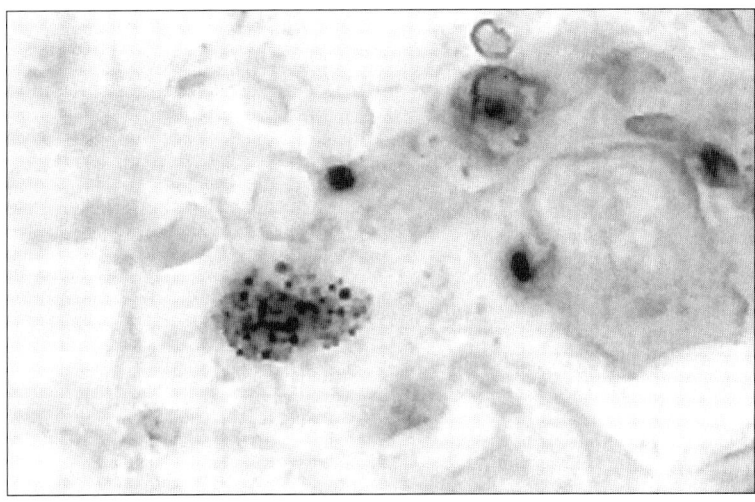

Fig. 2. Mast cell in atheromatous plaque (courtesy of George Youngberg, MD, East Tennessee State University).

histological applications of the aniline dyes. He presented his point of view that "aniline dyes displayed an absolutely characteristic behavior towards protoplasmic deposits of certain cells," which he called "mastzellen." He sought to distinguish these cells from the Waldeyer's "plasmazellen"—a heterogeneous category of cells described previously by Waldeyer *(1)*.

Ehrlich said that these anilophilic cells, from the descriptive point of view, should be most conveniently described as "granular cells of the connective tissue." He said that from a physiological standpoint, these cells might represent a "further development of the fixed cells of the connective tissue." He also provided a clarification to support his theory: aniline-reactive cells indeed "have a tendency to collect around developing preformed structures in the connective tissue." He said that granular cells are characterized by an "undetermined chemical substance" in the protoplasm with which the aniline dye reacts to give a typical metachromasia *(1)*. To this day, although by no means absolute, mast cells are recognized by the presence of metachromatic granules, when fixed and stained with toluidine blue. Further in his dissertation, Ehrlich provided an extremely accurate description of the microscopic features of the mast cell. He described that the typical aspect of these "granular cells" is mostly unstained protoplasm filled with numerous granules of varying size and a nucleus not mostly stainable, even in samples that otherwise display beautiful nuclear staining. Ehrlich strove to classify these cells using specific histochemical reactions rather than histology, a very progressive concept for his time.

A historically interesting aspect is how Ehrlich decided to call these cells the "mastzellen," or mast cell, as these were plump-appearing cells (well-fed cells). "Mast" may be derived from Greek, which meant breast or from the German "mastung" (from "masticate"). In today's research, mast cells are being increasingly recognized for their role in connective tissue remodeling and repair *(1)*. We now know that their granules contain many proteases and cytokines that are known to exert far reaching effects on other cells types, such as the smooth muscle, fibroblasts, and endothelial cells (much of this is reviewed in later chapters of this book).

Ehrlich also noted that mast cells sometimes localize far from the blood vessels and express a series of biological function not related to vascular functions. He also said that mast cells could be found around developing tissues. The close relationship between mast cell and tumor growth stems from this very same idea. Sadly, the original text of this remarkable work was destroyed in an air raid on Leipzig in 1943. Ehrlich subsequently moved to the Charité Hospital in Berlin, where he continued his work and wrote an influential thesis on the oxygen requirement of cells. In January 1879, the Physiological Society of Berlin reviewed the remarkable paper by Paul Ehrlich about the mast cells that he had discovered as a medical student 2 yr earlier. Ehrlich, in these papers, pointed out that mast cells exhibit a great avidity to basic dyes and characteristically altered the shade of the dye *(1)*.

In 1891 along with Westphal, one of his pupils, he showed another characteristic feature of the mast cell granules in many species, namely the water solubility. Almost 50 yr later, Michcals wrote that "uncounted pages of useless and misleading research have been a result of failure on the part of many investigators to heed the admonition originally given by Ehrlich and Westphal, that mast cell granules are soluble in water and that to preserve them, tissues must be fixed in 50% alcohol and stained in alcoholic thionine" *(1)*.

Ehrlich then studied the special affinity of leucocytes for various dyes. In 1891, he had discovered basophilic granular cells in human blood with myeloid leukemia. Ehrlich was quick to infer with his characteristic insight that, in higher species, especially humans, the human mast cells are actually leucocytes arising from precursor cells in the bone marrow. He believed that there were two types of mast cells: the first located in connective tissue and the second with their origin in the bone marrow and localized in the peripheral blood. In 1900, Jolly had established the bone marrow origin for the mast cells. Hence, by the time his textbook (Ehrlich and Lazarus, 1898) was revised in 1909, human mast cell origins were better understood. It is now accepted that mast cells arise from a pluripotent cell in the bone marrow that expresses CD43, *c-kit,* and CD13.

Ehrlich also led the way in observing mast cells in two pathological situations of utmost importance—chronic inflammation and neoplasia. He felt that in both these situations the tissue was "overnourished" because of lymph stasis and that there was an accumulation of tissue fluid rich in nutriments. This state led the mast cells to convert some of this abundant extracellular fluid to specific intracellular granules *(1)*. Thus, according to Ehrlich, mast cells served as an "indices for the nutritional status of the connective tissue," increased and decreased during periods of hypernutrition and starvation. Ehrlich and his pupil Westphal found that mast cells accumulated in many tumors, more so in the periphery of carcinomatous tumors than the substance of the tumor. Besides the discovery of the mast cell, Ehrlich made pioneering contributions to the method of staining the bacillus that causes tuberculosis, the development of a therapeutic antiserum against diphtheria, and to the concepts of antibodies and chemotherapy. Smoking 25 cigars a day, carrying around a pocketful of colored, precisely sharpened pencils, writing daily instructions to his research team, and possessing exceptional clinical knowledge characterized this great personality. On the 150th anniversary of his birth, we cannot help but admire the invaluable contribution he made to the science of immunology.

A chronology of developments in mast cell and immediate hypersensitivity research is provided below. This includes Paul Ehrlich's initial description, culminating in immunological, molecular, and genomic technologies that have accelerated our understanding of immediate hypersensitivity and relevant mast cell biology.

2. Chronology of Developments in Immediate Hypersensitivity and Relevant Mast Cell Research

3300-3640 BC: Allergic reaction to bee sting in a pharaoh is documented historically.

1878: Paul Ehrlich describes mast cells in his doctoral thesis at University of Leipzig and coins the term "mastzellen" derived from German word "mast" (breast *[1]*).

1879: Paul Ehrlich describes metachromasia *(1)*.

1891: Water solubility of mast cells demonstrated by Paul Ehrlich *(1)*.

1891: Description of cells with basophilic granules in leukemia by Paul Ehrlich *(1)*.

1898: Paul Ehrlich describes two types of cells with basophilic granules: one localized to tissue (tissue mast cells) and another derived from bone marrow and localized to blood (blood mast cell, basophil, mast leukocyte) *(1)*.

1900: Demonstration of bone marrow origin of mast cells by Jolly *(1)*.

1900: Paul Ehrlich describes antibody formation theory *(1)*.

1902: Description of "anaphylaxis" is made by Paul Portier and Charles Richet *(2)*.

1906: The term "allergy" is coined by Clemens von Pirquet.

1907: Histamine is synthesized by Windaus and Vogt *(3)*.

1908: Paul Ehrlich receives the Nobel Prize in Physiology or Medicine, along with Ilya Ilyich Metchnikov, for discoveries in immunology.

1910: Physiological functions of histamine described by Dale and Laidlaw *(3)*.

1913: Nobel Prize awarded to Charles Richet for discovery of "anaphylaxis" *(2,4–6)*.

1913: Schultz and Dale describe smooth muscle contraction in sensitized animals: Schultz used intestinal muscle whereas Dale used uterine muscle of guinea pigs *(7–9)*.

1921: Description of passive transfer of hypersensitivity with serum by Prausnitz, popularly known as the Prausnitz-Kustner reaction (P-K reaction *[10–12]*).

1948: Description of passive cutaneous anaphylaxis (i.e., PCA) by Ovary *(9)*.

1952: Discovery of "histamine" in mast cells by James Riley and Geoffrey West *(13)*.

1961: Ovary demonstrates the release of slow-reacting substance of anaphylaxis (i.e., SRS-A) from mast cells when activated by allergen *(9)*.

1961: Mast cells identified in the bronchial tissue in asthma.

1973: Putative receptor on mast cells for immunoglobulin E (IgE) recognized *(14)*.

1979: SRS-A identified in mast cells as a "leukotriene" *(15)*.

1988: Sir James Black awarded the Nobel Prize for discovery of histamine (H2) receptor antagonist *(16)*.

1967: Kimishige Ishizaka recognizes IgE as reaginic antibody *(17,18)*.

1985: Susumu Tonegawa receives the Nobel Prize for identification of immunoglobulin genes *(19–21)*.

1989: Plaut and Paul show mast cells are capable of secreting multiple lymphokines *(22)*.

1989: Cloning of canine mast cell tryptase is reported *(23)*.

1990: Cloning of human mast cell tryptase is reported *(24)*.

1990: Steel locus, kit ligand (KL) is identified as ligand for c-kit and reported to be involved in mast cell proliferation *(25,26)*.

1990: Cloning of canine mast cell chymase is reported *(27)*.

1991: Cloning of human mast cell chymase is reported *(28)*.

1994: Ability of mast cells to phagocytose bacteria is shown *(29)*.

1994: Murine mast cells are shown to present antigen to T cells *(30)*.

1994–1996: Dominant role for mast cells in the Arthus Reaction is demonstrated *(27,31,32)*.

1996: Mast cells are shown to be important in defense against *Escherichia coli* infection *(33)*.

2001: Transcriptome of human mast cells is analyzed *(34,35)*.

2001–2003: Toll-like receptors are described on mast cells *(36–38)*.

2003: Histamine deficiency induced by histidine decarboxylase gene targeting in mice reveals lower mast cell numbers and defective mast cell degranulation *(39)*.

2004: Expression of nitric oxide synthase and nitric oxide in human mast cells demonstrated *(40)*.

References

1. Crivellato, E., Beltrami, C., Mallardi, F., and Ribatti, D. (2003) Paul Ehrlich's doctoral thesis: a milestone in the study of mast cells. *Br. J. Haematol.* **123**, 19–21.

1a. Kasten, F. H. (1996) Paul Ehrlich: pathfinder in cell biology. 1. Chronicle of his life and accomplishments in immunology, cancer research, and chemotherapy. *Biotech. Histochem.* **71**, 2–37.

2. Kemp, S. F. and Lockey, R. F. (2002) Anaphylaxis: a review of causes and mechanisms. *J. Allergy Clin. Immunol.* **110**, 341–348.

3. Hill, S. J., Ganellin, C. R., Timmerman, H., et al. (1997) International Union of Pharmacology. XIII. Classification of histamine receptors. *Pharmacol. Rev.* **49**, 253–278.

4. Ring, J., Brockow, K., and Behrendt, H. (2004) History and classification of anaphylaxis. *Novartis. Found. Sympos.* **257**, 6–16.

5. Richet, G. and Estingoy, P. (2003) The life and times of Charles Richet. *Hist. Sci. Med.* **37**, 501–513.

6. Estingoy, P. (2003) On the creativity of the researcher: the work of Charles Richet. *Hist. Sci. Med.* **37**, 489–499.

7. Geiger, W. B. and Alpers, H. S. (1959) The mechanism of the Schultz-Dale reaction. *J. Allergy* **30**, 316–328.

8. Coulson, E. J. (1953) The Schultz-Dale technique. *J. Allergy* **24**, 458–473.

9. Ovary, Z. (1994) Immediate hypersensitivity. A brief, personal history. *Arerugi* **43**, 1375–1385.

10. Saint-Paul, M. and Millot, P. (1960) The Prausnitz-Kuestner reaction in experimental immunology. Its application to the study of tissue antigens and antibodies and in particular to autoantibodies in man and animal. *Pathol. Biol. (Paris)* **8**, 2223–2231.

11. Pisani, S., Poiron, J. M., Pisani, D. E., and Bocciolesi, L. (1953) Attempted passive transmission of food sensitivity; Prausnitz-Kustner technic. *Semin. Med.* **102**, 527–535.

12. Dogliotti, M. (1954) Prausnitz-Kuestner's passive transfer and gamma globulin. *Minerva Dermatol.* **29**, 383–387.

13. Riley, J. F. and West, G. B. (1952) Histamine in tissue mast cells. *J. Physiol.* **117**, 72P–73P.

14. Bach, M. K. and Brashler, J. R. (1973) On the nature of the presumed receptor for IgE on mast cells. II. Demonstration of the specific binding of IgE to cell-free particulate preparations from rat peritoneal mast cells. *J. Immunol.* **111**, 324–330.

15. Murphy, R. C., Hammarstrom, S., and Samuelsson, B. (1979) Leukotriene C: a slow-reacting substance from murine mastocytoma cells. *Proc. Natl. Acad. Sci. USA* **76,** 4275–4279.
16. Black, J. (1989) Nobel lecture in physiology or medicine—1988. Drugs from emasculated hormones: the principle of syntopic antagonism. *In Vitro Cell Dev. Biol.* **25,** 311–320.
17. Kishimoto, T. (2000) Immunology in the 20th century–progress made in research on infectious and immunological diseases. *Kekkaku* **75,** 595–598.
18. Woolcock, A. J. (1976) Immediate hypersensitivity: a clinical review. *Aust. N. Z. J. Med.* **6,** 158–167.
19. Tonegawa, S. (1993) The Nobel lectures in immunology. The Nobel Prize for Physiology or Medicine, 1987. Somatic generation of immune diversity. *Scand. J. Immunol.* **38,** 303–319.
20. Weltman, J. K. (1988) The 1987 Nobel Prize for physiology or medicine awarded to molecular immunogeneticist Susumu Tonegawa. *Allergy Proc.* **9,** 575–576.
21. Newmark, P. (1987) Nobel prize for Japanese immunologist. *Nature* **329,** 570.
22. Plaut, M., Pierce, J. H., Watson, C. J., Hanley-Hyde, J., Nordan, R. P., and Paul, W. E. (1989) Mast cell lines produce lymphokines in response to cross-linkage of Fc epsilon RI or to calcium ionophores. *Nature* **339,** 64–67.
23. Vanderslice, P., Craik, C. S., Nadel, J. A., and Caughey, G. H. (1989) Molecular cloning of dog mast cell tryptase and a related protease: structural evidence of a unique mode of serine protease activation. *Biochemistry* **28,** 4148–4155.
24. Miller, J. S., Westin, E. H., and Schwartz, L. B. (1989) Cloning and characterization of complementary DNA for human tryptase. *J. Clin. Invest.* **84,** 1188–1195.
25. Copeland, N. G., Gilbert, D. J., Cho, B. C., et al. (1990) Mast cell growth factor maps near the steel locus on mouse chromosome 10 and is deleted in a number of steel alleles. *Cell* **63,** 175–183.
26. Huang, E., Nocka, K., Beier, D. R., et al. (1990) The hematopoietic growth factor KL is encoded by the Sl locus and is the ligand of the c-kit receptor, the gene product of the W locus. *Cell* **63,** 225–233.
27. Caughey, G. H., Raymond, W. W., and Vanderslice, P. (1990) Dog mast cell chymase: molecular cloning and characterization. *Biochemistry* **29,** 5166–5171.
28. Caughey, G. H., Zerweck, E. H., and Vanderslice, P. (1991) Structure, chromosomal assignment, and deduced amino acid sequence of a human gene for mast cell chymase. *J. Biol. Chem.* **266,** 12,956–12,963.
29. Malaviya, R., Ross, E. A., MacGregor, J. I., et al. (1994) Mast cell phagocytosis of FimH-expressing enterobacteria. *J. Immunol.* **152,** 1907–1914.
30. Fox, C. C., Jewell, S. D., and Whitacre, C. C. (1994) Rat peritoneal mast cells present antigen to a PPD-specific T cell line. *Cell Immunol.* **158,** 253–264.
31. Smith, E. L. and Hainsworth, A. H. (1998) Acute effects of interleukin-1 beta on noradrenaline release from the human neuroblastoma cell line SH-SY5Y. *Neurosci. Lett.* **251,** 89–92.
32. Sylvestre, D. L. and Ravetch, J. V. (1996) A dominant role for mast cell Fc receptors in the Arthus reaction. *Immunity* **5,** 387–390.

33. Malaviya, R., Ikeda, T., Ross, E., and Abraham, S. N. (1996) Mast cell modulation of neutrophil influx and bacterial clearance at sites of infection through TNF-alpha. *Nature* **381,** 77–80.
34. Iida, M., Matsumoto, K., Tomita, H., et al. (2001) Selective down-regulation of high-affinity IgE receptor (FcepsilonRI) alpha-chain messenger RNA among transcriptome in cord blood-derived versus adult peripheral blood-derived cultured human mast cells. *Blood* **97,** 1016–1022.
35. Nakajima, T., Matsumoto, K., Suto, H., et al. (2001) Gene expression screening of human mast cells and eosinophils using high-density oligonucleotide probe arrays: abundant expression of major basic protein in mast cells. *Blood* **98,** 1127–1134.
36. Supajatura, V., Ushio, H., Nakao, A., et al. (2002) Differential responses of mast cell Toll-like receptors 2 and 4 in allergy and innate immunity. *J. Clin. Invest.* **109,** 1351–1359.
37. McCurdy, J. D., Lin, T. J., and Marshall, J. S. (2001) Toll-like receptor 4-mediated activation of murine mast cells. *J. Leukoc. Biol.* **70,** 977–984.
38. McCurdy, J. D., Olynych, T. J., Maher, L. H., and Marshall, J. S. (2003) Cutting edge: distinct Toll-like receptor 2 activators selectively induce different classes of mediator production from human mast cells. *J. Immunol.* **170,** 1625–1629.
39. Kozma, G. T., Losonczy, G., Keszei, M., et al. (2003) Histamine deficiency in gene-targeted mice strongly reduces antigen-induced airway hyper-responsiveness, eosinophilia and allergen-specific IgE. *Int. Immunol.* **15,** 963–973.
40. Gilchrist, M., McCauley, S. D., and Befus, A. D. (2004) Expression, localization and regulation of nitric oxide synthase (NOS) in human mast cell lines: effects on leukotriene production. *Blood* **104,** 462–469.

2

The Human Mast Cell

An Overview

Guha Krishnaswamy, Omar Ajitawi, and David S. Chi

Summary

Mast cells are fascinating, multifunctional, tissue-dwelling cells that have been tra-ditionally associated with the allergic response. However, recent studies suggest these cells may be capable of regulating inflammation, host defense, and innate immunity. The purpose of this review is to present salient aspects of mast cell biology in the con-text of mast cell function in physiology and disease. After their development from bone marrow-derived progenitor cells that are primed with stem cell factor, mast cells con-tinue their maturation and differentiation in peripheral tissue, developing into two well-described subsets of cells, MC_T and MC_{TC} cells. These cells can be distinguished on the basis of their tissue location, dependence on T lymphocytes, and their granule contents. Mast cells can undergo activation by antigens/allergens (acting via the high-affinity receptor for immunoglobulin E, also referred to as FcεRI), superoxides, complement proteins, neuropeptides, and lipoproteins. After activation, mast cells express histamine, leukotrienes, and prostanoids, as well as proteases, and many cytokines and chemokines. These mediators may be pivotal to the genesis of an inflammatory response. By virtue of their location and mediator expression, mast cells may play an active role in many diseases, such as allergy, parasitic diseases, atherosclerosis, malignancy, asthma, pul-monary fibrosis, and arthritis. Recent data also suggest that mast cells play a vital role in host defense against pathogens by elaboration of tumor necrosis factor alpha. Mast cells also express the Toll-like receptor, which may further accentuate their role in the immune-inflammatory response. This chapter summarizes the many well-known and novel functional aspects of human mast cell biology and emphasizes their unique role in the inflammatory response.

Key Words: Mast cells; immunoglobulin E; cytokine; gene expression; host defense; inflammation.

From: *Methods in Molecular Biology, vol. 315: Mast Cells: Methods and Protocols*
Edited by: G. Krishnaswamy and D. S. Chi © Humana Press Inc., Totowa, NJ

1. Introduction

Paul Ehrlich was the first researcher to describe cells in connective tissue that stained reddish–purple (referred to as metachromasia) with aniline dyes, calling them "mästzellen," a term that may have referred to feeding or could be interpreted as "well-fed" based on their granule contents *(1)*. The metachromasia exhibited by mast cells is caused by the interaction of dyes with acidic heparin, a well-known constituent of mast cell granules. The discovery of these cells by Paul Ehrlich and the historical development of mast cell research are described in greater detail in Chapter 1. Mast cells tend to be located perivascularly and in sentinel locations to respond to noxious stimuli as well as to allergens. The mast cell expresses the high-affinity receptor for immunoglobulin E (FcεRI) and the crosslinking of IgE occupying this receptor leads to mast cell activation and the manifestations of immediate-type hypersensitivity *(2–4)*. In some cases, other ligand–receptor interactions can lead to mast cell degranulation, which are summarized in **Fig. 1**.

2. Mast Cell Development and Differentiation

Mast cells develop from progenitor cells that in turn arise from uncommitted hematopoietic stem cells in the bone marrow *(5,6)*. These cells express the receptor for stem cell factor (SCF receptor or c-kit) that binds to SCF, the latter being a major growth factor for mast cells *(5–7)*. Researchers have described a $CD34^+$, $c-kit^+$, and $CD13^-$ precursor that develops into mast cells in the presence of specific growth factors *(8,9)*. Mast cell progenitors also have been described in peripheral blood by others, which may suggest the presence of a distinct pool of cells separate from leukocytes or mononuclear cells *(10)*. The interactions between SCF and c-kit and the subsequent signaling that follows are crucial for the growth and development of mast cells *(11)*. In humans, studies have demonstrated that mutations of c-kit and elevated levels of the c-kit proto-oncogene are associated with the development of the syndrome of mastocytosis, a condition characterized by mast cell infiltration of skin and other tissues *(12,13)*. SCF has multiple biological effects on mast cells, including modulating differentiation and homing, prolonging viability, inducing mast cell hyperplasia, and enhancing mediator production *(7)*. However, mast cells that have been deprived of SCF undergo programmed cell death (PCD) or apoptosis *(14)*. It is likely that PCD in mast cells is mediated by the modulation of Bcl-2 and Bcl-XL *(15)*. Interleukin 6 (IL-6), eotaxin, and nerve growth factor (NGF) also enhance mast cell development from hematopoietic stem cells, and the development of mast cells from stem cells derived from umbilical cord blood often requires SCF in conjunction with IL-6 *(5,16)*. Adventitial cells, including fibroblasts, contribute to further differentiation and maturation of mast cells in tissue by elaboration of SCF, NGF, or other mechanisms *(17,18)*. After tissue

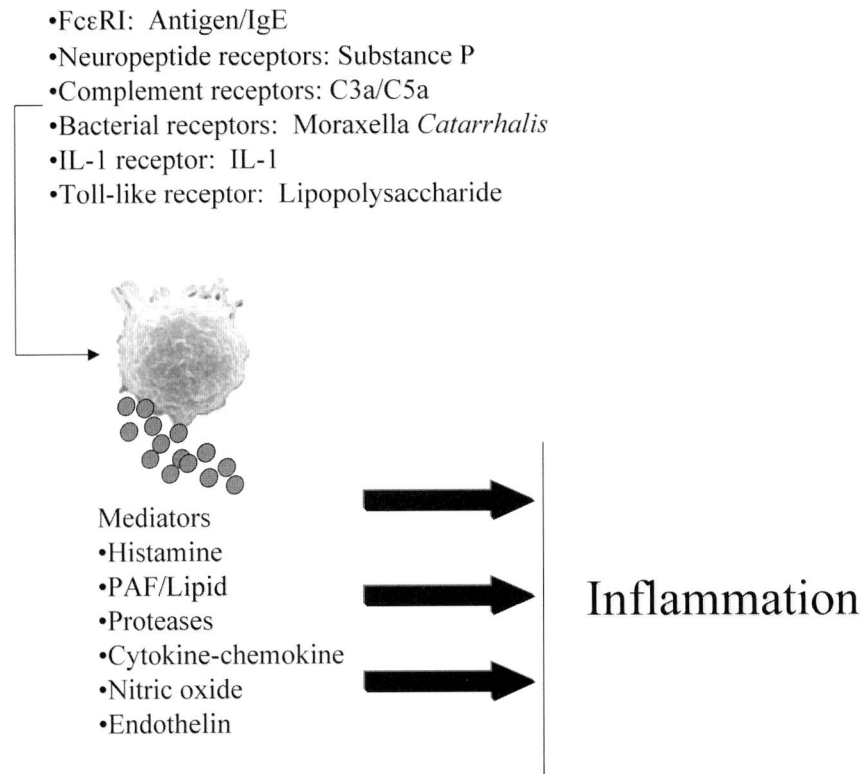

•FcεRI: Antigen/IgE
•Neuropeptide receptors: Substance P
•Complement receptors: C3a/C5a
•Bacterial receptors: Moraxella *Catarrhalis*
•IL-1 receptor: IL-1
•Toll-like receptor: Lipopolysaccharide

Mediators
•Histamine
•PAF/Lipid
•Proteases
•Cytokine-chemokine
•Nitric oxide
•Endothelin

Inflammation

Fig. 1. Mast cells undergo activation by IgE-dependent and IgE-independent stimuli, leading to release of a cascade of mediators culminating in the inflammatory response. Histamine, platelet-activating factor (PAF), lipid mediators (leukotrienes, prostanoids), proteases, cytokines, chemokines, nitric oxide, and endothelin may be released in the tissue, which can lead to inflammatory cell recruitment, endothelial activation, and cellular adhesion.

localization, mast cells can undergo further differentiation into distinct subsets. Two mast cell subtypes have been described in tissue—the mucosal (MC_T) or connective tissue (MC_{TC}) mast cell (**Table 1**). These subtypes are based on structural, biochemical, and functional differences and have been well characterized by several researchers *(3,19–21)*. Please *see* Chapter 4 for more information.

Distinctive features help differentiate the two subsets. For example, the MC_T mast cell predominantly expresses the protease tryptase (**Fig. 2A** demonstrates tryptase staining of mast cells derived from umbilical cord blood mononuclear cells). This subset usually is localized to mucosal surfaces, often in close prox-

Table 1
Mast Cell Subtypes

Feature	MC_{TC} cell	MC_T cell
Structural features		
Grating/lattice granule	++	–
Scroll granules	Poor	Rich
Tissue distribution		
Skin	++	–
Intestinal submucosa	++	+
Intestinal mucosa	+	++
Alveolar wall	–	++
Bronchi	+	++
Nasal mucosa	++	++
Conjunctiva	++	+
Mediator synthesized		
Histamine	+++	+++
Chymase	++	–
Tryptase	++	++
Carboxypeptidase	++	–
Cathepsin G	++	–
LTC_4	++	++
PGD_2	++	++
TNF-α	++	++
IL-4, IL-5, IL-6, IL-13	++	++

imity to T cells. These T lymphocytes are especially of the T-helper 2-type (Th2 secreting IL-4 and IL-5). This subset usually is seen in increased numbers infiltrating the mucosa in patients suffering from allergic and parasitic disease. Because of their unique T cell-dependence, the numbers of MC_T cells are diminished in individuals infected with human immunodeficiency virus (HIV) *(3)*. Structurally, granules from MC_T are scroll-rich (**Fig. 2B** demonstrates a typical scroll-like granule in mast cells developed from umbilical cord blood mononuclear cells).

The MC_{TC} mast cell, however, expresses tryptase, chymase, carboxypeptidase, and cathepsin G. It tends to predominate in the gastrointestinal tract as well as in skin, synovium, and subcutaneous tissue (**Table 1**). Increased numbers of MC_{TC} mast cells are seen in fibrotic diseases whereas its numbers are relatively unchanged in allergic or parasitic diseases and in HIV infection. The presence of these MC_{TC} cells could help explain why patients with HIV infection continue to have allergic reactions (e.g., to medications). MC_{TC} mast cells have lattice and grating structures and are scroll-poor.

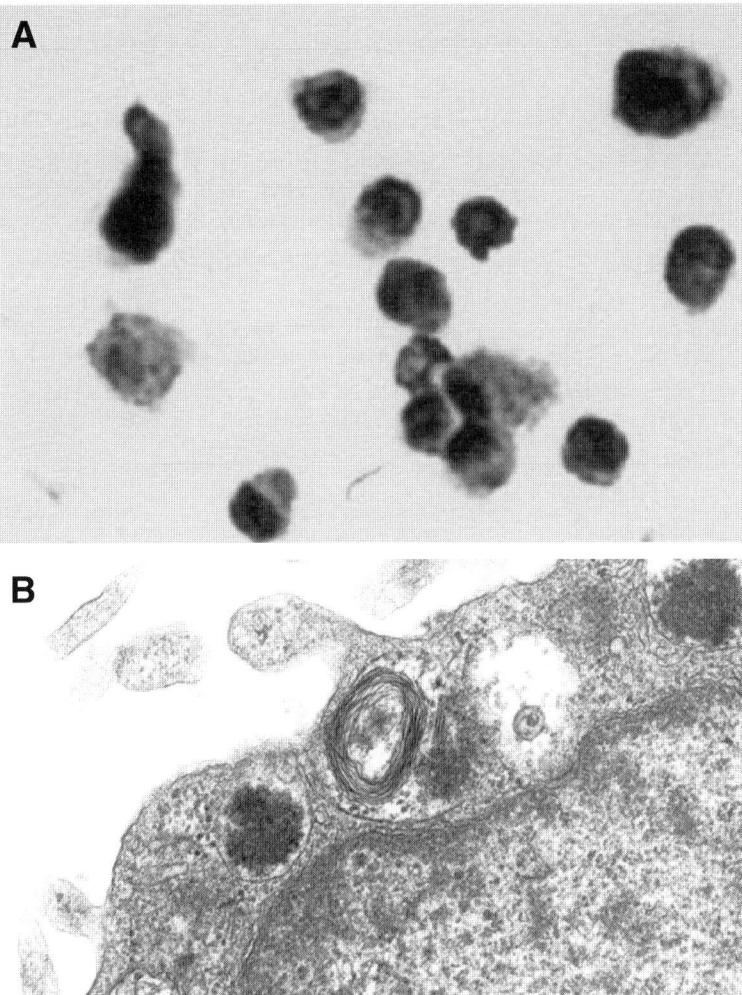

Fig. 2. (**A**) Tryptase immunostaining of human cord blood-derived mast cells (×400). In this specimen, more than 95% of human cord blood-derived mast cells expressed tryptase, with only 20% expressing chymase. (**B**) Ultrastructurally, mast cells demonstrate microvilli-like projections on the surface and typical granules. This picture demonstrates the presence of scroll-like granules within the mast cell derived from umbilical cord blood mononuclear cells.

3. Mast Cell Activation and Mediator Production

Human mast cells and basophils express the receptor for IgE, FcεRI *(2)*. FcεRI (in contrast to the other receptor for IgE, FcεRII) binds IgE with high affinity *(22)*. The other receptor for IgE, FcεRII, has been detected on eosinophils, mononuclear cells, lymphocytes, and platelets. FcεRI is a multimeric complex composed of four chains, designated as α (which has the IgE-binding domain), β, and the two disulfide-linked γ chains *(23,24)*. Typically, multivalent antigen binds to IgE, which in turn binds by the Fc portion to the α-chain of FcεRI, leading subsequently to receptor aggregation and internalization and culminating in receptor-mediated signaling. The β and γ chains of FcεRI possess the immune receptor tyrosine-based activation motifs, which are considered pivotal to signal transduction *(25)*. The bridging of two IgE molecules by multivalent antigen or by univalent antigen in presence of a carrier molecule results in activation of Lyn kinase, which then phosphorylates the β and γ chains *(22)*. The absence of Lyn has been associated with defective mast cell signaling in mice *(26)*. Syk kinase then becomes activated sequentially, followed by involvement of phospholipase C γ, mitogen-activated protein kinases (MAPK), and phosphoinositol-3 kinase *(27)*. The generation of inositol triphosphate and of diacylglycerol and other second messengers leads to release of calcium intracellularly as well as protein kinase C activation, events culminating in FcεRI-mediated secretion. Degranulation appears to be associated with activation of G proteins that cause actin polymerization and relocalization. These events also are accompanied by the transcription of several cytokine genes, leading to further evolution of the inflammatory cascade.

In a typical allergic reaction, antigen/allergen (for example, latex or peanut allergen) crosslinks two IgE molecules occupying FcεRI, resulting in a cascade of rapid sequence signaling events and leading to degranulation and elaboration of mediators *(28)*. Mast cells also can be activated to degranulate by a variety of stimuli including; opiates, components of the complement cascade *(29–31)*, neuropeptides (vasoactive intestinal peptide, calcitonin gene-related peptide, and substance P), superoxide anion, radio-contrast media, oxidized low-density lipoproteins, histamine releasing factors, chemokines (monocyte chemotactic proteins-1, -2, and -3 [MCP-1, -2, -3], and monocyte inflammatory peptide 1 α [MIP-1 α]), regulated upon activation normal T-cell-expressed and secreted (RANTES), connective tissue-activating peptide, pathogenic bacteria *(32,33)*, parasites *(34,35)*, enterotoxin B *(36)*, cholera toxin *(37)*, or changes in osmolality *(38,39)*. We have recently demonstrated that IL-1, catecholamines, and cell–cell interactions (e.g., mast cell-fibroblast contact) can enhance mast cell activation and cytokine expression *(40–43)*, which indicates the occurrence of multiple pathways of mast cell activation.

Mediators secreted by mast cells can be subdivided into preformed (secretory granule-associated) and others newly synthesized after cellular activation *(3,44)*. Preformed mediators (summarized in **Fig. 3**) include histamine, proteoglycans (heparin, chondroitin sulfate E), serotonin, proteases (such as tryptase, chymase, β-hexosaminidase, β-glucuronidase, β-D-galactosidase, cathepsin G,

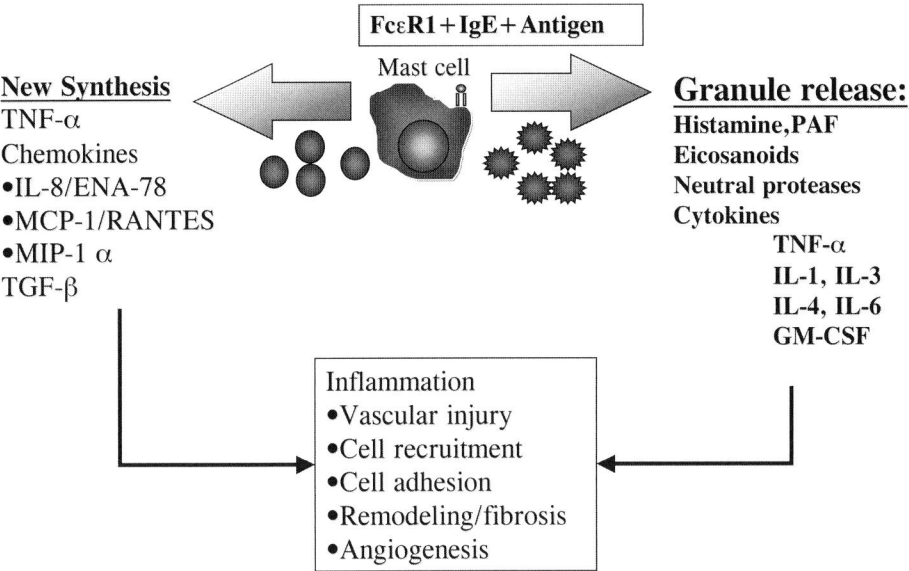

Fig. 3. After activation of mast cells by IgE and antigen, the release of preformed and newly synthesized mediators occurs, leading to acute and chronic inflammatory effects, mediated by vascular injury, cellular recruitment, and culminating in tissue remodeling and angiogenesis.

and carboxypeptidase), some cytokines (tumor necrosis factor [TNF]-α), and basic fibroblast growth factor (bFGF). The newly generated products include the lipid mediators (prostaglandin D_2 and leukotrienes, generated from arachidonic acid), thromboxanes, 5,12-hydroxy-eicosatetraenoic acid, nitrogen radicals, oxygen radicals, inflammatory cytokines, and several chemokines.

4. The Mediators Expressed by Mast Cells and Their Role in the Inflammatory Response

Plaut et al. *(45)* first demonstrated that murine mast cells were capable of expressing many cytokines. Since then, we and others have shown that human mast cells express a spectrum of cytokines and chemokines *(3,46,47)*. Both in vivo and in vitro studies have shown that human mast cells are capable of expressing pleiotropic cytokines and growth factors, such as TNF-α *(3,48–51)*, granulocyte macrophage colony-stimulating factor *(52)*, IL-3 and IL-4 *(36,53–59)*, IL-5 *(54–56,60)*, IL-6 *(55,56,61–64)*, IL-8 *(54,65,66)*, IL-10 *(67)*, IL-13 *(68–70)*, IL-16 *(71)*, MIP-1 α *(72)*, MIP-1 β *(73)*, regulated upon activation normal T-cell-expressed and -secreted *(3,73)*, and MCP-1 *(74,75)*. Human mast cells also are capable of expressing growth factors. Vascular endothelial growth factor (VEGF), a cytokine crucial to angiogenesis and the growth of blood vessels, and NGF *(76,77)*, are recognized products of mast cells. Autocrine production of SCF has been shown from mast cells *(78,79)*.

It is likely that heterogeneity of human mast cells exists in regards to cytokine expression in vivo and studies by Bradding et al. *(63)*, demonstrated this phenomenon in mast cells obtained from bronchial biopsies of patients suffering from asthma. By immunocytochemistry, these investigators noted that although MC_{TC} cells predominantly expressed IL-4, the MC_{TC} cells expressed both IL-5 and IL-6 *(63)*. In our studies, cord blood-derived mast cells expressed the eosinophil-active growth factors IL-5 and GM-CSF and the eosinophil chemotactic C-X-C chemokine, IL-8, after activation *(42)*. The production of these cytokines in cord blood-derived mast cells was further enhanced by the addition of the monokines IL-1β and TNF-α in a dose-dependent manner while dexamethasone inhibited production of these cytokines. How these various cytokines and chemokines interact with the inflammatory response is summarized below.

Mast cells have been incriminated in such diverse diseases as allergy, asthma, rheumatoid arthritis, atherosclerosis, interstitial cystitis, inflammatory bowel disease, progressive systemic sclerosis, chronic graft-vs-host disease, fibrotic diseases, sarcoidosis, asbestosis, ischemic heart disease, keloid scars, and malignancy *(3)*. The mediators released by mast cells can independently and, in synergy with macrophage- and T-cell-derived cytokines, induce much of the inflammatory pathology observed in inflammation and serve to orchestrate a complex immune response. Histamine, LTB_4, LTC_4, PAF, and PGD_2 may have multiple effects on inflammatory cell recruitment (eosinophils), smooth muscle hyperplasia, and vascular dilatation *(80,81)*. Tryptase, chymase, and TNF-α from mast cells activate fibroblasts, leading to collagen deposition and fibrosis. Mast cell-derived TNF-α regulates NF-κB-dependent induction of endothelial adhesion molecule expression on endothelial cells in vivo *(49)*. Mast cell granules and tryptase also can potentiate endotoxin-induced IL-6 production by endothelial cells. Mast cell-derived cytokines and chemokines further regulate IgE synthesis and cell migration, basophil histamine release, smooth muscle proliferation, and endothelial chemotaxis and proliferation. IL-4 and IL-13 can regulate adhesion molecule expression on endothelial cells but also can class switch B cells to synthesize IgE *(82,83)*. Data suggest that mast cells also can directly activate B cells to switch to IgE. IL-5, another product of mast cells, also can serve to activate eosinophils while accentuating IgA production from B cells. Chemokines (such as IL-8) and leukotrienes (specifically LTC_4) released by mast cells can recruit neutrophils and eosinophils to inflamed airways, which can further potentiate damage *(3)*. Mast cells also have been postulated to provide the IL-4 pulse that allows the development of Th2 cells that

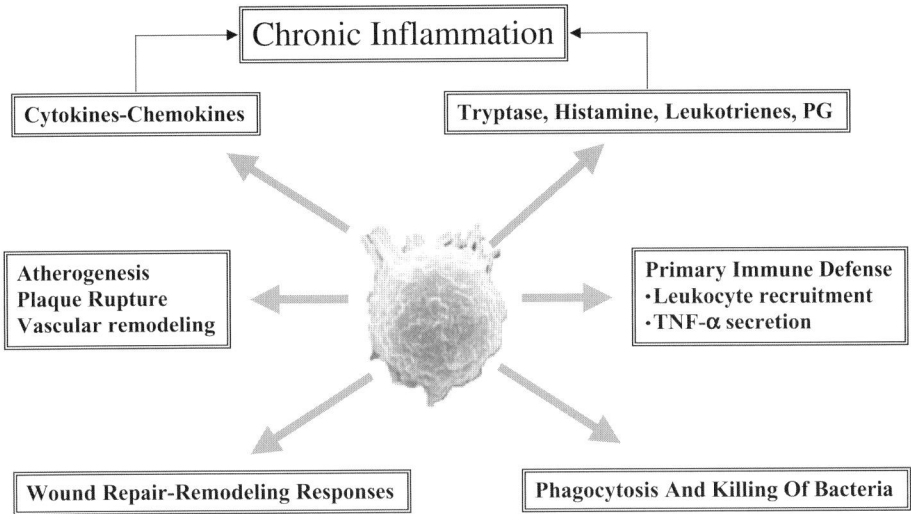

Fig. 4. Multiple roles of human mast cells in chronic disease states and immunophysiology or pathology.

selectively secrete IL-4 and IL-5 on activation *(84)*. Exciting recent data also suggest that certain mast cell-derived chemokines, especially MIP-1α, can potentiate a shift of T cells towards a Th1-phenotype, whereas others, such as MCP-1, can shift these cells functionally to a Th2-phenotype *(85)*. Thus, T cells and mast cells can complement the functions of each other and contribute to the "cytokine pool" that leads subsequently to chronic inflammation.

5. Functions of Mast Cells in Physiological and Pathological States

Mast cells may play crucial roles in various disease states, including vascular disease, fibrotic states, rheumatological disease, certain malignancies, and in host defense against infectious pathogens. The probable roles of the mast cell in human diseases are summarized in **Fig. 4**.

5.1. Vascular Disease

Mast cells are uniquely positioned around capillary vessels and may thus play crucial roles in vascular injury and atherosclerosis *(4)*. Mast cell granule components, released upon activation, could have both anticoagulant and thrombogenic functions *(86–88)*. On the other hand, mast cells may play several pathological roles in atherosclerosis. Increased numbers of mast cells have been found in the shoulders of atherosclerotic plaques, and here they appear to be associated with plaque rupture culminating in luminal thrombosis *(89)*. Kovanen et al. *(90)* found increased numbers of mast cells at the site of atheromatous rupture in patients who had died of acute myocardial infarction. Mast cell chymase and cathepsin G have been shown to convert angiotensin I to angiotensin II, which is a potent vasoconstrictor and can mediate several vascular, biological responses *(91,92)*. Mast cell chymase cleaves apolipoprotein B-100 of low-density lipoprotein, which facilitated lipid aggregation and foam cell development *(93)*, while at the same time also degrading apolipoprotein A of high-density lipoprotein, thereby reducing cholesterol efflux and increasing lipid deposition and thereby atherosclerosis *(94)*. On the other hand, mast cells have been reported to produce tissue plasminogen activator *(95)*, as well as plasminogen activator inhibitor-1 *(96)*. Mast cell tryptase also can cleave fibrinogen, thereby retarding coagulation *(97)*. One can therefore surmise multiple effects of mast cells on atherothrombotic disease, and the ultimate role of mast cells in any given situation may depend on the balance of these various effects.

5.2. Host Defense

Mast cells may play crucial roles in host defense by modulating both innate and adaptive immune responses *(38,44,98)*. Various functions of mast cells make them crucial players in host defense. First, these cells can directly phagocytose foreign particles (and bacteria) and also express receptors, such as intercellular adhesion molecule (ICAM)-1 and ICAM-3, CD 43, CD 80, CD 86, and CD 40L, allowing interaction with T and B lymphocytes. Second, they enhance the development of Th2 cells and allow B cells to class switch to IgE. A role as antigen presenting cells has also been proposed for mast cells *(99)*. By influencing both humoral and cell-mediated immune mechanisms, mast cells regulate host defense. Third, activated complement products (and neuropeptides), often generated during an innate immune response to an infectious event, induce mast cell degranulation, thereby integrating innate immunity and neuroimmune mechanisms. Fourth, mast cells are themselves capable of secreting a plethora of cytokines, chemokines, and other mediators that can activate lymphocytes and macrophages. These include the cytokines (TNF-α, IL-1 β, IL-4, IL-5, IL-8, and IL-13 *[32,100]*), lipid mediators, and histamine, which can have profound effects on vascular endothelium, including the alteration of vascular permeability and adhesiveness. This can allow other circulating inflammatory cells to adhere and emigrate into tissue. Thus, mast cells are key players in host defense, with a role in immune surveillance, phagocytosis, and immune activation.

5.3. Tissue Remodeling/Fibrosis

Mast cells are increased in numbers in many fibrotic diseases and may play a crucial role in the development of fibrosis *(101)*. The percentages of mast cells in bronchoalveolar lavage fluid from patients with sarcoidosis or interstitial fibrosis are greater than from control individuals *(102)*, and patients with idiopathic interstitial pulmonary fibrosis show evidence of mast cell degranulation and elevated mast cell numbers *(103)*. In the kidney tissue of patients with IgA nephropathy, mast cell numbers correlate with the degree of interstitial fibrosis and creatinine clearance. In these kidney tissues, mast cells express tryptase and bFGF *(104)*, which may be partially responsible for the fibrosis observed. The mast cell appears to be the dominant source of bFGF in some patients with pulmonary fibrosis *(105)*. Similarly, patients with pulmonary fibrosis associated with scleroderma show higher numbers of mast cells and quantities of histamine and tryptase in bronchoalveolar lavage fluid than patients with normal chest roentgenograms *(106)*. Mast cells also are found in intimate contact with myofibroblasts in keloid scars, suggesting they may play a role in fibroblast activation and scar formation *(107)*. Thus, it appears that mast cells play a pivotal role in fibrotic disorders *(108,109)*.

The mechanisms behind this relationship between mast cells and fibrosis/ tissue remodeling are unclear. Mast cell products, such as tryptase, TNF-α, and bFGF, induce fibroblast proliferation *(105,110,111)*. However, fibroblasts appear to enhance mast cell survival, suggesting the presence of a bidirectional relationship between these cell types *(3,112)*. Fibroblast expression of SCF and its interactions with c-kit on mast cells may provide one explanation for these observations. Fibroblasts, however, also are closely opposed to mast cells in fibrotic diseases, suggesting the additional possibility of cognate, cell–cell interaction such as that mediated by CD40–CD40L ligation *(113,114)*. To further complicate the picture, mast cells are themselves capable of laying down some forms of collagen and mast cell tryptase can activate collagenases capable of matrix degradation. These data suggest multiple mechanisms by which and multiple levels where mast cells can regulate tissue fibrosis and repair *(115)*.

5.4. Systemic Mastocytosis and Malignancy

A disorder characterized by excessive numbers of mast cells and tissue infiltration by these cells is systemic mastocytosis. In this condition, mutations of c-kit (Asp 816 Val mutation) occur *(11,116–118)*, and a subsequent pathological infiltration of affected tissue by mast cells may be seen, resulting in many of the manifestations *(119)*. The patients may present with skin lesions (pigmented macules that urticate with contact [Darrier's sign]) or systemic symptoms arising from mast cell infiltration of solid organs, such as the liver, spleen, lymph nodes, and bone marrow *(119,120)*. Cutaneous manifestations include urticaria pigmentosa, diffuse and erythematous mastocytosis, mastocytoma (mast cell deposits or tumors), and telangiectasia macularis eruptiva perstans *(121)*. Some patients have skin limited and indolent, slowly progressive disease, whereas others develop rapidly progressive and fatal mast cell leukemia, a feature especially found in some patients with the c-kit mutation *(13,122, 123)*. Osteoporosis is often a feature of mastocytosis, and mast cells may contribute to bone resorption *(124)*. Patients with mastocytosis may develop myeloproliferative syndromes, myelodysplasia, and/or lymphoreticular malignancy, the mechanisms of which are unknown *(125)*. Interestingly, the marker, α-tryptase is elevated in the serum of patients and provides us with an excellent diagnostic clinical tool *(126)*. By inducing angiogenesis, the secretion of VEGF and bFGF, and the elaboration of collagenases, mast cells can contribute to tumor pathology and invasiveness *(127–129)*.

5.5. HIV and Rheumatological Disease

A probable role for mast cells and IgE-mediated pathology has been reported in HIV infection *(130)*. The chemokine receptor, CCR3 is expressed on mast cells and may provide one explanation for the chemotactic effects of tat protein on mast cells *(130)*. In one study, increased adventitial mast cell numbers were noted in the arteries of patients dying of cocaine toxicity *(131,132)*, but the role of mast cells in HIV and cocaine-induced vascular pathology is unclear *(132)*.

Mast cells may play a role in various arthritides. For example, the release of mast cell mediators (α- and β-tryptase and histamine) has been demonstrated in the joint of various forms of inflammatory arthritis *(133,134)*. In osteoarthritis, a degenerative but potentially inflammatory disorder, mast cell counts and tryptase and histamine levels are elevated in synovial fluid *(135,136)*. Activated mast cells also are seen in the lesions present in patients with rheumatoid arthritis *(137–139)*, whereas mast cell chemotactic activity and their expression of VEGF have been demonstrated in rheumatoid synovium *(140,141)*. Mast cell infiltration of the minor salivary glands is observed in patients with Sjögren's syndrome, and this infiltration often is associated with fibrosis and c-kit expression *(142)*. Patients with fibromyalgia demonstrate higher dermal deposits of IgG and increased dermal mast cell numbers, but the role these play in pathogenesis of the disease is unknown *(143)*.

6. Conclusions

Mast cells are fascinating, multifunctional, bone marrow-derived, tissue-dwelling cells. They can be activated to degranulate in minutes, not only by IgE and antigen signaling via the high affinity receptor for IgE, but also by a diverse group of stimuli. These cells can release a wide variety of immune mediators, including an expanding list of cytokines, chemokines, and growth factors. Mast cells have been shown to play roles in allergic inflammation and, more recently, they have been shown to modulate coagulation cascades, host defense, and tissue remodeling. The role of mast cells in asthma, atherosclerosis, HIV, cocaine abuse, fibrotic disorders, and rheumatological disease is being actively studied. The availability of novel molecular tools, such as the chip array technology, should shed more light on these true biological roles of these ubiquitous cells.

Acknowledgments

The authors acknowledge the excellent secretarial assistance of Ms. Dolores Moore. This chapter was funded by NIH grants AI-43310 and HL-63070, the Rondal Cole Foundation and the Chair of Excellence in Medicine (State of Tennessee grant 20233), Cardiovascular Research Institute, AMGEN, Inc., and the Research Development Committee, East Tennessee State University.

References

1. Bloom, G. D. (1984) A short history of the mast cell. *Acta Otolaryngol. Suppl.* **414,** 87–92.
2. Metcalfe, D. D., Baram, D., and Mekori, Y. A. (1997) Mast cells. *Physiol. Rev.* **77,** 1033–1079.
3. Church, M. K. and Levi-Schaffer, F. (1997) The human mast cell. *J. Allergy Clin. Immunol.* **99,** 155–160.
4. Kelley, J. L., Chi, D. S., Abou-Auda, W., Smith, J. K., and Krishnaswamy, G. (2000) The molecular role of mast cells in atherosclerotic cardiovascular disease. *Mol. Med. Today* **6,** 304–308.
5. Valent, P. (1995) Cytokines involved in growth and differentiation of human basophils and mast cells. *Exp. Dermatol.* **4,** 255–259.
6. Valent, P., Sillaber, C., and Bettelheim, P. (1991) The growth and differentiation of mast cells. *Prog. Growth Factor Res.* **3,** 27–41.
7. Galli, S. J., Tsai, M., Wershil, B. K., Tam, S. Y., and Costa, J. J. (1995) Regulation of mouse and human mast cell development, survival and function by stem cell factor, the ligand for the c-kit receptor. *Int. Arch. Allergy Immunol.* **107,** 51–53.
8. Kirshenbaum, A. S., Goff, J. P., Semere, T., Foster, B., Scott, L. M., and Metcalfe, D. D. (1999) Demonstration that human mast cells arise from a progenitor cell population that is CD34(+), c-kit(+), and expresses aminopeptidase N (CD13). *Blood* **94,** 2333–2342.
9. Kirshenbaum, A. S., Kessler, S. W., Goff, J. P., and Metcalfe, D. D. (1991) Demonstration of the origin of human mast cells from CD34+ bone marrow progenitor cells. *J. Immunol.* **146,** 1410–1415.
10. Nilsson, G., Butterfield, J. H., Nilsson, K., and Siegbahn, A. (1994) Stem cell factor is a chemotactic factor for human mast cells. *J. Immunol.* **153,** 3717–3723.
11. Vliagoftis, H., Worobec, A. S., and Metcalfe, D. D. (1997) The protooncogene c-kit and c-kit ligand in human disease. *J. Allergy Clin. Immunol.* **100,** 435–440.
12. Nagata, H., Worobec, A. S., Semere, T., and Metcalfe, D. D. (1998) Elevated expression of the proto-oncogene c-kit in patients with mastocytosis. *Leukemia* **12,** 175–181.

13. Worobec, A. S., Semere, T., Nagata, H., and Metcalfe, D. D. (1998) Clinical correlates of the presence of the Asp816Val c-kit mutation in the peripheral blood mononuclear cells of patients with mastocytosis. *Cancer* **83,** 2120–2129.

14. Mekori, Y. A., Oh, C. K., and Metcalfe, D. D. (1995) The role of c-Kit and its ligand, stem cell factor, in mast cell apoptosis. *Int. Arch. Allergy Immunol.* **107,** 136–138.

15. Mekori, Y. A., Gilfillan, A. M., Akin, C., Hartmann, K., and Metcalfe, D. D. (2001) Human mast cell apoptosis is regulated through Bcl-2 and Bcl-XL. *J. Clin. Immunol.* **21,** 171–174.

16. Quackenbush, E. J., Wershil, B. K., Aguirre, V., and Gutierrez-Ramos, J. C. (1998) Eotaxin modulates myelopoiesis and mast cell development from embryonic hematopoietic progenitors. *Blood* **92,** 1887–1897.

17. Kirshenbaum, A. S., Goff, J. P., Albert, J. P., Kessler, S. W., and Metcalfe, D. D. (1994) Fibroblasts determine the fate of Fc epsilon RI+ cell populations in vitro by selectively supporting the viability of mast cells while internalizing and degrading basophils. *Int. Arch. Allergy Immunol.* **105,** 374–380.

18. Atkins, F. M., Friedman, M. M., Subba Rao, P. V., and Metcalfe, D. D. (1985) Interactions between mast cells, fibroblasts and connective tissue components. *Int. Arch. Allergy Appl. Immunol.* **77,** 96–102.

19. Schwartz, L. B. (1998) The mast cell, in *Textbook of Rheumatology* (Kelley, W. N., Harris, E. D., Ruddy, S., and Sledge, C. B., eds.), W.B. Saunders Company, Philadelphia, pp. 161–175.

20. Schwartz, L. B., Irani, A. M., Roller, K., Castells, M. C., and Schechter, N. M. (1987) Quantitation of histamine, tryptase, and chymase in dispersed human T and TC mast cells. *J. Immunol.* **138,** 2611–2615.

21. Kracmer, R. (1987) [Mechanisms of allergic reactions and potential therapeutic approach in childhood bronchial asthma] Mechanismen der allergischen Reaktion und mogliche therapeutische Ansatze beim kindlichen Asthma bronchiale. *Schweiz. Rundsch. Med. Prax.* **76,** 581–585.

22. Fung-Leung, W. P., Sousa-Hitzler, J., Ishaque, A., et al. (1996) Transgenic mice expressing the human high-affinity immunoglobulin (Ig) E receptor alpha chain respond to human IgE in mast cell degranulation and in allergic reactions. *J. Exp. Med.* **183,** 49–56.

23. Nadler, M. J., Matthews, S. A., Turner, H., and Kinet, J. P. (2000) Signal transduction by the high-affinity immunoglobulin E receptor Fc epsilon RI: coupling form to function. *Adv. Immunol.* **76,** 325–355.

24. Turner, H. and Kinet, J. P. (1999) Signalling through the high-affinity IgE receptor Fc epsilonRI. *Nature* **402,** B24-B30.

25. Daeron, M., Malbec, O., Latour, S., Espinosa, E., Pina, P., and Fridman, W. H. (1995) Regulation of tyrosine-containing activation motif-dependent cell signalling by Fc gamma RII. *Immunol. Lett.* **44,** 119–123.

26. Hibbs, M. L. and Dunn, A. R. (1997) Lyn, a src-like tyrosine kinase. *Int. J. Biochem. Cell Biol.* **29,** 397–400.

27. Suzuki, H., Takei, M., Yanagida, M., Nakahata, T., Kawakami, T., and Fukamachi, H. (1997) Early and late events in Fc epsilon RI signal transduction in human cultured mast cells. *J. Immunol.* **159,** 5881–5888.

28. Marone, G., Casolaro, V., Patella, V., Florio, G., and Triggiani, M. (1997) Molecular and cellular biology of mast cells and basophils. *Int. Arch. Allergy Immunol.* **114,** 207–217.

29. Schulman, E. S. (1993) The role of mast cells in inflammatory responses in the lung. *Crit. Rev. Immunol.* **13,** 35–70.

30. Schulman, E. S., Post, T. J., Henson, P. M., and Giclas, P. C. (1988) Differential effects of the complement peptides, C5a and C5a des Arg on human basophil and lung mast cell histamine release. *J. Clin. Invest.* **81,** 918–923.

31. Prodeus, A. P., Zhou, X., Maurer, M., Galli, S. J., and Carroll, M. C. (1997) Impaired mast cell-dependent natural immunity in complement C3-deficient mice. *Nature* **390,** 172–175.

32. Abraham, S. N. and Malaviya, R. (1997) Mast cells in infection and immunity. *Infect. Immun.* **65,** 3501–3508.

33. Malaviya, R. and Abraham, S. N. (1998) Clinical implications of mast cell-bacteria interaction. *J. Mol. Med.* **76,** 617–623.

34. Galli, S. J. and Wershil, B. K. (1996) The two faces of the mast cell. *Nature* **381,** 21–22.

35. Galli, S. J. (1993) New concepts about the mast cell. *N. Engl. J. Med.* **328,** 257–265.

36. Ackermann, L., Pelkonen, J., and Harvima, I. T. (1998) Staphylococcal enterotoxin B inhibits the production of interleukin-4 in a human mast-cell line HMC-1. *Immunology* **94,** 247–252.

37. McCloskey, M. A. (1988) Cholera toxin potentiates IgE-coupled inositol phospholipid hydrolysis and mediator secretion by RBL-2H3 cells. *Proc. Natl. Acad. Sci. USA* **85,** 7260–7264.

38. Galli, S. J., Maurer, M., and Lantz, C. S. (1999) Mast cells as sentinels of innate immunity. *Curr. Opin. Immunol.* **11,** 53–59.

39. Silber, G., Proud, D., Warner, J., et al. (1988) In vivo release of inflammatory mediators by hyperosmolar solutions. *Am. Rev. Respir. Dis.* **137,** 606–612.

40. Fitzgerald, S. M., Lee, S. A., Hall, H. K., Chi, D. S., and Krishnaswamy, G. (2004) Human lung fibroblasts express interleukin-6 in response to signaling after mast cell contact. *Am. J. Respir. Cell Mol. Biol.* **30,** 585–593.

41. Chi, D. S., Fitzgerald, S. M., Pitts, S., et al. (2004) MAPK-dependent regulation of IL-1- and beta-adrenoreceptor-induced inflammatory cytokine production from mast cells: implications for the stress response. *BMC Immunol.* **5,** 22.

42. Krishnaswamy, G., Hall, K., Youngberg, G., et al. (2002) Regulation of eosinophil-active cytokine production from human cord blood-derived mast cells. *J. Interferon Cytokine Res.* **22,** 379–388.

43. Lee, S. A., Fitzgerald, S. M., Huang, S. K., et al. (2004) Molecular regulation of interleukin-13 and monocyte chemoattractant protein-1 expression in human mast cells by interleukin-1beta. *Am. J. Respir. Cell Mol. Biol.* **31,** 283–291.

44. Abraham, S. N., Thankavel, K., and Malaviya, R. (1997) Mast cells as modulators of host defense in the lung. *Front. Biosci.* **2,** d78–d87.
45. Plaut, M., Pierce, J. H., Watson, C. J., Hanley-Hyde, J., Nordan, R. P., and Paul, W. E. (1989) Mast cell lines produce lymphokines in response to cross-linkage of Fc epsilon RI or to calcium ionophores. *Nature* **339,** 64–67.
46. Bradding, P. and Holgate, S. T. (1996) The mast cell as a source of cytokines in asthma. *Ann. N.Y. Acad. Sci.* **796,** 272–281.
47. Bradding, P. (1996) Human mast cell cytokines. *Clin. Exp. Allergy.* **26,** 13–19.
48. Malaviya, R., Ikeda, T., Ross, E., and Abraham, S. N. (1996) Mast cell modulation of neutrophil influx and bacterial clearance at sites of infection through TNF-alpha. *Nature* **381,** 77–80.
49. Walsh, L. J., Trinchieri, G., Waldorf, H. A., Whitaker, D., and Murphy, G. F. (1991) Human dermal mast cells contain and release tumor necrosis factor alpha, which induces endothelial leukocyte adhesion molecule 1. *Proc. Natl. Acad. Sci. USA* **88,** 4220–4224.
50. Bradding, P., Mediwake, R., Feather, I. H., et al. (1995) TNF alpha is localized to nasal mucosal mast cells and is released in acute allergic rhinitis. *Clin. Exp. Allergy* **25,** 406–415.
51. Anderson, W. H., Davidson, T. M., and Broide, D. H. (1996) Mast cell TNF mRNA expression in nasal mucosa demonstrated by *in situ* hybridization: a comparison of mast cell detection methods. *J. Immunol. Methods* **189,** 145–155.
52. Ackerman, V., Marini, M., Vittori, E., Bellini, A., Vassali, G., and Mattoli, S. (1994) Detection of cytokines and their cell sources in bronchial biopsy specimens from asthmatic patients. Relationship to atopic status, symptoms, and level of airway hyperresponsiveness. *Chest* **105,** 687–696.
53. Buckley, M. G., Williams, C. M., Thompson, J., et al. (1995) IL-4 enhances IL-3 and IL-8 gene expression in a human leukemic mast cell line. *Immunology* **84,** 410–415.
54. Krishnaswamy, G., Lakshman, T., Miller, A. R., et al. (1997) Multifunctional cytokine expression by human mast cells: regulation by T cell membrane contact and glucocorticoids. *J. Interferon. Cytokine. Res.* **17,** 167–176.
55. Bradding, P., Roberts, J. A., Britten, K. M., et al. (1994) Interleukin-4, -5, and -6 and tumor necrosis factor-alpha in normal and asthmatic airways: evidence for the human mast cell as a source of these cytokines. *Am. J. Respir. Cell Mol. Biol.* **10,** 471–480.
56. Bradding, P., Feather, I. H., Wilson, S., et al. (1993) Immunolocalization of cytokines in the nasal mucosa of normal and perennial rhinitic subjects. The mast cell as a source of IL- 4, IL-5, and IL-6 in human allergic mucosal inflammation. *J. Immunol.* **151,** 3853–3865.
57. Ying, S., Humbert, M., Barkans, J., et al. (1997) Expression of IL-4 and IL-5 mRNA and protein product by CD4+ and CD8+ T cells, eosinophils, and mast cells in bronchial biopsies obtained from atopic and nonatopic (intrinsic) asthmatics. *J. Immunol.* **158,** 3539–3544.

58. Ando, M., Miyazaki, E., Fukami, T., Kumamoto, T., and Tsuda, T. (1999) Interleukin-4-producing cells in idiopathic pulmonary fibrosis: an immunohistochemical study. *Respirology* **4,** 383–391.

59. Barata, L. T., Ying, S., Meng, Q., et al. (1998) IL-4- and IL-5-positive T lymphocytes, eosinophils, and mast cells in allergen-induced late-phase cutaneous reactions in atopic subjects. *J. Allergy Clin. Immunol.* **101,** 222–230.

60. Okayama, Y., Petit-Frere, C., Kassel, O., et al. (1995) IgE-dependent expression of mRNA for IL-4 and IL-5 in human lung mast cells. *J. Immunol.* **155,** 1796–1808.

61. Lippert, U., Kruger-Krasagakes, S., Moller, A., Kiessling, U., and Czarnetzki, B. M. (1995) Pharmacological modulation of IL-6 and IL-8 secretion by the H1-antagonist decarboethoxy-loratadine and dexamethasone by human mast and basophilic cell lines. *Exp. Dermatol.* **4,** 272–276.

62. Bradding, P., Feather, I. H., Wilson, S., Holgate, S. T., and Howarth, P. H. (1995) Cytokine immunoreactivity in seasonal rhinitis: regulation by a topical corticosteroid. *Am. J. Respir. Crit. Care Med.* **151,** 1900–1906.

63. Bradding, P., Okayama, Y., Howarth, P. H., Church, M. K., and Holgate, S. T. (1995) Heterogeneity of human mast cells based on cytokine content. *J. Immunol.* **155,** 297–307.

64. Kruger-Krasagakes, S., Grutzkau, A., Krasagakis, K., Hoffmann, S., and Henz, B. M. (1999) Adhesion of human mast cells to extracellular matrix provides a co-stimulatory signal for cytokine production. *Immunology* **98,** 253–257.

65. Grutzkau, A., Kruger-Krasagakes, S., Kogel, H., Moller, A., Lippert, U., and Henz, B. M. (1997) Detection of intracellular interleukin-8 in human mast cells: flow cytometry as a guide for immunoelectron microscopy. *J. Histochem. Cytochem.* **45,** 935–945.

66. Hultner, L., Kolsch, S., Stassen, M., et al. (2000) In activated mast cells, IL-1 up-regulates the production of several Th2-related cytokines including IL-9. *J. Immunol.* **164,** 5556–5563.

67. Ishizuka, T., Okayama, Y., Kobayashi, H., and Mori, M. (1999) Interleukin-10 is localized to and released by human lung mast cells. *Clin. Exp. Allergy* **29,** 1424–1432.

68. Burd, P. R., Thompson, W. C., Max, E. E., and Mills, F. C. (1995) Activated mast cells produce interleukin 13. *J. Exp. Med.* **181,** 1373–1380.

69. Toru, H., Pawankar, R., Ra, C., Yata, J., and Nakahata, T. (1998) Human mast cells produce IL-13 by high-affinity IgE receptor cross-linking: enhanced IL-13 production by IL-4-primed human mast cells. *J. Allergy Clin. Immunol.* **102,** 491–502.

70. Kanbe, N., Kurosawa, M., Yamashita, T., Kurimoto, F., Yanagihara, Y., and Miyachi, Y. (1999) Cord-blood-derived human cultured mast cells produce interleukin 13 in the presence of stem cell factor. *Int. Arch. Allergy Immunol.* **119,** 138–142.

71. Rumsaeng, V., Cruikshank, W. W., Foster, B., et al. (1997) Human mast cells produce the CD4+ T lymphocyte chemoattractant factor, IL-16. *J. Immunol.* **159,** 2904–2910.

72. Yano, K., Yamaguchi, M., de Mora, F., et al. (1997) Production of macrophage inflammatory protein-1alpha by human mast cells: increased anti-IgE-dependent secretion after IgE- dependent enhancement of mast cell IgE-binding ability. *Lab. Invest.* **77,** 185–193.

73. Selvan, R. S., Butterfield, J. H., and Krangel, M. S. (1994) Expression of multiple chemokine genes by a human mast cell leukemia. *J. Biol. Chem.* **269,** 13,893–13,898.

74. Trautmann, A., Toksoy, A., Engelhardt, E., Brocker, E. B., and Gillitzer, R. (2000) Mast cell involvement in normal human skin wound healing: expression of mono-cyte chemoattractant protein-1 is correlated with recruitment of mast cells which synthesize interleukin-4 in vivo. *J. Pathol.* **190,** 100–106.

75. Baghestanian, M., Hofbauer, R., Kiener, H. P., et al. (1997) The c-kit ligand stem cell factor and anti-IgE promote expression of monocyte chemoattractant protein-1 in human lung mast cells. *Blood* **90,** 4438–4449.

76. Yamada, T., Sawatsubashi, M., Yakushiji, H., et al. (1998) Localization of vascu-lar endothelial growth factor in synovial membrane mast cells: examination with "multi-labelling subtraction immunostainin." *Virchows Arch.* **433,** 567–570.

77. Nilsson, G., Forsberg-Nilsson, K., Xiang, Z., Hallbook, F., Nilsson, K., and Metcalfe, D. D. (1997) Human mast cells express functional TrkA and are a source of nerve growth factor. *Eur. J. Immunol.* **27,** 2295–2301.

78. De Paulis, A., Minopoli, G., Arbustini, E., et al. (1999) Stem cell factor is localized in, released from, and cleaved by human mast cells. *J. Immunol.* **163,** 2799–2808.

79. Zhang, S., Anderson, D. F., Bradding, P., et al. (1998) Human mast cells express stem cell factor. *J. Pathol.* **186,** 59–66.

80. Krishnaswamy, G., Mukkamala, R., Yerra, L., and Smith, J. K. (1999) Molecular therapies for asthma. *Fed. Pract.* **2,** 16–26.

81. Byrd, R. P., Krishnaswamy, G., and Roy, T. M. (2000) Difficult-to-manage asthma. How to pinpoint the exacerbating factors. *Postgrad. Med.* **108,** 37–51.

82. Gauchat, J. F., Henchoz, S., Mazzei, G., et al. (1993) Induction of human IgE synthesis in B cells by mast cells and basophils. *Nature* **365,** 340–343.

83. Stadler, B. M. and Gauchat, D. (1987) [Current concepts in immunoregulation and its significance for allergies] Concepts nouveaux de l'immuno-regulation et leur signification pour l'allergie. *Rev. Med. Suisse Romande* **107,** 289–293.

84. Paul,W. E. and Seder, R. A. (1994) Lymphocyte responses and cytokines. *Cell* **76,** 241–251.

85. Karpus, W. J., Lukacs, N. W., Kennedy, K. J., Smith, W. S., Hurst, S. D., and Barrett, T. A. (1997) Differential CC chemokine-induced enhancement of T helper cell cytokine production. *J. Immunol.* **158,** 4129–4136.

86. Szczeklik, A. (2000) Atopy and sudden cardiac death. *Lancet* **355,** 2254.

87. Szczeklik, A., Sladek, K., Szczerba, A., and Dropinski, J. (1988) Serum immuno-globulin E response to myocardial infarction. *Circulation* **77,** 1245–1249.

88. Kauhanen, P., Kovanen, P. T., Reunala, T., and Lassila, R. (1998) Effects of skin mast cells on bleeding time and coagulation activation at the site of platelet plug formation. *Thromb. Haemost.* **79,** 843–847.

89. Jeziorska, M., McCollum, C., and Woolley, D. E. (1997) Mast cell distribution, activation, and phenotype in atherosclerotic lesions of human carotid arteries. *J. Pathol.* **182,** 115–122.

90. Kovanen, P. T., Kaartinen, M., and Paavonen, T. (1995) Infiltrates of activated mast cells at the site of coronary atheromatous erosion or rupture in myocardial infarction. *Circulation* **92,** 1084–1088.

91. Reilly, C. F., Schechter, N. B., and Travis, J. (1985) Inactivation of bradykinin and kallidin by cathepsin G and mast cell chymase. *Biochem. Biophys. Res. Commun.* **127,** 443–449.

92. Uehara, Y., Urata, H., Sasaguri, M., et al. (2000) Increased chymase activity in internal thoracic artery of patients with hypercholesterolemia. *Hypertension* **35,** 55–60.

93. Paananen, K. and Kovanen, P. T. (1994) Proteolysis and fusion of low density lipoprotein particles independently strengthen their binding to exocytosed mast cell granules. *J. Biol. Chem.* **269,** 2023–2031.

94. Lindstedt, L., Lee, M., Castro, G. R., Fruchart, J. C., and Kovanen, P. T. (1996) Chymase in exocytosed rat mast cell granules effectively proteolyzes apolipoprotein AI-containing lipoproteins, so reducing the cholesterol efflux-inducing ability of serum and aortic intimal fluid. *J. Clin. Invest.* **97,** 2174–2182.

95. Sillaber, C., Baghestanian, M., Bevec, D., et al. (1999) The mast cell as site of tissue-type plasminogen activator expression and fibrinolysis. *J. Immunol.* **162,** 1032–1041.

96. Cho, S. H., Tam, S. W., Demissie-Sanders, S., Filler, S. A., and Oh, C. K. (2000) Production of plasminogen activator inhibitor-1 by human mast cells and its possible role in asthma. *J. Immunol.* **165,** 3154–3161.

97. Schwartz, L. B., Bradford, T. R., Littman, B. H., and Wintroub, B. U. (1985) The fibrinogenolytic activity of purified tryptase from human lung mast cells. *J. Immunol.* **135,** 2762–2767.

98. Henz, B. M., Maurer, M., Lippert, U., Worm, M., and Babina, M. (2001) Mast cells as initiators of immunity and host defense. *Exp. Dermatol.* **10,** 1–10.

99. Mekori, Y. A. and Metcalfe, D. D. (1999) Mast cell-T cell interactions. *J. Allergy Clin. Immunol.* **104,** 517–523.

100. Arock, M., Ross, E., Lai-Kuen, R., Averlant, G., Gao, Z., and Abraham, S. N. (1998) Phagocytic and tumor necrosis factor alpha response of human mast cells following exposure to gram-negative and gram-positive bacteria. *Infect. Immun.* **66,** 6030–6034.

101. Levi-Schaffer, F. and Rubinchik, E. (1995) Mast cell role in fibrotic diseases. *Isr. J. Med. Sci.* **31,** 450–453.

102. Chlap, Z., Jedynak, U., and Sladek, K. (1998) [Mast cell: its significance in bronchoalveolar lavage fluid cytologic diagnosis of bronchial asthma and interstitial lung disease] Komorka tuczna: znaczenie w diagnostyce cytologicznej plynu oskrzelowo-pecherzykowego w astmie oskrzelowej i chorobach srodmiazszowych pluc. *Pneumonol. Alergol. Pol.* **66,** 321–329.

103. Hunt, L. W., Colby, T. V., Weiler, D. A., Sur, S., and Butterfield, J. H. (1992) Immunofluorescent staining for mast cells in idiopathic pulmonary fibrosis: quantification and evidence for extracellular release of mast cell tryptase. *Mayo Clin. Proc.* **67,** 941–948.

104. Ehara, T. and Shigematsu, H. (1998) Contribution of mast cells to the tubulointerstitial lesions in IgA nephritis. *Kidney Int.* **54,** 1675–1683.

105. Inoue, Y., King, T. E., Jr., Tinkle, S. S., Dockstader, K., and Newman, L. S. (1996) Human mast cell basic fibroblast growth factor in pulmonary fibrotic disorders. *Am. J. Pathol.* **149,** 2037–2054.

106. Chanez, P., Lacoste, J. Y., Guillot, B., et al. (1993) Mast cells' contribution to the fibrosing alveolitis of the scleroderma lung. *Am. Rev. Respir. Dis.* **147,** 1497–1502.

107. Lee, Y. S. and Vijayasingam, S. (1995) Mast cells and myofibroblasts in keloid: a light microscopic, immunohistochemical and ultrastructural study. *Ann. Acad. Med. Singapore* **24,** 902–905.

108. Pesci, A., Bertorelli, G., Gabrielli, M., and Olivieri, D. (1993) Mast cells in fibrotic lung disorders. *Chest* **103,** 989–996.

109. Jordana, M. (1993) Mast cells and fibrosis—who's on first? *Am. J. Respir. Cell Mol. Biol.* **8,** 7–8.

110. Yamashita, Y., Nakagomi, K., Takeda, T., Hasegawa, S., and Mitsui, Y. (1992) Effect of heparin on pulmonary fibroblasts and vascular cells. *Thorax* **47,** 634–639.

111. Jordana, M., Befus, A. D., Newhouse, M. T., Bienenstock, J., and Gauldie, J. (1988) Effect of histamine on proliferation of normal human adult lung fibroblasts. *Thorax* **43,** 552–558.

112. Levi-Schaffer, F., Kelav-Appelbaum, R., and Rubinchik, E. (1995) Human foreskin mast cell viability and functional activity is maintained ex vivo by coculture with fibroblasts. *Cell Immunol.* **162,** 211–216.

113. Heard, B. E., Dewar, A., and Corrin, B. (1992) Apposition of fibroblasts to mast cells and lymphocytes in normal human lung and in cryptogenic fibrosing alveolitis. Ultrastructure and cell perimeter measurements. *J. Pathol.* **166,** 303–310.

114. Adawi, A., Zhang, Y., Baggs, R., et al. (1998) Blockade of CD40-CD40 ligand interactions protects against radiation-induced pulmonary inflammation and fibrosis. *Clin. Immunol. Immunopathol.* **89,** 222–230.

115. Williams, C. M. and Galli, S. J. (2000) The diverse potential effector and immunoregulatory roles of mast cells in allergic disease. *J. Allergy Clin. Immunol.* **105,** 847–859.

116. Worobec, A. S., Akin, C., Scott, L. M., and Metcalfe, D. D. (1998) Cytogenetic abnormalities and their lack of relationship to the Asp816Val c-kit mutation in the pathogenesis of mastocytosis. *J. Allergy Clin. Immunol.* **102,** 523–524.

117. Nagata, H., Okada, T., Worobec, A. S., Semere, T., and Metcalfe, D. D. (1997) c-kit mutation in a population of patients with mastocytosis. *Int. Arch. Allergy Immunol.* **113,** 184–186.

118. Akin, C., Kirshenbaum, A. S., Semere, T., Worobec, A. S., Scott, L. M., and Metcalfe, D. D. (2000) Analysis of the surface expression of c-kit and occurrence of the c-kit Asp816Val activating mutation in T cells, B cells, and myelomonocytic cells in patients with mastocytosis. *Exp. Hematol.* **28,** 140–147.

119. Metcalfe, D. D. and Akin, C. (2001) Mastocytosis: molecular mechanisms and clinical disease heterogeneity. *Leuk. Res.* **25,** 577–582.

120. Hartmann, K. and Henz, B. M. (2001) Mastocytosis: recent advances in defining the disease. *Br. J. Dermatol.* **144,** 682–695.

121. Soter, N. A. (2000) Mastocytosis and the skin. *Hematol. Oncol. Clin. North Am.* **14,** 537–55, vi.

122. Horny, H. P., Ruck, P., Krober, S., and Kaiserling, E. (1997) Systemic mast cell disease (mastocytosis). General aspects and histopathological diagnosis. *Histol. Histopathol.* **12,** 1081–1089.

123. Pullarkat, V. A., Pullarkat, S. T., Calverley, D. C., and Brynes, R. K. (2000) Mast cell disease associated with acute myeloid leukemia: detection of a new c-kit mutation Asp816His. *Am. J. Hematol.* **65,** 307–309.

124. Lehmann, T., Beyeler, C., Lammle, B., et al. (1996) Severe osteoporosis due to systemic mast cell disease: successful treatment with interferon alpha-2B. *Br. J. Rheumatol.* **35,** 898–900.

125. Parker, R. I. (2000) Hematologic aspects of systemic mastocytosis. *Hematol. Oncol. Clin. North Am.* **14,** 557–568.

126. Schwartz, L. B., Sakai, K., Bradford, T. R., et al. (1995) The alpha form of human tryptase is the predominant type present in blood at baseline in normal subjects and is elevated in those with systemic mastocytosis. *J. Clin. Invest.* **96,** 2702–2710.

127. Dabbous, M. K., Woolley, D. E., Haney, L., Carter, L. M., and Nicolson, G. L. (1986) Host-mediated effectors of tumor invasion: role of mast cells in matrix degradation. *Clin. Exp. Metastasis* **4,** 141–152.

128. Duncan, L. M., Richards, L. A., and Mihm, M. C., Jr. (1998) Increased mast cell density in invasive melanoma. *J. Cutan. Pathol.* **25,** 11–15.

129. Le Querrec, A., Duval, D., and Tobelem, G. (1993) Tumour angiogenesis. *Baillieres Clin. Haematol.* **6,** 711–730.

130. Marone, G., Florio, G., Triggiani, M., Petraroli, A., and De Paulis, A. (2000) Mechanisms of IgE elevation in HIV-1 infection. *Crit. Rev. Immunol.* **20,** 477–496.

131. Kolodgie, F. D., Virmani, R., Cornhill, J. F., Herderick, E. E., and Smialek, J. (1991) Increase in atherosclerosis and adventitial mast cells in cocaine abusers: an alternative mechanism of cocaine-associated coronary vasospasm and thrombosis. *J. Am. Coll. Cardiol.* **17,** 1553–1560.

132. Kelley, J., Chi, D. S., Henry, J., Stone, W. L., Smith, J. K., and Krishnaswamy, G. (2000) HIV- and cocaine-induced cardiovascular disease: pathogenesis and clinical implications. *Cardiovasc. Rev. Rep.* **XXI,** 365–370.

133. Buckley, M. G., Walters, C., Wong, W. M., et al. (1997) Mast cell activation in arthritis: detection of alpha- and beta-tryptase, histamine and eosinophil cationic protein in synovial fluid. *Clin. Sci. (Colch.)* **93,** 363–370.

134. Mican, J. M. and Metcalfe, D. D. (1990) Arthritis and mast cell activation. *J. Allergy Clin. Immunol.* **86,** 677–683.

135. Renoux, M., Hilliquin, P., Galoppin, L., Florentin, I., and Menkes, C. J. (1996) Release of mast cell mediators and nitrites into knee joint fluid in osteoarthritis—comparison with articular chondrocalcinosis and rheumatoid arthritis. *Osteoarthritis Cartilage* **4,** 175–179.

136. Renoux, M., Hilliquin, P., Galoppin, L., Florentin, J., and Menkes, C. J. (1995) Cellular activation products in osteoarthritis synovial fluid. *Int. J. Clin. Pharmacol. Res.* **15,** 135–138.

137. Woolley, D. E. and Tetlow, L. C. (2000) Mast cell activation and its relation to proinflammatory cytokine production in the rheumatoid lesion. *Arthritis Res.* **2,** 65–74.

138. He, S., Gaca, M. D., and Walls, A. F. (2001) The activation of synovial mast cells: modulation of histamine release by tryptase and chymase and their inhibitors. *Eur. J. Pharmacol.* **412,** 223–229.

139. Bridges, A. J., Malone, D. G., Jicinsky, J., et al. (1991) Human synovial mast cell involvement in rheumatoid arthritis and osteoarthritis. Relationship to disease type, clinical activity, and antirheumatic therapy. *Arthritis Rheum.* **34,** 1116–1124.

140. Olsson, N., Ulfgren, A. K., and Nilsson, G. (2001) Demonstration of mast cell chemotactic activity in synovial fluid from rheumatoid patients. *Ann. Rheum. Dis.* **60,** 187–193.

141. Yamada, T., Sawatsubashi, M., Yakushiji, H., et al. (1998) Localization of vascular endothelial growth factor in synovial membrane mast cells: examination with "multi-labelling subtraction immunostaining." *Virchows Arch.* **433,** 567–570.

142. Skopouli, F. N., Li, L., Boumba, D., et al. (1998) Association of mast cells with fibrosis and fatty infiltration in the minor salivary glands of patients with Sjogren's syndrome. *Clin. Exp. Rheumatol.* **16,** 63–65.

143. Enestrom, S., Bengtsson, A., and Frodin, T. (1997) Dermal IgG deposits and increase of mast cells in patients with fibromyalgia—relevant findings or epiphenomena? *Scand. J. Rheumatol.* **26,** 308–313.

3

Mast Cells in Allergy and Autoimmunity

Implications for Adaptive Immunity

Gregory D. Gregory and Melissa A. Brown

Summary

As in the fashion industry, trends in a particular area of scientific investigation often are fleeting but then return with renewed and enthusiastic interest. Studies of mast cell biology are good examples of this. Although dogma once relegated mast cells almost exclusively to roles in pathological inflammation associated with allergic disease, these cells are emerging as important players in a number of other physiological processes. Consequently, they are quickly becoming the newest "trendy" cell, both within and outside the field of immunology. As sources of a large array of pro- and anti-inflammatory mediators, mast cells also express cell surface molecules with defined functions in lymphocyte activation and trafficking. Here, we provide an overview of the traditional and newly appreciated contributions of mast cells to both innate and adaptive immune responses.

Key Words: Mast cells; allergy; asthma; autoimmune disease; mast cell-deficient mice (W/W^v); c-kit, activation.

1. Introduction

Mast cells are finally becoming recognized for their potent influence in many physiologic responses outside the realm of allergy. This long-overdue recognition is the result of several factors. First, mast cells contribute to many of the initiating and subsequent events in allergic disease *(1)*. Given allergies cause considerable rates of morbidity in society, most mast cell biologists previously have focused their energy on studying the consequences of mast cell activation in immediate hypersensitivity responses, late-phase allergic inflammation, and chronic inflammation associated with diseases such as asthma. Second, there are considerable difficulties in isolating and analyzing mast cells populations directly ex vivo. Thus, most early studies of mast cells relied on the use of

From: *Methods in Molecular Biology, vol. 315: Mast Cells: Methods and Protocols*
Edited by: G. Krishnaswamy and D. S. Chi © Humana Press Inc., Totowa, NJ

transformed mast cells *(2–5)*. Although such cells have been instrumental in delineating mast cell signaling pathways and in revealing the surprising potential of mast cells to express a wide variety of cytokines and chemokines, they are not useful for assessing in vivo function.

2. Key Discoveries Have Enabled the Current Revolution in Mast Cell Biology

2.1. Identification of Methods to Grow Mast Cells In Vitro

Unlike lymphocytes and monocytes, mast cells do not circulate but remain relatively fixed and dispersed in tissues under basal conditions. Thus, there is no good repository of fully mature mast cells from which to draw to study their function ex vivo. The secondary lymphoid organs normally contain mast cell residents. However, even in inflammatory settings in which additional mast cells migrate to the lymph nodes, the relative scarcity of cells, when compared with T cells or B cells, for example, precludes easy functional analysis. The definition of mast cell differentiation factors, in particular, interleukin (IL)-3 and stem cell factor (SCF), that can act on hematopoietic stem cells present in bone marrow or fetal liver have made it possible to grow large numbers of committed mast cell precursors *(6–11)*. These cells express high levels of c-kit and the high-affinity immunoglobulin E (IgE) receptor (FcεRI), contain preformed mediators that are present in the characteristic granules, and express some of the inducible mast cell mediators associated with more mature tissue mast cells *(11)*. Importantly, bone marrow-derived mast cells (BMDMCs) remain growth factor-dependent, are nontransformed, and thus provide a better model to study mast cell biology.

2.2. Use of Mast Cell-Deficient Mice to Study In Vivo Contributions of Mast Cells

A major breakthrough in mast cell biology was the discovery of several distinct and naturally occurring mutations in the *c-kit* locus, some of which have profound effects on murine mast cell development. Mast cell precursors require the expression of c-kit, a transmembrane receptor with intrinsic tyrosine kinase activity, for the normal response to SCF, a major migration, proliferation, maturation, and survival factor (reviewed in *[12–14]*). SCF is expressed in the variety of tissue microenvironments in which mast cells normally develop. The *c-kit* mutations result in receptors that either fail to be expressed on the cell surface or have markedly deficient tyrosine kinase activity. The most commonly used c-kit-mutant mouse for studies of mast cell function is designated WBB6/F1-*c-kit^W/c-kit^{Wv}* (often referred to as *W/W^v*). W/W^v mice have two distinct mutations in the c-kit receptor locus (which is allelic with the W [white spotting] locus, hence the designation) that result in severe impairment of SCF signaling. The *W* mutation is a loss of function mutation, resulting from a 234 basepair in frame deletion in the c-kit coding sequence resulting in the loss of the transmembrane domain and the N-terminal amino acids of the kinase domain. *c-kit^W* mutations lead to an inability of c-kit to be expressed on the cell surface, and homozygous *c-kit^W* mice exhibit perinatal lethality. The *W^v* mutation results in a leaky, loss-of-function phenotype as the result of a single missense mutation within the canonical kinase sequence resulting in an 80–90% reduction in autophosphorylation of c-kit. *c-kit^{Wv/Wv}* homozygous mice express normal cell surface levels of c-kit and are not mast cell-deficient. However, a cross between *c-kit^{W/+}* and *c-kit^{Wv/+}* mice yields W/W^v heterozygous progeny that are viable and virtually lack mast cells *(15)*. These mice also are deficient in skin melanocytes, are anemic, and are sterile *(12)*. Another mutation, W^{sh}, also results in a mast cell-deficient phenotype. W^{sh}/W^{sh} (W-sash) mice are gaining popularity for use in studies of mast cell function. These mice are viable, fertile, and do not have the anemia that occurs in W/W^v mice *(16–20)*. Although the *sh* mutation in the *c-kit* gene is not yet genetically defined, these mice offer a future alternative to W/W^v mice for mast cell function studies.

An advantage of the c-kit-mutant mouse model for in vivo studies of mast cell function is that normal mast cell populations can be restored to many tissues by the transfer of a population of BMDMCs *(11)*. Reconstitution with BMDMCs leads to a *selective* correction of the mast cell defect (the anemia associated with the *c-kit* mutation is not corrected), allowing a direct assessment of the contribution of mast cells to a given phenotypic outcome.

2.3. Characterization of Other Modes of Mast Cell Activation

A hallmark of mast cells is the cell surface expression of FcεRI *(21)*. The strong interaction of this receptor with IgE molecules confers mast cells with an antigen-specific receptor that can activate the cell immediately upon antigen crosslinking. IgG also is an effective mast cell activator that acts through low-affinity Fcγ receptors *(22–24)*. It is now clear that mast cells can be activated by several Ig-independent routes as well. Mast cells express a number of Toll-like receptors, a highly conserved family of pattern-recognition receptors that are activated by interaction with microbial products *(25)*. Complement, neuropeptides, and several cytokines also elicit degranulation and/or new gene expression *(26–30)*. This finding has implications for understanding mast cells in the context of both allergic and nonallergic events. If an adaptive immune response that elicits IgG and IgE is not necessary for initial mast cell activation, this implies that mast cells can exert their effects much earlier in an immune response than originally proposed, before antigen-specific lymphocyte responses are initiated. Indeed there is evidence that mast cells directly influence the initiation of both T- and B-cell responses.

3. Roles of Mast Cells in Immediate-Type Hypersensitivity

Although allergies can cause extreme discomfort and alter quality of life, they also have the potential to be life threatening. Allergic responses generally are classified as immediate, occurring within minutes of allergen exposure; late phase, occurring within hours; or chronic, during which symptoms can relapse and remit over time, as is the case with asthma *(1)*. These responses generally occur locally at mucosal surfaces, such as the airway passages and the gut, as well as in the skin, where mast cells are prevalent. Although there are differences in the particular manifestations of immediate-type allergic reactions at various sites, all pathology is the direct result of inflammation that gives rise to itch, redness, edema, and cellular influx. When allergen is encountered systemically, anaphylaxis occurs, resulting in rapid onset of these symptoms at several sites simultaneously *(31)*. The precipitous drop in blood pressure can be deadly in this circumstance.

Mast cells are the central effector cells in the early events associated with allergic inflammatory responses. Poised at the interface of the external environment in the skin and at mucosal surfaces, mast cells are situated to be among the first cells to encounter antigens that elicit allergic reactions *(32)*. The high-affinity IgE receptor that associates with IgE through its Fc region forms a stable antigen receptor that shares a remarkably similar downstream signaling pathway with the transmembrane T-cell receptor complex. Interaction of multivalent allergen with cell-bound IgE results in: (1) the immediate release of contents of mast cell secretory granules, which includes preformed mediators such as histamine, neutral proteases, some cytokines, and proteoglycans; and (2) newly synthesized mediators include the products of endogenous arachidonic acid metabolism, such as prostaglandin D and leukotrienes (e.g., LTB_4 and LTC_4). The inducible expression of a large array of cytokines and chemokines also occurs. Collectively, these mediators initiate rapid vascular permeability, leading to plasma extravasation and tissue edema, bronchoconstriction, mucous overproduction, and leukocyte recruitment. Mast cells also are implicated in the late-phase responses. A prolonged secretion of chemoattractive and immunomodulatory molecules contributes to the continuing tissue edema, cellular influx, and inflammation observed hours after initial mast cell activation. Using the mast cell-deficient mouse model, it has been shown that all of the tissue swelling, increased vascular permeability, intersitial clotting, and neutrophil recruitment in both immediate and late phases of an IgE-mediated cutaneous inflammatory response are dependent on mast cells *(13)*.

Although mast cells have an established role in these processes, what is not known is where mast cells first exert their influence. The classic model purports that mast cells are players in immediate-type hypersensitive responses only after the adaptive immune response is established *(33)*. In many respects, an allergic response is very similar to responses to conventional antigens. T cells must be primed (sensitized) via antigen presentation by dendritic cells in the lymph nodes. In allergic responses, this process is thought to be dominated by the generation of Th2 cells, which express IL-4, IL-5, and IL-10 among other cytokines. This Th2 "milieu" has effects on developing B cells, inducing class switching to IgE production, primarily by IL-4 and IL-13. Allergen-specific IgE binds to mast cells and only upon secondary exposure to allergen are the mast cells triggered. However, new findings suggest that mast cells can have a more direct influence on very early events and thus contribute to shaping the character of the adaptive immune response. Evidence to support this comes from studies showing that B cells can undergo isotype switching, leading to the production of IgE in the absence of T cells *(34)*. This switching is dependent on the expression of CD40L (CD154) and IL-4 by mast cells. T-cell responses, as assessed by interferon-γ production and activation markers such as CD44 and CD11a, also are attenuated in mast cell-deficient mice after immunization with peptide and adjuvant (Robbie-Ryan and Brown, unpublished results). Finally, mast cells express IL-4 and IL-12, as well as histamine, molecules that regulate T-helper cell fate decisions. Histamine may exert its effects on T cells, either directly during initial antigen encounter in the lymph node or indirectly through effects on dendritic cells at sites of antigen entry (**Fig. 1.** *[35–38]*).

How mast cells are activated through Ig-independent modes in initial phases of an allergic response is still a matter of speculation. Evidence exists that allergens, many of which are serine proteases, can directly activate mast cells, as has been demonstrated for eosinophils *(39,40)*. As discussed previously in this chapter, a multitude of nonmicrobial agonists of mast cells exist, including neuropeptides, cytokines, and stress hormones, that could also have an influence on mast cell activation in this setting.

4. Roles of Mast Cells in Asthma

Allergic asthma is a chronic disease of the respiratory tract *(41)*. It is characterized by relapsing–remitting episodes of reversible airway obstruction. Clinical symptoms include shortness of breath, wheezing, chest discomfort, and coughing, which can lead to respiratory failure. Eosinophilia, lung inflammation, elevated serum IgE, mucus hypersecretion, and hyperreactive airways are typical. Like immediate hypersensitive responses, allergens elicit the initial symptoms, and mast cell mediators promote early bronchial constriction, airway edema, and mucus plugging as well as recruitment of eosinophils. Lymphocytes and eosinophils are recruited within 24 h and contribute to the disordered airway physiology and early remodeling. Because mast cell-stabi-

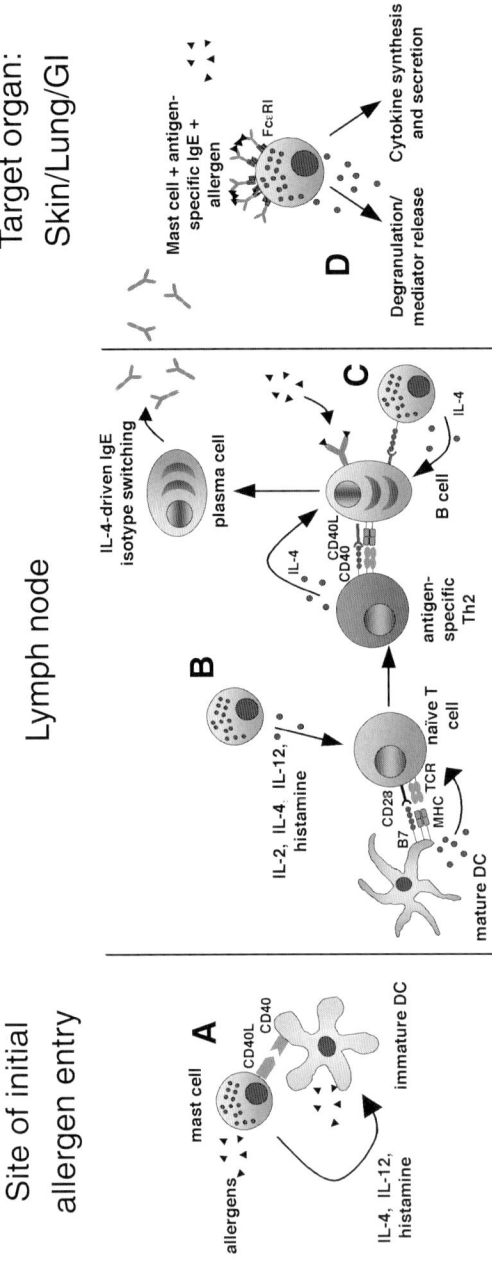

Fig. 1. Mast cells act at multiple sites to modulate allergic inflammation. (**A**) Mast cells may be directly activated by allergen and through the release of mediators and interaction with dendritic cell (DC) CD40 alter DC maturation and migration. (**B**) In the lymph node, cytokines such as IL-4, expressed by mast cells or histamine, directly influence the differentiation of naive allergen-specific T-helper cells upon antigen (allergen) presentation by DCs and promote the differentiation of Th2 cells capable of IL-4 and IL-13 secretion. (**C**) Activated Th2 cells, in conjunction with allergen, can stimulate allergen-specific B cells and promote B cell isotype switching to IgE. Mast cells may also have a direct role in inducing IgE production via IL-4 and interaction with CD40 on B cells. (**D**) Within the target organ (e.g., lung, skin, or gastrointestinal tract), allergen-specific IgE binds to the high-affinity FcεRI receptor expressed on resident mast cells. Crosslinking of the FcεRI/IgE complexes on mast cells by subsequent exposure to allergen leads to mast cell degranulation and release of proinflammatory mediators.

lizing drugs have little value in treating chronic asthma, it has been assumed that mast cells do not contribute to later events in the pathophysiology of this disease.

However, recent data from human studies strongly suggest that mast cells are intimately involved. Mast cells are prevalent within the bronchial smooth muscle, and their density correlates with indices of bronchial hyperresponsiveness. Tryptase, a mast cell specific mediator, induces airway smooth muscle hyperplasia and also affects lung epithelial cells by promoting fibrosis. Long-term effects likely include the irreversible alterations in airway anatomy and decline in lung function with time. Animal models of asthma are limited in their ability to recapitulate chronic asthma and, thus, an in vivo demonstration of the effects of mast cells on chronic asthma has not been established.

5. Roles of Mast Cells in Autoimmune Inflammation

Autoimmune diseases comprise a group of diverse disorders *(42)*. Although they differ in effector mechanisms and site of tissue damage, they are all characterized by immune reactivity to self-antigens. The ensuing inflammation leads to destruction of specific cells or tissues. Clonally expanded populations of self-reactive B or T lymphocytes may initiate some of the inflammatory events, but other immune cells also are essential for the full manifestation of disease. It is not surprising, given the potent proinflammatory capability of mast cells, that mast cells have been implicated in these processes. A wealth of correlative data is available that implicate mast cells in the inflammation that is associated with autoimmune disease. For example, multiple sclerosis is a CD4$^+$ T-cell-mediated autoimmune disease characterized by inflammation in the central nervous system (CNS *[43,44]*). It is associated with an early breach of the blood–brain barrier, focal perivascular mononuclear cell infiltrates, gliosis, and demyelination of the CNS white matter *(44–46)*. A major autoimmune response appears to occur against myelin proteins and/or myelin-producing cells of the CNS (i.e., oligodendrocytes), leading to demyelination, a hallmark of these diseases. More than 100 yr ago, Neuman observed that mast cells were associated with CNS plaques in patients with multiple sclerosis (MS *[47]*). This finding has been confirmed in several subsequent studies. In both the murine model of MS, experimental allergic encephalomyelitis (EAE) and the human disease, it was shown that sites of inflammatory demyelination are also sites of mast cell accumulation in brain and spinal cord *(48–50)*. In acute EAE, the percentage of degranulated mast cells increases with the clinical onset of disease symptoms *(51)*. Tryptase, a mast cell-specific proteolytic enzyme, is elevated in the cerebrospinal fluid of patients with MS *(52)*, and mast cell-derived proteases can degrade myelin in vitro *(53,54)*. Myelin can directly stimulate mast cell degranulation as well *(49,51,55)*. Differences in disease susceptibility may be influenced by genetically determined mast cell numbers. Indeed, the classic EAE-susceptible murine strain, SJL/J, has increased numbers of mast cells compared to the resistant C3H strain *(56)*. Mast cell-stabilizing drugs used to treat both human disease and experimental demyelinating diseases in rodents have met with some success *(57–60)*. Finally, compelling data linking mast cells and MS were very recently obtained in microarray analyses of MS plaques. Transcripts encoding the histamine 1 receptor as well as mast cell-specific genes, including tryptase and FcεRI, are increased significantly in plaques from patients with chronic MS compared with normal control patients *(61)*.

Rheumatoid arthritis, a chronic inflammatory disease of the diarthrodial joints, appears to be exacerbated by mast cells. In collagen-induced arthritis, mast cells accumulate in the swollen paws of mice and are subject to degranulation as disease progresses *(62)*. Mast cells also are implicated in a model of spontaneous disease observed in K/BxN mice *(63)*. Like the human disease, the symptoms appear to be initiated by T cells, but B cells also are required. IgG antibodies to a ubiquitous cytoplasmic enzyme, glucose-6-phospate isomerase, are able to transfer disease in a strain-independent fashion *(64–69)*. These antibodies aggregate as immune complexes with the enzyme at the articular cavity. One of the first events is the degranulation of local mast cells in the joint. In humans, mast cells accumulate in the synovial tissue and fluids of affected joints *(70)*.

Many other examples of the connection between mast cells and autoimmunity exist. Mast cell infiltrates are prevalent in the salivary glands of patients with Sjögren's syndrome, an inflammatory disorder of the tear ducts and salivary glands *(71)*. Bullous pemphigoid, a blistering skin disease, is characterized by degranulated mast cells in the blisters and high concentrations of mast cell-derived chemoattractants in blister fluids *(72–75)*. Mast cell involvement is also suspected in experimental vasculitis and thyroid eye disease *(76,77)*. Because mast cells are located within the pancreatic ducts and implicated in other inflammatory conditions of the pancreas *(78–82)*, there exists a likely role for mast cells in the islet cell destruction associated with type I diabetes. In vivo proof of a role for mast cells has been shown for EAE, serum-induced rheumatoid arthritis, and bullous pemphigoid using mast cell-deficient mice *(63,83,84)*. Although this proof does not definitely prove mast cells alter the course of the human disease counterparts, the features of mast cells, including their widespread distribution, their ability to migrate during an immune response, and the nature of the mediators they produce, make it likely that they do make an important contribution.

It is likely that the details of mast cell activation and their mode of action are somewhat different in these various disease syndromes. Mast cells may be activated relatively late in the inflammatory process by the self-reactive antibodies

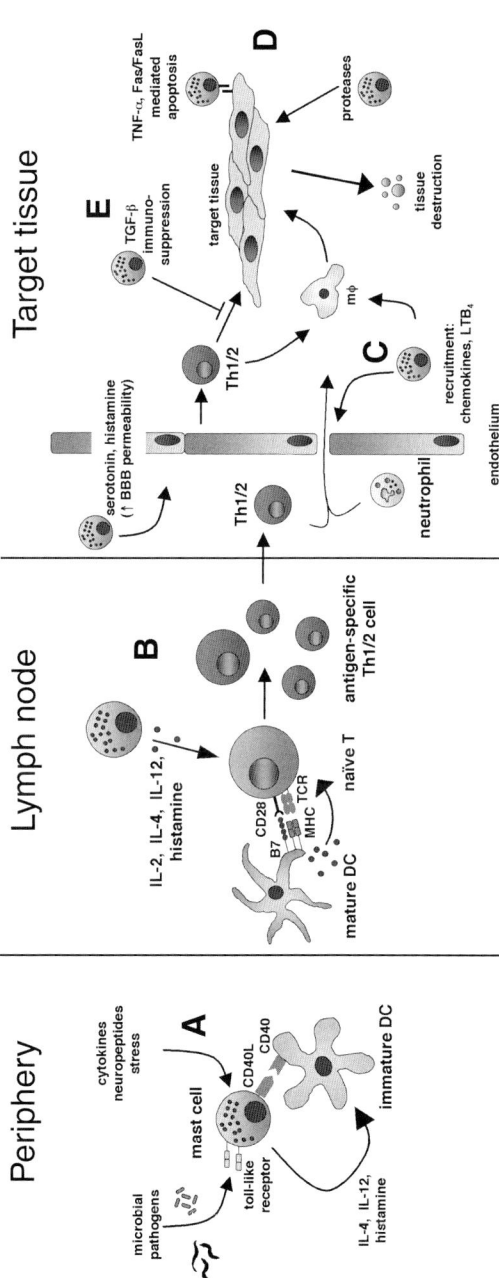

Fig. 2. Mast cell exacerbates the inflammation associated with autoimmunity. (**A**) Mast cells activated by microbial pathogens, cytokines, neuropeptides, or stress may release mediators that could differentially mature/activate dendritic cells (DCs). This release may be particularly relevant in settings in which infection-associated autoimmunity is important. (**B**) In the lymph nodes, resident or newly recruited mast cells can become activated by cytokines, neuropeptides, or stress hormones to release IL-4, IL-12, histamine, and influence the polarization of T cells by directly affecting T cells. (**C**) Mast cells activated at sites of inflammation will secrete a number of chemotactic factors, including MIP1β and LTB$_4$, that can selectively recruit lymphocytes and granulocytes. Histamine and serotonin increase vascular permeability. (**D**) Mast cells also are present at sites of inflammation and may directly damage tissue via release of proteases and TNF-α. (**E**) In contrast to proinflammatory roles, mast cells also may have a protective effect by suppressing inflammation through release of transforming growth factor (TGF)-β and IL-10.

43

observed in rheumatoid arthritis, MS, and systemic lupus erythematosus (SLE) or by complement or cytokines that are present locally. In MS, this can contribute to the activation of CNS antigen-presenting cells and direct destruction of the myelin sheath. Likewise, mast cell products may be directly involved in joint destruction in RA. Mast cell chemokines, particularly IL-8, that recruit neutrophils appear to be important in bullous pemphigus *(84)*. As proposed for mast cells in allergic responses, these cells also may have influence during the inductive phase of disease. The influence of mast cells on dendritic cells at the site of antigen entry may regulate dendritic cell function or T-cell development directly **(Fig. 2)**.

6. Conclusion

Scientists have only begun to understand the place that mast cells have in both immunity and disease. Our understanding of the contribution of mast cells to bacterial immunity *(85,86)*, wound healing *(87)*, angiogenesis *(88)*, cardiac function *(89–91)*, and cancer *(92–95)* is still in its infancy. Although traditionally considered players in Th2 type responses that are dominated by IL-4, IL-13, and IL-10, there is much strain-specific heterogeneity in murine mast cell cytokine responses. In some settings, mast cells that produce high levels of these "anti-inflammatory cytokines" may actually downregulate the immune response. These genetically based differences also are likely to exist in humans and can profoundly affect the magnitude or quality of a response. It is possible that these observations explain, in part, why mast cell mediators do not promote severe allergic responses in some individuals.

References

1. Galli, S. J. and Lantz, C. S. (1999) Allergy, in *Fundamental Immunology, 4th ed.* (Paul, W. E., ed.), Lippincott-Raven Press, Philadelphia. pp. 1127-1174.
2. Taurog, J. D., Mendoza, G. R., Hook, W. A., Siraganian, R. P., and Metzger, H. (1977) Noncytotoxic IgE-mediated release of histamine and serotonin from murine mastocytoma cells. *J. Immunol.* **119,** 1757–1761.
3. Barsumian, E. L., McGivney, A., Basciano, L. K., and Siraganian, R. P. (1985) Establishment of four mouse mastocytoma cell lines. *Cell Immunol.* **90,** 131–141.
4. Siraganian, R. P. (2003) Mast cell signal transduction from the high-affinity IgE receptor. *Curr. Opin. Immunol.* **15,** 639–646.
5. Pierce, J. H., Di Fiore, P. P., Aaronson, S. A., et al. (1985) Neoplastic transformation of mast cells by Abelson-MuLV: abrogation of IL-3 dependence by a nonautocrine mechanism. *Cell* **41,** 685–693.
6. Keller, G., Kennedy, M., Papayannopoulou, T., and Wiles, M. V. (1993) Hematopoietic commitment during embryonic stem cell differentiation in culture. *Mol. Cell Biol.* **13,** 473–486.
7. Ishizaka, T., Adachi, T., Chang, T. H., and Ishizaka, K. (1977) Development of mast cells in vitro. II. Biologic function of cultured mast cells. *J. Immunol.* **118,** 211–217.

8. Valent, P., Sillaber, C., and Bettelheim, P. (1991) The growth and differentiation of mast cells. *Prog. Growth Factor Res.* **3,** 27–41.

9. Denburg, J. A. (1990) Cytokine-induced human basophil/mast cell growth and differentiation in vitro. *Springer Semin. Immunopathol.* **12,** 401–414.

10. Iemura, A., Tsai, M., Ando, A., Wershil, B. K., and Galli, S. J. (1994) The c-kit ligand, stem cell factor, promotes mast cell survival by suppressing apoptosis. *Am. J. Pathol.* **144,** 321–328.

11. Nakano, T., Sonoda, T., Hayashi, C., et al. (1985) Fate of bone marrow-derived cultured mast cells after intracutaneous, intraperitoneal, and intravenous transfer into genetically mast cell-deficient *W/W^v* mice. *J. Exp. Med.* **162,** 1025–1043.

12. Galli, S. J. and Kitamura, Y. (1987) Genetically mast-cell-deficient W/W^v and Sl/Sl^d mice: their value for the analysis of the roles of mast cells in biologic responses in vivo. *Am. J. Pathol.* **127,** 191–198.

13. Galli, S. J., Tsai, M., Gordon, J. R., Geissler, E. N., and Wershil, B. K. (1992) Analyzing mast cell development and function using mice carrying mutations at W/c-kit or Sl/MGF (SCF) loci. *Ann. N. Y. Acad. Sci.* **664,** 69–88.

14. Nocka, K., Tan, J. C., Chiu, E., et al. (1990) Molecular bases of dominant negative and loss of function mutations at the murine c-kit/white spotting locus: W^{37}, W^v, W^{41} and *W. EMBO J.* **9,** 1805–1813.

15. Kitamura, Y., Go, S., and Hatanaka, K. (1978) Decrease of mast cells in *W/W^v* mice and their increase by bone marrow transplantation. *Blood* **52,** 447–452.

16. Duttlinger, R., Manova, K., Berrozpe, G., et al. (1995) The Wsh and Ph mutations affect the c-kit expression profile: c-kit misexpression in embryogenesis impairs melanogenesis in Wsh and Ph mutant mice. *Proc. Natl. Acad. Sci. USA* **92,** 3754–3758.

17. Yamazaki, M., Tsujimura, T., Morii, E., et al. (1994) C-kit gene is expressed by skin mast cells in embryos but not in puppies of Wsh/Wsh mice: age-dependent abolishment of c-kit gene expression. *Blood* **83,** 3509–3516.

18. Duttlinger, R., Manova, K., Chu, T. Y., et al. (1993) W-sash affects positive and negative elements controlling c-kit expression: ectopic c-kit expression at sites of kit-ligand expression affects melanogenesis. *Development* **118,** 705–717.

19. Tono, T., Tsujimura, T., Koshimizu, U., et al. (1992) C-kit gene was not transcribed in cultured mast cells of mast cell-deficient Wsh/Wsh mice that have a normal number of erythrocytes and a normal c-kit coding region. *Blood* **80,** 1448–1453.

20. Besmer, P., Manova, K., Duttlinger, R., et al. (1993) The kit-ligand (steel factor) and its receptor c-kit/W: pleiotropic roles in gametogenesis and melanogenesis. *Dev. Suppl.* 125–137.

21. Scharenber, A. M. and Kinet J. P. (1995) Early events in mast cell signal transduction, in *Human Basophils and Mast Cells: Biological Aspects* (Marone, G., ed.), Karger, Basel, pp. 72–87.

22. Okayama, Y., Tkaczyk, C., Metcalfe, D. D., and Gilfillan, A. M. (2003) Comparison of Fc epsilon RI- and Fc gamma RI-mediated degranulation and TNF-alpha synthesis in human mast cells: selective utilization of phosphatidylinositol-3-kinase for Fc gamma RI-induced degranulation. *Eur J. Immunol.* **33,** 1450–1459.

23. Sylvestre, D. L. and Ravetch, J. V. (1996) A dominant role for mast cell Fc receptors in the Arthus reaction. *Immunity* **5,** 387–390.

24. Daeron, M., Malbec, O., Latour, S., Arock, M., and Fridman, W. H. (1995) Regulation of high-affinity IgE receptor-mediated mast cell activation by murine low-affinity IgG receptors. *J. Clin. Invest.* **95,** 577–585.

25. Marshall, J. S., McCurdy, J. D., and Olynych, T. (2003) Toll-like receptor-mediated activation of mast cells: implications for allergic disease? *Int. Arch. Allergy Immunol.* **132,** 87–97.

26. el-Lati, S. G., Dahinden, C. A., Church, M. K., Dahinden, C. A., and Church, M. K. (1994) Complement peptides C3a- and C5a-induced mediator release from dissociated human skin mast cells. *J. Invest. Dermatol.* **102,** 803–806.

27. Fuereder, W., Agis, H., Willheim, M., et al. (1995) Differential expression of complement receptors on human basophils and mast cells. *J. Immunol.* **155,** 3152–3160.

28. Wotja, J., Kaun, C., Zorn, G., et al. (2002) C5a stimulates production of plasminogen activator inhibitor-1 in human mast cells and basophils. *Blood* **100,** 517–523.

29. Ansel, J. C., Brown, J. R., Payan, D. G., and Brown, M. A. (1993) Substance P selectively activates TNF-alpha gene expression in murine mast cells. *J. Immunol.* **150,** 4478–4485.

30. Galli, S. J. (1997) The mast cell: a versatile effector cell for a challenging world. *Int. Arch. Allergy Immunol.* **113,** 14–22.

31. Kemp, S. F. and Lockey, R. F. (2002) Anaphylaxis: a review of causes and mechanisms. *J. Allergy Clin. Immunol.* **110,** 341–348.

32. Galli, S. and Wershil, B. (1996) The two faces of the mast cell. *Nature* **381,** 21–22.

33. Wills-Karp, M. and Hershey, G. K. K. (2003) Immunological mechanisms of allergic disorders, in *Fundamental Immunology* (Paul, W E., ed.), Lippincott Williams and Wilkins, Philadelphia, pp. 1439–1479.

34. Gauchat, J. F., Henchoz, S., Mazzei, G., et al. (1993) Induction of human IgE synthesis in B cells by mast cells and basophils. *Nature* **365,** 340–343.

35. Jutel, M., Klunker, S., Akdis, M., et al. (2001) Histamine upregulates Th1 and downregulates Th2 responses due to different patterns of surface histamine 1 and 2 receptor expression. *Int. Arch. Allergy Immunol.* **124,** 190–192.

36. Jutel, M., Watanabe, T., Klunker, S., et al. (2001) Histamine regulates T-cell and antibody responses by differential expression of H1 and H2 receptors. *Nature* **413,** 420–425.

37. Mazzoni, A., Young, H. A., Spitzer, J. H., Visintin, A., and Segal, D. M. (2001) Histamine regulates cytokine production in maturing dendritic cells, resulting in altered T cell polarization. *J. Clin. Invest.* **108,** 1865–1873.

38. Teuscher, C., Poynter, M. E., Offner, H., et al. (2004) Attenuation of Th1 effector cell responses and susceptibility to experimental allergic encephalomyelitis in histamine H2 receptor knockout mice is due to dysregulation of cytokine production by antigen-presenting cells. *Am. J. Pathol.* **164,** 883–892.

39. Montealegre, F., Quinones, C., Torres, N., and Goth, K. (2002) Detection of serine proteases in extracts of the domestic mite Blomia tropicalis. *Exp. Appl. Acarol.* **26,** 87–100.

40. Miike, S. and Kita, H. (2003) Human eosinophils are activated by cysteine proteases and release inflammatory mediators. *J. Allergy Clin. Immunol.* **111,** 704–713.

41. Bradding, P. (2003) The role of the mast cell in asthma: a reassessment. *Curr. Opin. Allergy Clin. Immunol.* **3,** 45–50.

42. Marrack, P., Kappler, J., and Kotzin, B. L. (2001) Autoimmune disease: why and where it occurs. *Nat. Med.* **7,** 899–905.

43. Martin, R., McFarland, H. F., and McFarlin, D. E. (1992) Immunological aspects of demyelinating diseases. *Ann. Rev. Immunol.* **10,** 153–187.

44. Steinman, L. (1996) Multiple sclerosis: a coordinated immunological attack against myelin in the central nervous system. *Cell* **85,** 299–302.

45. French-Constant, C. (1994) Pathogenesis of multiple sclerosis. *Lancet* **343,** 271–275.

46. Kermode, A. G. (1990) Breakdown of the blood-brain barrier precedes symptoms and other MRI signs of new lesions in multiple sclerosis. *Brain* **113,** 1477–1489.

47. Neuman, J. (1890) Ueber das Vorkommen der sogneannten "Mastzellen" bei pathologischen Veraenderungen des Gehirns. *Arch. Pathol. Anat. Physiol. Virchows* **122,** 378–381.

48. Bebo, B. F., Jr., Yong, T., Orr, E. L., and Linthicum, D. S. (1996) Hypothesis: a possible role for mast cells and their inflammatory mediators in the pathogenesis of autoimmune encephalomyelitis. *J. Neurosci. Res.* **45,** 340–348.

49. Orr, E. L. (1988) Presence and distribution of nervous system-associated mast cells that may modulate experimental autoimmune encephalomyelitis. *Ann. N.Y. Acad. Sci.* **540,** 723–726.

50. Ibrahim, M. Z., Reder, A. T., Lawand, R., Takash, W., and Sallouh-Khatib, S. (1996) The mast cells of the multiple sclerosis brain. *J. Neuroimmunol.* **70,** 131–138.

51. Brenner, T., Soffer, D., Shalit, M., and Levi-Schaffer, F. (1994) Mast cells in experimental allergic encephalomyelitis: characterization, distribution in the CNS and in vitro activation by myelin basic protein and neuropeptides. *J. Neurol. Sci.* **122,** 210–213.

52. Rozniecki, J. J., Hauser, S. L., Strein, M., Lincoln, R., and Theoharides, T. C. (1995) Elevated mast cell tryptase in cerebrospinal fluid of multiple sclerosis patients. *Ann. Neurol.* **37,** 63–66.

53. Dietsch, G. N. and Hinrichs, D. J. (1991) Mast cell proteases liberate stable encephalitogenic fragments from intact myelin. *Cell. Immunol.* **135,** 541–548.

54. Johnson, D., Seeldrayers, P. A., and Weiner, H. L. (1988) The role of mast cells in demyelination. 1. Myelin proteins are degraded by mast cell proteases and myelin basic protein and P2 can stimulate mast cell degranulation. *Brain Res.* **44,** 195–198.

55. Johnson, D., Weiner, H. L., and Seeldrayers, P. A. (1988) Role of mast cells in peripheral nervous system demyelination. *Ann. N.Y. Acad. Sci.* **540,** 727–731.

56. Johnson, D., Yasui, D., and Seeldrayers, P. (1991) An analysis of mast cell frequency in the rodent nervous system: Numbers vary between different strains and can be reconstituted in mast cell-deficient mice. *J. Neuropath. Exp. Neurol.* **50,** 227–234.

57. Brosnan, C. F. and Tansey, F. A. (1984) Delayed onset of experimental allergic neuritis in rats treated with reserpine. *J. Neuropathol. Exp. Neurol.* **43,** 84–93.

58. Dietsch, G. N. and Hinrichs, D. J. (1989) The role of mast cells in the elicitation of experimental allergic encephalomyelitis. *J. Immunol.* **142,** 1476–1481.
59. Seeldrayers, P. A., Yasui, D., Weiner, H. L., and Johnson, D. (1989) Treatment of experimental allergic neuritis with nedocromil sodium, an anti-inflammatory drug with mast cell stabilizing properties. *J. Neuroimmunol.* **25,** 221–226.
60. Pedotti, R., Mitchell, D., Wedemeyer, J., et al. (2001) An unexpected version of horror autotoxicus: anaphylactic shock to a self-peptide. *Nat. Immunol.* **2,** 216–222.
61. Lock, C., Hermans, G., Pedotti, R., et al. (2002) Gene microarray analysis of multiple sclerosis lesions yield new targets validated in autoimmune encephalomyelitis. *Nat. Med.* **8,** 500–508.
62. Malfait, A. M., Malik, A. S., Marinova-Mutafchieva, L., Butler, D. M., Maini, R. N., and Feldmann, M. (1999) The beta2-adrenergic agonist salbutamol is a potent suppressor of established collagen-induced arthritis: mechanisms of action. *J. Immunol.* **162,** 6278–6283.
63. Lee, D. M., Friend, D. S., Gurish, M. F., Benoist, C., Mathis, D., and Brenner, M. B. (2002) Mast cells: a cellular link between autoantibodies and inflammatory arthritis. *Science* **297,** 1689–1692.
64. Matsumoto, I., Lee, D. M., Goldbach-Mansky, R., et al. (2003) Low prevalence of antibodies to glucose-6-phosphate isomerase in patients with rheumatoid arthritis and a spectrum of other chronic autoimmune disorders. *Arthritis Rheum.* **48,** 944–954.
65. Maccioni, M., Zeder-Lutz, G., Huang, H., et al. (2002) Arthritogenic monoclonal antibodies from K/BxN mice. *J. Exp. Med.* **195,** 1071–1077.
66. Ji, H., Ohmura, K., Mahmood, U., et al. (2002) Arthritis critically dependent on innate immune system players. *Immunity* **16,** 157–168.
67. Benoist, C. and Mathis, D. (2001) Autoimmunity provoked by infection: how good is the case for T cell epitope mimicry? *Nat. Immunol.* **2,** 797–801.
68. Matsumoto, I., Staub, A., Benoist, C., and Mathis, D. (1999) Arthritis provoked by linked T and B cell recognition of a glycolytic enzyme. *Science* **286,** 1732–1735.
69. Ji, H., Korganow, A. S., Mangialaio, S., et al. (1999) Different modes of pathogenesis in T-cell-dependent autoimmunity: clues from two TCR transgenic systems. *Immunol. Rev.* **169,** 139–146.
70. Wolley, D. E. and Tetlow, L. C. (2000) Mast cell activation and its relation to proinflammatory cytokine production in the rheumatoid lesion. *Arthritis Res.* **2,** 65–74.
71. Skopouli, F. N., Li, L., Boumba, D., et al. (1998) Association of mast cells with fibrosis and fatty infiltration in the minor salivary glands of patients with Sjogren's syndrome. *Clin. Exp. Rheumatol.* **16,** 63–65.
72. Baba, T., Sonozaki, H., Seki, K., Uchiyama, M., Ikesawa, Y., and Toriisu, M. (1976) An eosinophil chemotactic factor present in blister fluids of bullous pemphigoid patients. *J. Immunol.* **116,** 112–116.
73. Goldstein, S. M., Wasserman, S. I., and Wintroub, B. U. (1989) Mast cell and eosinophil mediated damage in bullous pemphigoid. *Immunol. Ser.* **46,** 527–545.
74. Wintroub, B. U., Mihm, M. C., Jr., Goetzl, E. J., Soter, N. A., and Austen, K. F. (1978) Morphologic and functional evidence for release of mast-cell products in bullous pemphigoid. *N. Engl. J. Med.* **298,** 417–421.

75. Katayama, I., Doi, T., and Nishioka, K. (1984) High histamine level in the blister fluid of bullous pemphigoid. *Arch. Dermatol. Res.* **276,** 126–127.
76. Ludgate, M. and Baker, G. (2002) Unlocking the immunological mechanisms of orbital inflammation in thyroid eye disease. *Clin. Exp. Immunol.* **127,** 193–198.
77. Kiely, P. D., Pecht, I., and Oliveira, D. B. (1997) Mercuric chloride-induced vasculitis in the Brown Norway rat: alpha beta T cell-dependent and -independent phases: role of the mast cell. *J. Immunol.* **159,** 5100–5106.
78. Esposito, I., Friess, H., Kappeler, A., et al. (2001) Mast cell distribution and activation in chronic pancreatitis. *Hum. Pathol.* **32,** 1174–1183.
79. Esposito, I., Kleeff, J., Bischoff, S. C., et al. (2002) The stem cell factor-c-kit system and mast cells in human pancreatic cancer. *Lab. Invest.* **82,** 1481–1492.
80. Dib, M., Zhao, X., Wang, X., and Andersson, R. (2002) Mast cells contribute to early pancreatitis-induced systemic endothelial barrier dysfunction. *Pancreatology* **2,** 396–401.
81. Dib, M., Zhao, X., Wang, X. D., and Andersson, R. (2002) Role of mast cells in the development of pancreatitis-induced multiple organ dysfunction. *Br. J. Surg.* **89,** 172–178.
82. Zimnoch, L., Szynaka, B., and Puchalski, Z. (2002) Mast cells and pancreatic stellate cells in chronic pancreatitis with differently intensified fibrosis. *Hepatogastroenterology* **49,** 1135–1138.
83. Secor, V. H., Secor, W. E., Gutekunst, C. A., and Brown, M. A. (2000) Mast cells are essential for early onset and severe disease in a murine model of multiple sclerosis. *J. Exp. Med.* **191,** 813–822.
84. Chen, R., Ning, G., Zhao, M. L., et al. (2001) Mast cells play a key role in neutrophil recruitment in experimental bullous pemphigoid. *J. Clin. Invest.* **108,** 1151–1158.
85. Echtenacher, B., Mannel, D. N., and Hultner, L. (1996) Critical protective role of mast cells in a model of acute septic peritonitis. *Nature* **381,** 75–77.
86. Malaviya, R., Ikeda, T., Ross, E., and Abraham, S. N. (1996) Mast cell modulation of neutrophil influx and bacterial clearance at sites of infection through TNF-α. *Nature* **381,** 77–80.
87. Garbuzenko, E., Nagler, A., Pickholtz, D., et al. (2002) Human mast cells stimulate fibroblast proliferation, collagen synthesis and lattice contraction: a direct role for mast cells in skin fibrosis. *Clin. Exp. Allergy* **32,** 237–246.
88. Hiromatsu, Y. and Toda, S. (2003) Mast cells and angiogenesis. *Microsc. Res. Tech.* **60,** 64–69.
89. Gavrisheva, N. A. and Tkachenko, S. B. (2003) Mast cells in normal and diseased heart. *Kardiologiia* **43,** 59–65.
90. Shiota, N., Rysa, J., Kovanen, P. T., Ruskoaho, H., Kokkonen, J. O., and Lindstedt, K. A. (2003) A role for cardiac mast cells in the pathogenesis of hypertensive heart disease. *J. Hypertens.* **21,** 1935–1944.
91. Ren, G., Dewald, O., and Frangogiannis, N. G. (2003) Inflammatory mechanisms in myocardial infarction. *Curr. Drug Targets Inflamm. Allergy* **2,** 242–256.
92. Iamaroon, A., Pongsiriwet, S., Jittidecharaks, S., Pattanaporn, K., Prapayasatok, S., and Wanachantararak, S. (2003) Increase of mast cells and tumor angiogenesis in oral squamous cell carcinoma. *J. Oral Pathol. Med.* **32,** 195–199.

93. Samoszuk, M. and Corwin, M. A. (2003) Mast cell inhibitor cromolyn increases blood clotting and hypoxia in murine breast cancer. *Int. J. Cancer* **107,** 159–163.
94. Le Querrec, A., Duval, D., and Tobelem, G. (1993) Tumour angiogenesis. *Baillieres Clin. Haematol.* **6,** 711–730.
95. Ranieri, G., Passantino, L., Patruno, R., et al. (2003) The dog mast cell tumour as a model to study the relationship between angiogenesis, mast cell density and tumour malignancy. *Oncol. Rep.* **10,** 1189–1193.

II

IDENTIFICATION OF MAST CELLS IN CULTURE AND IN TISSUE

4

Analysis of MC$_T$ and MC$_{TC}$ Mast Cells in Tissue

Lawrence B. Schwartz

Summary

The MC$_{TC}$ and MC$_T$ types of human mast cells initially were recognized on the basis of the protease compositions of their secretory granules, with tryptase, chymase, carboxypeptidase A3, and cathepsin G in the former and only tryptase in the latter. Antibodies against chymase and tryptase traditionally have been used to distinguish these mast cell types from one another. Antitryptase antibodies label all mast cells; antichymase labels only the MC$_{TC}$ type. To identify both types in a tissue section, a sequential double-labeling scheme was developed to first stain chymase-positive cells, thereby blocking their recognition by the antitryptase antibody, which will label only the chymase-negative mast cells. In general, these immunocytochemical techniques are more sensitive and specific than classical histochemical techniques for detecting mast cells.

Key Words: Mast cells; tryptase; chymase.

1. Introduction

Mast cells in humans are primary effector cells in immediate hypersensitivity reactions, such as systemic anaphylaxis, urticaria, atopic asthma, atopic rhinitis, and atopic conjunctivitis. Mast cell involvement in atopic diseases provides neither a teleologic justification for their existence through evolution nor a rationale for their existence in nonatopic individuals. In rodents, mast cells may play a protective role. Rodent mast cells participate in the innate immune response against bacteria and viruses (*1–3*) and also against certain parasites (*4,5*). Rodent mast cells play key roles in the pathogenesis of non-immunoglobulin E (IgE)-mediated hypersensitivity disorders (*6–8*). Mast cells occupy sentinel positions in tissues where noxious substances might attempt entry, and immediate-type hypersensitivity reactions typically begin.

Mast cells in human tissues have been divided into two major types based on the protease content of their secretory granules (*9*). Those cells with tryptase

From: *Methods in Molecular Biology, vol. 315: Mast Cells: Methods and Protocols*
Edited by: G. Krishnaswamy and D. S. Chi © Humana Press Inc., Totowa, NJ

together with chymase, carboxypeptidase, and cathepsin G are called MC_{TC} cells; those with only tryptase are called MC_T cells *(10–12)*. These two phenotypes of mast cells have been studied by electron and light microscopy. Immunogold labeling with antichymase and antitryptase MAbs illustrates the protease phenotypes described above, whereas the scroll-rich granules being more apparent in MC_T cells and grating/lattice substructures in MC_{TC} cells *(13)*. Ultrastructural studies of immature mast cells in tissues suggest that these protease phenotypes appear at the time granules first form *(14)*. MC_{TC} cells are the predominant mast cell type in normal and urticaria pigmentosa skin, perivascular sites, cardiac tissue, and in small bowel submucosa, whereas MC_T cells are the predominant type found in the small bowel mucosa and in the normal airway, where they also appear to be selectively recruited to the surface epithelium of the airway during seasonal allergic disease. In asthmatics, concentrations of MC_{TC} cells in airway smooth muscle increase dramatically and correlate with methacholine-induced bronchial hyperreactivity *(15)*. Of further interest is the selective attenuation of the numbers of MC_T cells in the small bowel of patients with end-stage immunodeficiency diseases *(16)*, a finding that suggests the recruitment, development, or survival of MC_T cells is somehow dependent on the presence of functional T lymphocytes.

Basophils normally reside in the circulation but enter tissues at sites of inflammation, particularly during the late phase of IgE-mediated immediate-hypersensitivity reactions and during the early phase of cell-mediated delayed-type hypersensitivity reactions. Although basophils differ from mast cells by lineage and by a number of morphologic and functional features, they also express tryptase, albeit in much smaller quantities than mast cells *(17)*. Mast cells from different tissues, irrespective of their protease phenotype, and basophils exhibit functional differences in their response to non-IgE-dependent activators and pharmacologic modulators of activation.

Although all mast cells degranulate when FcεRI is cross-linked, skin-derived MC_{TC} cells also respond to C5a and Compound 48/80, whereas MC_T cells from lung do not *(18)*. The ability of MC_{TC} cells to be activated by agents not associated with FcεRI and IgE suggest this cell type may have a greater role in innate immunity by responding to either innate or microbial danger molecules.

Substantial amounts of both PGD_2 and LTC_4 are secreted by FcεRI-stimulated lung-derived MC_T cells, whereas skin-derived MC_{TC} cells make primarily PGD_2 *(19)*. Cord blood-derived mast cells exhibit this same lipid profile as skin-derived mast cells, but when primed with interleukin (IL)-4 and IL-5, their ability to secrete LTC_4 is induced *(20)*.

The functional differences between MC_T and MC_{TC} cells may depend in part upon the properties of the proteases uniquely expressed in the latter cell type *(21)*. For example, the ability of chymase to activate angiotensinogen/ angiotensin I to angiotensin II (independent of angiotensin converting enzyme) and endothelin suggest the potential for mast cells to locally regulate the circulation. Chymase also can process procollagen to a collagen fibril-like material, potentially affecting fibrosis. Finally, the ability of chymase to stimulate mucus production may be important in disorders of the airway, such as asthma.

Another interesting feature that distinguishes MC$_T$ from MC$_{TC}$ cells is their response to IL-4. MC$_T$, but not MC$_{TC}$ cells, undergo apoptosis when treated with IL-4 if IL-6 has been neutralized *(22)*. Otherwise, IL-6 protects MC$_T$ cells from IL-4-induced apoptosis. Also of interest is the ability of MC$_{TC}$ cells from skin to proliferate in serum-free media *(23)*. In contrast, MC$_T$ cells from lung do not proliferate under these conditions. These distinguishing properties may provide pathways for regulating the relative levels of these two mast cell types in tissues. **Subheadings 2.** and **3.** will focus on the detection of these two mast cell types in tissues.

2. Materials

1. Biotin-conjugated or free B7 monoclonal antibody (MAb) against chymase, alkaline phosphatase-conjugated or free G3 MAb against tryptase (Chemicon International, Temecula, CA; *see* **Note 1**).
2. 3-amino-9-ethyl-carbazole, Fast Blue RR and naphthol AS-MX phosphoric acid (Sigma, St. Louis, MO).
3. D-Val-Leu-Arg-4-methoxy-2-naphthylamide (MNA), Z-Ala-Ala-Lys-MNA, and Suc-Ala-Ala-Phe-MNA (Enzyme Systems Products, Livermore, CA).

3. Methods

Although chymase and carboxypeptidase appear to be uniquely expressed by MC$_{TC}$ cells, to date, a unique marker for the MC$_T$ cell has not been reported. Thus, current detection techniques are based on experiments that show all mast cells contain tryptase, while a distinct subset contains chymase.

3.1. Enzyme Histochemistry

Because of the high levels of tryptic activity in all human mast cells and of chymotryptic activity in a portion of these cells, enzyme histochemical substrates have been used to detect MC$_T$ and MC$_{TC}$ cells *(24,25)*. These substrates can be used on cryostat sections of unfixed or formalin-fixed (with or without glutaraldehyde) tissues as well as on sections of paraffin-embedded Carnoy's fluid-fixed tissues. Tissues fixed in aldehydes should be washed overnight at 4°C in 0.05 *M* cacodylate buffer, pH 7.2, containing 7.5% sucrose before being stored at –70°C.

MNA (0.2–0.4 m*M*) and Z-Ala-Ala-Lys-MNA (0.2–0.4 m*M*) have been used successfully for the detection of tryptase activity, whereas Suc-Ala-Ala-Phe-

MNA (0.4 m*M*) can be used for chymase detection. Each MNA substrate is applied in 0.15 *M* of phosphate buffer at an optimal pH (6.5–8.0) containing Fast Blue B salt zinc chloride complex (3.2 m*M*) as a capture reagent at 37°C for a time interval of up to 2 h. Sections are then washed in distilled water, dehydrated with ethanol, cleared and mounted (*see* **Note 2**).

3.2. Immunocytochemistry

3.2.1. Specimen Preparation

1. Carnoy's fluid (ethanol:chloroform:acetic acid, 6:3:1 v/v) originally was reported as an optimal fixative for cytocentrifuged preparations of dispersed mast cells and for tissues. However, fixation of cytocentrifuged preparations with methanol containing 0.6% H_2O_2 and of tissue sections and cytocentrifuged preparations with neutral-buffered formalin also has been performed.
2. Tissue sections that are paraffin embedded should be dewaxed with graded ethanol solutions (100%, 95%, 80%, 70%, 50%, 0%), and nonspecific staining can be reduced by incubation with an appropriate dilution of heat-inactivated serum that corresponds to the species of the secondary antibody.
3. Fixed cells or tissue sections are blocked by incubation with 0.6% H_2O_2 in methanol for 30 min at room temperature if peroxidase is to be used for color development.
4. Cells are then washed with 50 m*M* Tris-HCl, pH 7.6, containing 0.05% Tween-20 and 0.15 *M* NaCl (TTBS).

3.2.2. Single Labeling

1. Anti-tryptase (G3 MAb, 1.5 µg/mL), anti-chymase (B7 MAb, 1.5 µg/mL) or negative control mouse MAb in phosphate-buffered saline (PBS) containing 10% heat-inactivated serum from the species of the secondary detector antibody are incubated with the cells or tissues overnight at 4°C. The optimal MAb concentration must be determined empirically. Shorter incubation periods at room temperature or 37°C may be possible.
2. After washing the cells or tissue section with TTBS, peroxidase-conjugated goat anti-mouse IgG (Fc-specific) is added at an appropriate dilution for 1 h at room temperature.
3. Samples are then washed with TTBS and incubated with a freshly-prepared solution of 3-amino-9-ethyl carbazole (0.2 mg/mL in 0.1 *M* acetated buffer, pH 5.2) containing 0.01% H_2O_2 for 5–10 min at room temperature.
4. The slides are washed with distilled water and then mounted in a 90% glycerol solution. Positively stained cells become reddish brown. Biotinylated primary Ab also can be used and developed with Streptavidin-peroxidase and peroxidase substrate as above. Finally, primary labeling with alkaline phosphatase-conjugated G3 MAb (0.7 µg/mL) followed by Fast Blue RR (1 mg/mL) in 0.1 *M* Tris-HCl, pH 8.2, containing naphthol AS-MX phosphate (0.2 mg/mL) stains tryptase-containing cells blue (*see* **Note 3**).

3.2.3. Simultaneous Double-Labeling

The double-labeling technique in which antitryptase and anti-chymase MAbs are added simultaneously to show that chymase resides in mast cells that also contain tryptase (**9**).

1. Endogenous peroxidase in cytospins and tissue sections is inhibited as previously mentioned.
2. Cells are incubated with a mixture of anti-chymase (biotin-B7, 4 µg/mL) and anti-tryptase (alkaline phosphatase-G3, 0.7 µg/mL) MAbs overnight at 4°C.
3. Tryptase-positive mast cells are stained blue by addition of Fast Blue RR and naphthol AS-MX phosphate, mounted in 90% glycerol, and photographed on a calibrated stage.
4. Cover slips are then floated off and chymase-positive cells are labeled with Streptavidin-peroxidase. By examining the same fields as those photographed after the alkaline phosphatase stage, one can see that chymase-positive cells convert from blue to reddish brown after addition of 3-amino-9-ethyl carbazole. Tryptase-positive mast cells without chymase remain blue (*see* **Note 4**).

3.2.4. Sequential Double-Labeling

Sequential double-labeling with anti-chymase MAb and then anti-tryptase MAb is used to display differentially stained MC_T and MC_{TC} cells in the same tissue section or cytospin (**9,10**).

1. Tissue sections or cytospins prepared as above are incubated first with biotin-B7 MAb (4 µg/mL) overnight a 4°C followed by streptavidin-peroxidase and naphthol AS-MX phosphate.
2. Mast cells with tryptase but not chymase are then labeled with alkaline phosphatase-G3 (0.7 µg/mL), which can then be visualized by deposition of a blue dye, Fast Blue RR, thereby showing chymase⁻ mast cells. Deposition of the reddish-brown naphthol AS-MX phosphate dye on chymase⁺ mast cells blocks subsequent labeling by alkaline phosphatase-conjugated anti-tryptase MAb. When this sequential double-labeling technique has been completed, MC_T cells appear blue and MC_{TC} cells appear brown (*see* **Note 5**).

3.2.5. Immunogold Electron Microscopy

Labeling of chymase and tryptase at an ultrastuctural resolution provides a more detailed analysis of their subcellular locations (**13,14,26**).

3.2.5.1. Single-Labeling

1. Fresh surgical tissue at 4°C is fixed in a solution of in 0.1 *M* of cacodylate buffer, pH 7.2, containing 2% paraformaldehyde and 1.5% glutaraldehyde for 2 h, washed in cacodylate buffer containing 5% sucrose, and postfixed with 1% osmium tetroxide in cacodylate buffer for 1 h. Osmication improves ultrastructural resolution without appreciably affecting immunogold staining.

2. Specimens are then dehydrated in graded ethanol, transferred through propylene oxide, and embedded in araldite obtained from Fluka Durcupan ACM.

3. Thick sections (1 μm) are cut first, stained with toluidine blue and examined for orientation and histologic quality.

4. Then thin sections of 60–100 nm are cut with an ultramicrotome.

5. Thin sections are placed on uncoated 200HH mesh ultrahigh transmission Thinline nickel grids and allowed to dry overnight. Each section fills the entire grid opening of about 1.3 mm in diameter. This viewing area permits viewing of approx 10 mast cells in skin, 15 mast cells in basal intestinal mucosa and superficial submucosa, and 5 mast cells in alveolar wall.

6. Sections on grids are placed upon drops of reagents in cavities of porcelain color plates, etched for 70 min in saturated aqueous sodium metaperiodate solution, and finally washed in microfiltered deionized water.

7. Each grid is washed in PBS and incubated with normal goat serum for 1 h at room temperature. Etching times that were only 15–30 min yielded less immunogold staining, whereas longer etching times produced no apparent change in the distribution or intensity of staining. Use of hydrogen peroxide as an etching agent proved to be suboptimal.

3.2.5.2. DOUBLE-LABELING

1. For double immunogold labeling, grids are placed overnight at 4°C and for 2 h at 25°C onto 20-μL drops of mixtures of each primary Ab. Anti-tryptase (48 μg/mL of the G3 mouse MAb) and anti-chymase (45 or 90 μg/mL of rabbit IgG anti-chymase pAb) antibodies are diluted in PBS containing 0.1% bovine serum albumin (BSA).

2. Sections are then washed sequentially for 5-min intervals in 0.05 M Tris-HCl buffer at pH 7.2, 0.05 M Tris-HCl buffer pH 7.2 containing 0.2% BSA, and 0.05 M Tris-HCl buffer at pH 8.2 containing 1% BSA.

3. Gold-labeled goat IgG anti-mouse IgG and goat IgG anti-rabbit IgG are incubated with the grids for 1 h at room temperature and then sequentially washed in Tris-HCl buffer at pH 7.2 containing 0.2% BSA, Tris-buffered saline, and deionized water. Controls should include omission of the primary antibodies and utilization of comparable concentrations of nonimmune control mouse and rabbit primary antibodies.

4. Sections labeled with the antibodies should be sequentially counterstained with uranyl acetate for approx 5–30 s, depending on the tissue, and then with lead citrate for 45–90 s and examined by transmission electron microscopy. Using this technique one concludes that MC_{TC} cells store tryptase and chymase in the same secretory granules, whereas MC_T cells lack chymase in all secretory granules.

3.3. Flow Cytometry

3.3.1. Lung-Derived Mast Cells

Fresh surgical specimens of human lung are mechanically minced and digested with proteases to disperse cells *(27)*.

1. Samples should be minced in a balanced salt buffer such as Hank's balanced salt solution without calcium (HBSS⁻), and incubated with type 2 collagenase (1.5 mg/mL) and hyaluronidase (0.5 mg/mL) at 37°C for 60 min with gentle agitation (2–5 mL of protease solution per gram of lung).
2. Dispersed cells are separated from residual tissue by washing them through a no. 80 mesh sieve.
3. Proteases are then removed by washing the cells in HBSS⁻.
4. Residual tissue is digested up to three more times to disperse retained mast cells.
5. The dispersed cells are combined, filtered, layered onto a 65–70% (v/v) Percoll cushion and centrifuged at 700g for 20 min at room temperature. Erythrocytes and tissue debris pass through the cushion while nucleated cells are collected from the HBSS⁻/Percoll interface. Typically 0.2 to 1 × 10⁶ mast cells of 5–15% purity are obtained per gram of lung.

3.3.2. Skin-Derived Mast Cells

1. Fresh samples of surgical skin are cleaned of subcutaneous fat by blunt dissection, and residual tissue is cut into 1- to 2-mm fragments and digested with type 2 collagenase (1.5 mg/mL), hyaluronidase (0.7 mg/mL), and type 1 DNase (0.3 mg/mL) in HBSS⁻ for 2 h at 37°C *(23)*.
2. The dispersed cells are collected by filtering through a no. 80 mesh sieve and are then resuspended in HBSS containing 1% FCS and 10 mM 4-(2-hydroxyethyl)-1-piperazine-ethanesulfonic acid (HEPES).
3. Resuspended cells are layered over a 70–75% Percoll cushion and centrifuged at 700g at room temperature for 20 min. Nucleated cells are collected from the buffer/Percoll interface, while erythrocytes sediment to the bottom of the tube (*see* **Note 5**).
4. Skin-derived mast cells can be cultured at a concentration of 1 × 10⁶ cells/mL in serum-free AIM-V medium (Life Technologies, Rockville, MD) containing 100 ng/mL of recombinant human stem cell factor at 37°C in 6% CO$_2$. The culture medium should be changed weekly and cells are split when they reach a concentration of approx 2 × 10⁶ cells/mL. The percentages of mast cells can be assessed cytochemically by metachromatic staining with toluidine blue, immunocytochemistry with anti-tryptase and anti-chymase Abs and by flow cytometry with anti-Kit (YB5.B8) and anti-FcεRI (22E7) MAbs. The protease phenotype of cultured cells can be examined by immunocytochemistry with anti-tryptase and anti-chymase MAbs *(10)*. Typically, mature mast cells approaching 100% purity are obtained by 4 wk of culture, and these cells divide about every 5–7 d for 2–3 mo.

4. Notes

1. Alternative mouse monoclonal antibodies against chymase (CC1) and tryptase (AA1) (Calbiochem, San Diego, CA) are also available.
2. Although mast cells in general are readily distinguished from other cell types because of their large content of proteases, these substrates are not specific for tryptase and chymase. Consequently, other cell types with trypsin-like and chy-

motrypsin-like proteases will be labeled. In contrast, antibodies against these enzymes can provide greater specificity.

3. All human mast cells are stainable with the anti-tryptase MAb, whereas only a subset is stainable with the anti-chymase MAb. Basophils, which contain much less tryptase than mast cells *(17)*, often are stained after indirect immunocytochemistry but not with the less-sensitive alkaline phosphatase-G3 technique described in **Note 2** *(28)*.

4. Although basophils from healthy subjects do not express chymase, one study indicated that those from patients with asthma or drug allergic reactions may do so *(29)*, whereas another study found that basophils from asthmatics do not express chymase *(30)*. Also, transient expression of chymase in a human bone marrow-derived cell of uncertain lineage also has been reported *(31)*.

5. The precise conditions for sequential double-labeling to effectively distinguish chymase-positive from chymase-negative mast cells must be determined empirically. The advantage of the technique is that blue MC_T cells and reddish brown MC_{TC} cells can be visualized in the same field. However, because tryptase resides in both cell types, the success of the technique requires relatively intense staining for chymase such that the anti-tryptase MAb is blocked from recognizing tryptase in those cells.

6. Cells from lung and skin that have been enriched by Percoll density-dependent sedimentation are suitable for activation and tissue culture. To reduce the likelihood of any microbial contamination, cells are typically layered over a solution of PBS containing 20% human AB serum (Sigma) and centrifuged at low speed (500g) for 20 min at room temperature. Further purification of the mast cells can be achieved by cell sorting or magnetic bead techniques using anti-Kit antibody. However, this technique does not separate MC_T from MC_{TC} cells.

References

1. Malaviya, R. and Georges, A. (2002) Regulation of mast cell-mediated innate immunity during early response to bacterial infection. *Clin. Rev. Allergy Immunol.* **22,** 189–204.

2. Marone, G., Florio, G., Petraroli, A., Triggiani, M., and De Paulis, A. (2001) Role of human Fc epsilon RI+ cells in HIV-1 infection. *Immunol. Rev.* **179,** 128–138.

3. Marshall, J. S., King, C. A., and McCurdy, J. D. (2003) Mast cell cytokine and chemokine responses to bacterial and viral infection. *Curr. Pharm. Des.* **9,** 11–24.

4. Urban, J. F., Schopf, L., Morris, S. C., et al. (2000) Stat6 signaling promotes protective immunity against Trichinella spiralis through a mast cell- and T cell-dependent mechanism. *J. Immunol.* **164,** 2046–2052.

5. Knight, P. A., Wright, S. H., Lawrence, C. E., Paterson, Y. Y., and Miller, H. R. (2000) Delayed expulsion of the nematode Trichinella spiralis in mice lacking the mucosal mast cell-specific granule chymase, mouse mast cell protease-1. *J. Exp. Med.* **192,** 1849–1856.

6. Sylvestre, D. L. and Ravetch, J. V. (1996) A dominant role for mast cell Fc receptors in the Arthus reaction. *Immunity* **5,** 387–390.

7. Lee, D. M., Friend, D. S., Gurish, M. F., Benoist, C., Mathis, D., and Brenner, M. B. (2002) Mast cells: a cellular link between autoantibodies and inflammatory arthritis. *Science* **297**, 1689–1692.

8. Robbie-Ryan, M., Tanzola, M. B., Secor, V. H., and Brown, M. A. (2003) Cutting edge: both activating and inhibitory Fc receptors expressed on mast cells regulate experimental allergic encephalomyelitis disease severity. *J. Immunol.* **170**, 1630–1634.

9. Irani, A. A., Schechter, N. M., Craig, S. S., DeBlois, G., and Schwartz, L. B. (1986) Two types of human mast cells that have distinct neutral protease compositions. *Proc. Natl. Acad. Sci. USA* **83**, 4464–4468.

10. Irani, A.-M. A., Bradford, T. R., Kepley, C. L., Schechter, N. M., and Schwartz, L. B. (1989) Detection of MC$_T$ and MC$_{TC}$ types of human mast cells by immunohistochemistry using new monoclonal anti-tryptase and anti-chymase antibodies. *J. Histochem. Cytochem.* **37**, 1509–1515.

11. Schechter, N. M., Irani, A.-M. A., Sprows, J. L., Abernethy, J., Wintroub, B., and Schwartz, L. B. (1990) Identification of a cathepsin G-like proteinase in the MC$_{TC}$ type of human mast cell. *J. Immunol.* **145**, 2652–2661.

12. Irani, A.-M. A., Goldstein, S. M., Wintroub, B. U., Bradford, T., and Schwartz, L. B. (1991) Human mast cell carboxypeptidase: selective localization to MC$_{TC}$ cells. *J. Immunol.* **147**, 247–253.

13. Craig, S. S., Schechter, N. M., and Schwartz, L. B. (1988) Ultrastructural analysis of human T and TC mast cells identified by immunoelectron microscopy. *Lab. Invest.* **58**, 682–691.

14. Craig, S. S., Schechter, N. M., and Schwartz, L. B. (1989) Ultrastructural analysis of maturing human T and TC mast cells *in situ*. *Lab. Invest.* **60**, 147–157.

15. Brightling, C. E., Bradding, P., Symon, F. A., Holgate, S. T., Wardlaw, A. J., and Pavord, I. D. (2002) Mast-cell infiltration of airway smooth muscle in asthma. *N. Engl. J. Med.* **346**, 1699–1705.

16. Irani, A. M., Craig, S. S., DeBlois, G., Elson, C. O., Schechter, N. M., and Schwartz, L. B. (1987) Deficiency of the tryptase-positive, chymase-negative mast cell type in gastrointestinal mucosa of patients with defective T lymphocyte function. *J. Immunol.* **138**, 4381–4386.

17. Jogie-Brahim, S., Min, H. K., Fukuoka, Y., Xia, H. Z., and Schwartz, L. B. (2004) Expression of alpha-tryptase and beta-tryptase by human basophils. *J. Allergy Clin. Immunol.* **113**, 1086–1092.

18. Oskerittian, C. A., Zhao, W., Min, H., et al. (2005) Surface CD88 functionally distinguishes the MC$_{tc}$ type of human lung mast cell. *J. Allergy Clin. Immunol.*, In Press.

19. Lawrence, I. D., Warner, J. A., Cohan, V. L., Hubbard, W. C., Kagey-Sobotka, A., and Lichtenstein, L. M. (1987) Purification and characterization of human skin mast cells. *J. Immunol.* **139**, 3062–3069.

20. Hsieh, F. H., Lam, B. K., Penrose, J. F., Austen, K. F., and Boyce, J. A. (2001) T helper cell type 2 cytokines coordinately regulate immunoglobulin E-dependent cysteinyl leukotriene production by human cord blood-derived mast cells: Pro-

found induction of leukotriene C-4 synthase expression by interleukin 4. *J. Exp. Med.* **193,** 123–133.

21. Schwartz, L. B. (2002) Mast cells and basophils, in *Inflammatory Mechanisms in Allergic Diseases*, (Zweiman, B. and Schwartz, L. B., eds.), Marcel Dekker, New York, pp. 3–42.

22. Oskeritzian, C. A., Zhao, W., Pozez, A. L., Cohen, N. M., Grimes, M., and Schwartz, L. B. (2004) Neutralizing endogenous IL-6 renders mast cells of the MCT type from lung, but not the MCTC type from skin and lung, susceptible to human recombinant IL-4-induced apoptosis. *J. Immunol.* **172,** 593–600.

23. Kambe, N., Kambe, M., Kochan, J. P., and Schwartz, L. B. (2001) Human skin-derived mast cells can proliferate while retaining their characteristic functional and protease phenotypes. *Blood* **97,** 2045–2052.

24. Osman, I. A. R., Garrett, J. R., and Smith, R. E. (1989) Enzyme histochemical discrimination between tryptase and chymase in mast cells of human gut. *J. Histochem. Cytochem.* **37,** 415–421.

25. Harvima, I. T., Naukkarinen, A., Harvima, R. J., and Fraki, J. E. (1988) Immunoperoxidase and enzyme-histochemical demonstration of human skin tryptase in cutaneous mast cells in normal and mastocytoma skin. *Arch. Dermatol. Res.* **280,** 363–370.

26. Craig, S. S. and Schwartz, L. B. (1990) Human MC$_{TC}$ type of mast cell granule: the uncommon occurrence of discrete scrolls associated with focal absence of chymase. *Lab. Invest.* **63,** 581–585.

27. Xia, H. Z., Kepley, C. L., Sakai, K., Chelliah, J., Irani, A. M., and Schwartz, L. B. (1995) Quantitation of tryptase, chymase, FcεRIα, and FcεRIgamma mRNAs in human mast cells and basophils by competitive reverse transcription-polymerase chain reaction. *J. Immunol.* **154,** 5472–5480.

28. Castells, M. C., Irani, A. M., and Schwartz, L. B. (1987) Evaluation of human peripheral blood leukocytes for mast cell tryptase. *J. Immunol.* **138,** 2184–2189.

29. Li, L. X., Li, Y., Reddel, S. W., et al. (1998) Identification of basophilic cells that express mast cell granule proteases in the peripheral blood of asthma, allergy, and drug-reactive patients. *J. Immunol.* **161,** 5079–5086.

30. Foster, B., Schwartz, L. B., Devouassoux, G., Metcalfe, D. D., and Prussin, C. (2002) Characterization of mast-cell tryptase-expressing peripheral blood cells as basophils. *J. Allergy Clin. Immunol.* **109,** 287–293.

31. Shimizu, Y., Suga, T., Maeno, T., et al. (2004) Detection of tryptase-, chymase+ cells in human CD34 bone marrow progenitors. *Clin. Exp. Allergy* **34,** 1719–1724.

5

Mast Cell Ultrastructure and Staining in Tissue

Shruti A. Shukla, Ranjitha Veerappan, Judy S. Whittimore, Lou Ellen Miller, and George A. Youngberg

Summary

Mast cells are bone marrow-derived cells that are widely distributed in the tissue. They are found predominantly in the subepithelial tissue near blood vessels and nerves and usually are sprinkled diffusely without forming clusters. In tissue sections stained with hematoxylin and eosin, normal mast cells usually display a round-to-oval nucleus with clumped chromatin and indistinct or no nucleoli. They have moderately abundant cytoplasm and are oval, spindle, or polygonal in shape. The cytoplasm is amphophilic, and sometimes small slightly eosinophilic granules may be visible. Hematoxylin and eosin staining is not a specific or reliable method for detecting mast cells in tissue sections because of variable cellular morphology. For confirmation of mast cells, special stains, such as mast cell tryptase or CD117, are required.

Key Words: Mast cell; hematoxylin and eosin; toluidine blue; mast cell tryptase and chymase; Leder stain; CD117 (*c-kit*); ultrastructure.

1. Introduction

Identification of mast cells in tissue can be performed by routine staining methods that allow visualization of cellular morphology by using special stains that are more specific for mast cells or by performing ultrastructural examination. In this chapter, methods to prepare tissue for ultrastructural examination, along with procedures to perform different stains that are commonly used to identify mast cells, are described. The methods described in this chapter are well established and are obtained from the listed references. Hematoxylin and eosin, which is the most common stain used for tissue sections in pathology, is not a very specific or reliable method to demonstrate mast cells. Other histochemical and immunohistochemical stains, such as toluidine blue, mast cell tryptase and chymase, Leder stain, and CD117 (*c-kit*), are more specific for mast cells.

From: *Methods in Molecular Biology, vol. 315: Mast Cells: Methods and Protocols*
Edited by: G. Krishnaswamy and D. S. Chi © Humana Press Inc., Totowa, NJ

Mast cells also can be identified on electron microscopy. Ultrastructurally, the mast cell nucleus is small with a round-to-oval shape. The cell surface shows slender filiform cytoplasmic projections or folds. Numerous membrane-bound mast cell granules are present in the cytoplasm in addition to rough endoplasmic reticulum, Golgi vesicles, free ribosomes, mitochondria, lysosomes, filaments, microtubules, and lipid bodies. The mast cells can be of two subtypes depending on the scroll-rich or scroll-poor morphologies displayed by the granules *(1)*. Both morphologies may demonstrate granules with amorphous material, finely granular electron-dense material, nondiscrete scroll formations that merge with one another, loosely organized internal lamellae, or some peripheral coiled parallel lamellae. The scroll-rich variant has granules containing multiple discrete complete membranous scroll formations that are usually loosely wound and may enclose cores of central electron dense material. Some granules may display tightly wound scrolls. Granules with discrete scrolls are generally absent in mast cells with scroll-poor morphology. Crystalloid substructures with a grating or lattice appearance may be seen in some of the electron-dense granules that are present in cells with scroll-poor morphology.

The substructures can demonstrate variable periodicities. Granules associated with the scroll-poor morphology tend to be more numerous, larger, and more uniform in shape. Lipid bodies, large round nonmembrane-bound cytoplasmic structures with internal lucencies, are less frequent in cells with scroll-poor morphology. The scroll-rich and the scroll-poor morphology (grating or lattice patterns), along with varying content of chymase and tryptase, further divide the mast cells into the MC_T (tryptase-positive only) and MC_{TC} (tryptase- and chymase-positive) subtypes, respectively. Effects of fixation and variable planes of sectioning cause difficulties in the interpretation of granule morphology. Mast cells cultured from peripheral blood have been shown to have minimal chymase activity in presence of a scroll-poor ultrastructure. Mast cell ultrastructure can be affected by the degree of maturity and by degranulation. Immature mast cells demonstrate a smaller size and a higher nuclear cytoplasmic ratio with fewer granules. Granules with dense central nucleoids embedded in granule matrix may be present *(1,2)*.

In regard to staining methods, hematoxylin, the most widely used nuclear stain, is extracted from logwood known as campeache wood. Fresh-cut wood is colorless but converted to dark reddish brown when exposed to atmospheric oxidation; the oxidized dye is hematein *(3)*. Hematoxylin and its counterstain eosin are the most commonly used stains for routine histologic examination of tissue sections.

The classic histochemical stains used to demonstrate mast cells are the metachromatic stains like toluidine blue. The membrane-bound granules in the mast cell cytoplasm contain biologically active mediators, including acidic proteoglycans, which bind basic dyes, such as toluidine blue. Because stained granules typically acquire a color that is different from that of a native dye, they are referred to as metachromatic granules. Metachromatic stains are strongly recommended as routine stains for mast cells *(4).*

The most specific method for identification of mast cells in tissue is immunohistochemical staining for mast cell tryptase. It has been recently demonstrated that tryptase is present in both major subtypes of human mast cells that have been described so far: T mast cells, predominantly found in the lung and containing only tryptase, and TC mast cells, predominantly found in the skin and bowel and containing chymase in addition to tryptase. Tryptase alone is useful in the identification of mast cells, whereas the addition of the chymase stain helps in subtyping the mast cell population. Rare human mast cells may contain only chymase *(5–7).*

Esterases are enzymes that are capable of hydrolyzing aliphatic and aromatic bonds. They have been classified as specific or nonspecific esterases depending on their preference for certain substrates. Chloacetate esterase is found in granulocytes and mast cells. Specimens containing mast cells are incubated with naphthol AS-D chloracetate in the presence of freshly formed diazonium salt. Enzymatic hydrolysis of ester linkages liberates free naphthol compounds. These couple with the diazonium salt forming highly colored deposits at the site of enzyme activity *(8,9).*

CD117 (*c-kit*) is a tyrosine kinase receptor found in various normal cells, including interstitial cells of Cajal, germ cells, bone marrow stem cells, melanocytes, breast epithelium, and mast cells. It also can be found in a wide variety of tumors, such as follicular and papillary carcinoma of the thyroid; adenocarcinoma of the endometrium, lung, ovary, pancreas, and breast; malignant melanoma; endodermal sinus tumor; and small cell carcinoma, and has been particularly useful in identifying gastrointestinal stromal tumors *(10–13).* Several other stains have been used to identify mast cells or mast cell subsets, including berberine and Alcian blue. CD34 is used in the proper context to identify mast cell precursors.

2. Materials

2.1. Tissue Preparation for Electron Microscopy

1. Tissue fixative: 3% glutaraldehyde in cacodylate buffer and 1% osmium tetroxide in cacodylate buffer.
2. 70% ethanol.
3. 100% ethanol.
4. 100% propylene oxide.
5. Araldite 502.
6. Dodecenyl succinic anhydride (DDSA; HY 964).
7. 2,4,6-tris (dimethylaminomethyl) phenol; (DMP-30; DY 064).
8. Uranyl acetate in 50% ethanol.

9. 10 *N* sodium hydroxide.
10. Embedding medium (*see* **Note 1**): 20 mL of araldite 502, 22 mL of DDSA, and 0.63–0.84 mL of DMP-30.
11. Lead citrate solution: add 0.3 g of lead citrate and 0.5 mL of 10 *N* sodium hydroxide to 10 mL of distilled water in a centrifuge tube. Shake the tube until the lead citrate is dissolved.

2.2. Tissue Preparation for Paraffin-Embedded Tissue

1. Alcoholic formalin (10% formalin, 65% alcohol).
2. 95% alcohol.
3. Absolute alcohol.
4. Xylene.
5. Paraffin.
6. The paraffin embedded specimens are cut at 4–5 µ and appropriate sections are used for hematoxylin and eosin stain, toluidine blue stain, mast cell tryptase and chymase stain, Leder stain, and CD117 stain.
7. Control sections can be obtained from paraffin-embedded sections of neurofibromas with mast cells for the toluidine blue stain, Leder stain, and CD117 stain. Paraffin-embedded sections of skin, colon, or lung can be used for mast cell tryptase and chymase stains.

2.3. Hematoxylin and Eosin Staining

1. Harris hematoxylin: 5 g of hematoxylin, 50 mL of absolute ethyl alcohol, 100 g of ammonium aluminum sulfate (aluminum works as mordant), 1000 mL of distilled water, and 2.5 g of mercuric oxide (ripening agent).
2. Eosin solution: 200 mL of eosin Y (1% aqueous solution), 600 mL of 95% ethyl alcohol, and 4 mL of acetic acid glacial. (This solution must be acidic, best staining occurs at pH 4.6–5.0, to develop the appropriate charge on protein.)

2.4. Toluidine Blue Staining

1. 0.5% toluidine blue stain: 0.5 g of toluidine blue O (CI no. 52040 Certistain®, Merck, cat. no. 1.15930) and 100 mL of distilled water.

2.5. Mast Cell Tryptase and Chymase Staining

1. 0.05 *M* Tris-buffered saline (DAKO® TBS, cat. no. S3001), pH 7.2–7.6.
2. DAKO EnVision® system, peroxidase (K1390) includes: peroxidase blocking reagent, labeled polymer, buffered substrate solution, pH 7.5, and DAB chromogen.
3. Absorbent wipes.
4. Ammonium hydroxide, 15 *M* diluted to 37 m*M*.
5. Harris hematoxylin.
6. 95% and absolute ethanol.
7. Anti-human tryptase monoclonal antibodies (Promega, cat. no. G3361).

2.6. Leder Stain (Naphthol-AS-D Chloracetate Esterase) Staining (see *Note 2*)

1. The commercially available Sigma Kit (no. 91C) includes: Naphthol AS-D chloracetate solution, Fast Blue BB base solution, Trizmal concentrate pH −7.6 ± 0.15, sodium nitrite solution, citrate solution and Gill No.3 hematoxylin solution.
2. Acetone.
3. 37% formaldehyde.

2.7. CD117 (C-Kit) Staining

1. Electric pressure cooker (Cell Marque™, cat. no. CMM977).
2. One pair of plastic staining dishes and slide rack (Cell Marque, cat. no. CMM960).
3. Declere by Cell Marque (cat. no. CMX633-P) or Trilogy™ by Cell Marque (cat. no. CMX833-P).
4. Anti-CD117 antibody (Cell Marque) is available as 1, 6, or 15 mL prediluted antibodies that are ready to use and as 0.05, 0.5, or 1 mL concentrate, which can be diluted 1:10 or 1:30 before using. Five slides per pack of positive control slides are available.

3. Methods

The methods described in **Subheadings 3.1.–3.7.** outline: (1) tissue preparation for electron microscopy; (2) tissue preparation for paraffin-embedded tissue; (3) hematoxylin and eosin staining; (4) toluidine blue staining; (5) mast cell chymase and tryptase staining; (6) Leder staining; and (7) CD117 staining in tissue sections.

3.1. Tissue Preparation for Electron Microscopy

The procedure for tissue preparation includes fixation, dehydration, infiltration, embedding, and staining. Araldite 502 is an epoxy resin embedding medium that is used in our laboratory. Tissues to be embedded in araldite 502 can be dehydrated with commonly used organic solvents such as propylene oxide, because epoxy resins are more soluble in propylene oxide *(14–16)*.

3.1.1. Fixation

Tissues can be fixed in a wide range of fixatives. The tissue is diced into small fragments to achieve better fixation and infiltration. One of the most commonly used fixation method is utilizing glutaraldehyde followed by osmium tetroxide. The procedure used in our laboratory is given below:

1. Tissue is fixed with 3% glutaraldehyde in cacodylate buffer for 3 h.
2. Replace the glutaraldehyde solution with 1% osmium tetroxide in cacodylate buffer and let the tissue fix for 1 h.

3.1.2. Dehydration

Many different dehydration schedules can be followed. The procedure used in our institution is as follows:

1. Replace the fixative with 70% ethanol for 10 min.
2. Replace the solution with 95% ethanol for 10 min.
3. Replace the solution with 100% ethanol for 10 min.
4. Replace the solution with 100% ethanol for 15 min.
5. Replace the solution with 100% propylene oxide for 15 min.
6. Replace the solution with 100% propylene oxide for 15 min.

3.1.3. Infiltration

For all of the infiltration steps, a specimen rotator is used to ensure continuous mixing *(17)*.

1. Drain the tissue of most of the propylene oxide, leaving a little so that the tissue does not dry out.
2. Replace the solvent with a 1:1 solution of propylene oxide: embedding medium, and allow it to stand for at least 4 h at room temperature.
3. Remove the mixture, replace it with 100% embedding medium and leave for 6–12 h at room temperature.

3.1.4. Embedding

This may be done in EMS embedding capsules (EMS, cat. no. 70020) or a flat embedding mold (EMS, cat. no. 70900).

1. Transfer each sample to a dry capsule or mold and fill the mold with embedding medium.
2. Cure the medium overnight or for 48 h in an oven at 60°C.
3. Blocks can be trimmed and sectioned after they return to room temperature.
4. The sections are then placed on copper grids (EMS, cat. no. FF100-Cu) for double stained using uranyl acetate and lead citrate.

3.1.5. Staining

The staining method used in our laboratory is the double-staining method. The sections are first stained with saturated uranyl acetate in 50% ethanol, followed by staining with lead citrate. Stock solutions of lead citrate can be prepared and stored before use. The lead citrate stock solution in our laboratory is prepared by the Venable and Coggeshall method. The double-staining procedure used in our laboratory is as follows *(18)*:

1. Place a piece of filter paper at the bottom of a Petri dish and place a piece of premarked dental wax sheet on top of the filter paper. Prepare two such Petri dishes.

2. Pipet out and place drops of the uranyl acetate stain on the dental wax paper.
3. With the help of tweezers, place the grids with the section side down on a drop of uranyl acetate stain and leave it for 10–15 min.
4. Remove the grids from the first Petri dish and wash with 10 mL of 70% ethanol followed by 10 mL of distilled water.
5. Pipet out and place drops of lead citrate stain on the dental wax paper in the second Petri dish.
6. With the help of tweezers, place the grids with the section side down on a drop of the lead citrate stain and leave it for 10 min.
7. Remove the grid and wash with 20 mL of distilled water, twice.
8. The sections now are ready to be visualized using a transmission electron microscope.

3.2. Tissue Preparation for Paraffin-Embedded Tissue

Formalin-fixed tissue is processed with a standard procedure, which includes dehydration, clearing, infiltration, and embedding. Dehydration is necessary in the preparation of tissue blocks for embedding in a nonaqueous medium, such as paraffin, celloidin, and some plastics. These media will not infiltrate tissue that contains water. There are two ways in which the dehydrating agents act to remove water. Some reagents are hydrophilic and attract water from tissue, whereas other reagents dehydrate by repeated dilution of the aqueous tissue fluids. Most dehydrating agents are alcohols (e.g., ethyl alcohol, methyl alcohol, isopropyl alcohol, and butyl alcohol). Acetone is a very rapid-acting and less-expensive dehydrator.

Clearing agents also are referred to as dealcoholization agents; their primary purpose is to remove alcohol used for dehydration and to make the tissue receptive to the infiltration medium. Xylene is the most widely used clearing agent. Xylene is a flammable reagent and is considered a hazardous substance, so the waste product must be either recycled or disposed of in an appropriate manner.

After dehydration and clearing, tissue must be infiltrated with a supporting medium, which also is called embedding medium. Paraffin wax is the most popular medium because the tissue blocks may be processed in comparatively short period of time, serial sections are easily taken and routine and most special stains are easily done. Water-soluble waxes, celloidin, plastics, agar and gelatin and 30% sucrose are examples of other embedding media *(19,20)*.

A wide variety of processors are available. The two major systems used by processors are the open system and the closed system. The open system does not use vacuum, whereas the closed system uses heat and vacuum. The closed system is computerized and can be programmed to change the solutions at desired intervals. The following is an example of solutions and times for routine overnight processing with a closed system that is used in our laboratory utilizing the Thermo Shandon Hypercenter XP processor (*see* **Note 3**):

1. A total of 3 h in alcoholic formalin.
2. 40 min each in six changes of dehydrant.
3. 40 min each in three changes of clearing agent.
4. 1 h in paraffin.
5. 1.5 h in paraffin.

3.3. Staining Tissue With Hematoxylin and Eosin

Harris hematoxylin stains specimens rapidly with very good results. A commonly used stain is 4 mL of glacial acetic acid added to every 96 mL of Harris hematoxylin (*see* **Note 4**). In the progressive method, slides are first stained with hematoxylin, which stains only the nucleus, then rinsed and stained with eosin *(21–23)*. The regressive method uses a stronger hematoxylin dye that stains the entire cell and an acid alcohol solution is used to remove the excess stain such that only the nucleus remains stained *(21–23)*.

3.3.1. The Progressive Method

1. Dip in three changes of xylene for 2 min each.
2. 10 dips in absolute alcohol.
3. 10 dips each in two changes of 95% alcohol.
4. Rinse under tap water until water runs off evenly.
5. Dip for 1–3 min in Harris hematoxylin with acetic acid.
6. 10 dips each in two changes of tap water (*see* **Note 5**).
7. Dip in 0.25% ammonia water or 0.5% lithium carbonate until blue.
8. 10 dips each in two changes of tap water or running water may be used.
9. 10–20 dips in eosin or 1–3 min in eosin-phloxine.
10. 10–15 dips in two changes of 95% alcohol.
11. 10–15 dips each in three changes of absolute alcohol.
12. 10–15 dips each in three changes of xylene and let slides remain in the last container until a cover slip is applied.
13. The result from a representative section stained with hematoxylin and eosin is shown in **Fig. 1A**.

3.3.2. The Regressive Method

1. Dip in three changes xylene for 2 min each.
2. 10 dips in absolute alcohol.
3. 10 dips each in two changes of 95% alcohol.
4. Rinse under tap water until water runs off evenly.
5. 10–15 min in Harris hematoxylin without acetic acid.
6. 10 dips each in two changes of tap water.
7. 5–10 dips in 1% hydrochloric acid in 70% alcohol.
8. Wash well under running water.
9. Dip for 30 s in 0.25% ammonia water without agitating (*see* **Note 6**).
10. 10 dips each in two changes of tap water.
11. 10–20 dips in eosin.

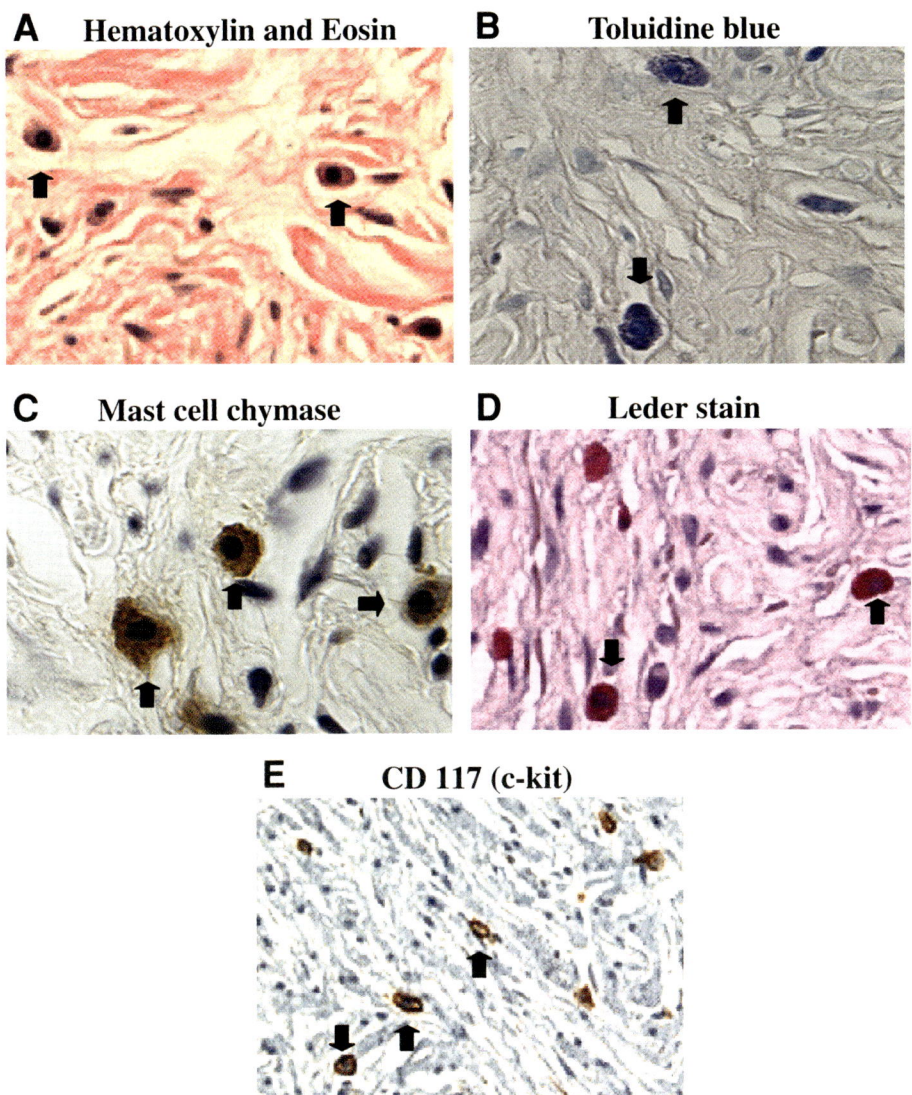

Fig. 1. (**A**) Hematoxylin and eosin-stained tissue section (×400) shows round-to-oval mast cell nuclei that stain blue and the cytoplasm stains pink and very faint pink granules are visible in the cytoplasm, as indicated by the arrows. (**B**) Toluidine blue-stained tissue section (×1000) shows the presence of metachromatic granules in mast cells that appear red–purple and the orthochromatic background that stains blue, as indicated by the arrows. (**C**) Chymase-stained tissue sections (×1000) show brown staining in the mast cell cytoplasm, as indicated by the arrows. (**D**) Mast cell granules are stained red with Leder stain (×1000), as indicated by the arrows. (**E**) Mast cell cytoplasmic membrane is stained brown with CD117 (*c-kit*) (×1000), as indicated by the arrows.

12. 10 dips each in two changes of 95% alcohol.
13. 10 dips each in three changes of absolute alcohol.
14. 10 dips each in three changes xylene and let slides remain in last container until a cover slip is applied.

3.4. Staining Tissue Section With Toluidine Blue

The procedure used in our laboratory is as follows *(4)*:

1. Bring the section to tap water and rinse for 5 min.
2. Stain in 0.5% toluidine blue solution for 5 min.
3. Rinse quickly in two changes of 95% ethyl alcohol for 1 min each.
4. Place in two changes of absolute ethyl alcohol for 1 min each.
5. Clear in xylene.
6. Mount with permaslip.
7. The result from a representative section stained with toluidine is shown in **Fig. 1B.** Toluidine blue stains mast cells red–purple (metachromatic staining) and the background blue (orthochromatic staining).

3.5. Staining Tissue Section With Mast Cell Tryptase and Chymase

The procedure used in our laboratory is as follows *(24)*:

1. Rehydrate tissue to distilled water.
2. Place tissue in TBS for 2 min.
3. Wipe off TBS and incubate the specimen for 5 min with the peroxidase blocking reagent. This will quench any endogenous peroxidase activity.
4. Rinse gently with TBS.
5. Wipe off TBS and incubate the specimen and positive control with the primary antibody, and the negative control with TBS. Incubate for 15–20 min.
6. Rinse gently with TBS.
7. Wipe off TBS and incubate with labeled polymer for 15–20 min.
8. Rinse gently with TBS.
9. Wipe off TBS and incubate with the substrate–chromogen solution for 5–10 min. (*see* **Note 7**).
10. Rinse gently with TBS and distilled water.
11. Immerse slides in a bath of Harris hematoxylin for 6 s.
12. Rinse slides with distilled water.
13. "Blue" slides with 0.25% ammonia.
14. Rinse slides with distilled water for 2–5 min.
15. Dehydrate, clear, and mount with Cytoseal.
16. The result from a representative section stained with mast cell chymase is shown in **Fig. 1C.** The mast cell cytoplasm stains brown.

3.6. Staining Tissue Section With Leder Stain (Naphthol-AS-D Chloracetate Esterase) (8,9)

1. Prewarm sufficient deionized water for substrate use to 37°C. Check the temperature before use.

2. Immediately before fixation, add 1 mL of sodium nitrate solution to 1 mL of fast red violet LB base solution in a test tube. Mix gently by inversion and allow standing 2 min. Active evolution of gas bubbles should be avoided.
3. Add solution from **step 2** to 40 mL of prewarmed deionized water.
4. Add 5 mL of TRIZMAL, pH 6.3, buffer concentrate.
5. Add 1 mL of Naphthol AS-D chloracetate solution (*see* **Note 8**). The solution should turn red. Mix well and pour into Coplin jar.
6. Bring citrate-acetone formaldehyde solution to room temperature (23–26°C) and fix the slides by immersing in this solution for 30 s (*see* **Note 9**).
7. Rinse slides thoroughly in running water for 45–60 s and then place in solution from **step 5**. Do not allow slides to dry.
8. Incubate for 30 min at 37°C protected from light.
9. After 30 min, remove slides and rinse thoroughly in running deionized water for at least 2 min.
10. Counter stain 2 min in hematoxylin solution, Gill no. 3.
11. Rinse in tap water and air dry.
12. Evaluate microscopically. If cover slipping is required use only aqueous mounting media.
13. The result from a representative section stained with chloracetate esterase is shown in **Fig. 1D**. The mast cell cytoplasmic granules stain red with Leder stain.

3.7. Staining Tissue Section With CD117 (C-Kit)

The immunohistochemical staining for CD117 includes: (1) paraffin specimen preparation, (2) pretreatment, and (3) staining.

3.7.1. Paraffin Specimen Preparation

1. For the most optimal results, use Paraffin-embedded tissue that has been fixed in neutral formalin (preferably) or other fixative for 6–24 h.
2. Dry overnight at 37°C or 2–4 h at 58°C, and the slides are ready for pretreatment.

3.7.2. Pretreatment Options

The preferred method of pretreatment is the use of HIER (Heat Induced Epitope Retrieval) technique using Cell Marque's Declere with citrate or Trilogy with ethylene diamine tetraacetic acid. This method allows for simultaneous deparaffinization, rehydration, and epitope retrieval and is as follows *(25)*:

1. Fill two staining dishes with 200 mL of Declere or Trilogy and place them in the pressure cooker.
2. Put a slide rack containing the slides to be stained in one of the staining dishes and cover the staining dishes with their lids.
3. Lock the pressure cooker lid and make sure vent is in the closed position.
4. Set the pressure mode for "high" and move "up" arrow until 15 is reached; then, press the "start" button.
5. The timer will start when the correct pressure and temperature is reached.
6. Wait approx 5 min, then push "rapid release" tab.

7. Red pin will descend when all the pressure is released so you can remove the lid.
8. Transfer slides from the first container to hot rinse.
9. Agitate slides and let sit it for 5 min.
10. Rinse slides in IHC Wash Buffer and proceed with IHC protocol.

3.7.3. Staining

The Ventana NexES IHC–Full system is used for automated CD117 staining in our laboratory. A manual staining method can be used if required. The recommended manual staining procedure is as follows (26):

1. Place slides in peroxide block for 10–15 min; rinse with deionized water.
2. Apply the antibody and incubate for 60 min at room temperature; rinse with deionized water.
3. Apply link, incubate for 10 min at room temperature; rinse with deionized water.
4. Apply ample amount of chromogen and incubate for 1–10 min at room temperature.
5. Rinse with four to five changes of deionized water.
6. Counterstain and cover slip.
7. The result from a representative section stained with CD117 is shown in **Fig. 1E**. The mast cell cytoplasmic membrane stains brown.

4. Notes

1. a) For better penetration and stability, benzyldimethylamine (BDMA) is recommended in place of DMP-30 as an accelerator. The quantity of BDMA required is 1–1.2 mL. Slight variations of the accelerator (DMP-30 or BDMA) will drastically affect the color and brittleness of the block. b) Before measuring and mixing the resin, the anhydride should be warmed (60°C) to reduce the viscosity. Thorough mixing is necessary to be able to achieve uniform blocks. The final block can be made harder by replacing some of the DDSA with NMA (0.5 mL of nadic methyl anhydride (NMA) for each 1.0 mL of DDSA). c) Although the mixture can be stored for up to 6 mo at 40°C, it is highly recommended that freshly prepared embedding medium always be used. If the mixture is stored, it should be warmed thoroughly prior to adding the accelerator (17).
2. Store the Naphthol AS-D chloracetate solution, Fast Blue BB base solution, Trizmal concentrate pH −7.6 ± 0.15, sodium nitrite solution, and citrate solution in refrigerator at 4°C. Store acetone in flammable cabinet.
3. The cassettes in which the tissue is placed must be completely immersed in the solution. The reagents must be changed as frequently as required depending on the workload.
4. Mix the ammonium aluminium sulfate dissolved in water by heating and the hematoxylin dissolved in alcohol and ring it to a boil rapidly. Remove from heat and slowly add the mercuric oxide. Reheat the solution until it turns dark purple and cool it by immediately plunging the container in a basin of ice (21).
5. Change water frequently. Where two changes are indicated, one container should be changed after each basket. Rotate the containers so that the clean water is in the second container.

6. Do not agitate in the ammonia water, as most section loss will occur at this point. This step requires 10–30 s, and the solution should be changed when it becomes discolored.
7. Prepare the substrate–chromogen solution: combine 1 mL of the buffered substrate and 1 drop of the DAB chromogen, and mix immediately. This solution is stable for approx 5 d when stored at 2–8°C. Rinse the test tube thoroughly after use.
8. If the substrate appears turbid bring to room temperature and mix well.
9. To prepare citrate–acetone-formaldehyde fixative, add 65 mL of acetone and 8 mL of 37% formaldehyde to 25 mL of citrate solution. Store in refrigerator and bring to room temperature before use.

References

1. Krishnaswamy, G., Kelley, J., Johnson, D., et al. (2001) The human mast cell: functions in physiology and disease. *Front. Biosci.* **6**, D1109–D1127.
2. Craig , S. S., Schechter, N. M., and Schwartz, L. B. (1988) Ultrastructural analysis of human T and TC mast cells identified by immunoelectron microscopy. *Lab. Invest.* **58**, 682–691.
3. Meloan, S. N. and Puchtler, H. (1987) Harris hematoxylin: what Harris really wrote and mechanism of hemalum stains. *J. Histotechnol.* **10**, 257.
4. Haas, E. (1981) *50 Diagnostic Special Stains for Surgical Pathology.* J. B. Lippincott and Company, Philadelphia.
5. Peeker, R., Enerback.L., Fall, M., and Aldenborg, F. (2000) Recruitment, distribution and phenotypes of mast cells in interstitial cystitis. *Urology* **163**, 1009–1015.
6. Nakagami, T., Murakami, A., Okisaka, S., and Ebihara, N. (1999) Mast cells in pterygium: number and phenotype. *Jpn. J. Opthamol.* **43**, 75–79.
7. Irani, A. M., Bradford, T. R., Keply, C. L., Schechter, N. M., and Schwartz, L. B. (1989) Detection of MCT and MCTC types of human mast cells by immunohistochemistry using new monoclonal anti- tryptase and anti-chymase antibodies. *J. Histochem. Cytochem.* **37**, 1509–1515.
8. Moloney, W. C., McPherson, K., and Fliegerman, L. (1960) Esterase activity in leukocyte demonstrated by the use of naphthol AS-D chloroacetate substrate. *J. Histochem. Cytochem.* **8**, 200–207.
9. Yam, L. T., Li, C. Y., and Crosby, W. H. (1972) Cytochemical identification of monocyte and granulocytes. *Am. J. Clin. Pathol.* **55**, 283–290.
10. Miettinen, M., and Sarloma-Rikala, M. (2000) Esophageal stromal tumors: a clinicopathologic, immunohistochemical, and molecular genetic study of 17 cases and comparison with esophageal leiomyomas and leiomyosarcomas. *Am. J. Surg Pathol.* **24**, 211–222.
11. Miettinen, M. and Monihan, J. M. (1999) Gastrointestinal stromal tumors/smooth muscle tumors (GISTs) primary in the omentum and mesentery: clinicopathologic and immunohistochemical study of 26 cases. *Am. J. Surg. Pathol.* **23**, 1109–1118.
12. Sircar, K., Hewlett , B. R., Huizinga, J. D., Chorneyko, K., Berezin, I., and Riddell, R. H. (1999) Interstitial cells of Cajal as precursors of gastrointestinal stromal tumors. *Am. J. Surg. Pathol.* **23**, 377–389.

13. Arber, D. A., Tamayo, R., and Weiss, L. M. (1998) Paraffin section detection of the c-kit gene product (CD117) in human tissues: value in the diagnosis of mast cell disorders. *Hum. Pathol.* **29,** 498–504.

14. Finck, H. (1960) Epoxy resins in electron microscopy. *J. Biophys. Biochem. Cytol.* **7,** 27–30.

15. Luft, J. H. (1961) Improvements in epoxy resin embedding methods. *J. Biophys. Biochem. Cytol.* **9,** 409–414.

16. Glauert, A. M. (1991) Epoxy resins: an update on their selection and use. *Microscopy and Analysis.* September; 15–20.

17. Araldite 502 kit, Technical data sheet. Electron microscopy Sciences. Available at: http://www.emsdiasum.com/microscopy/technical/techdata/54.aspx; Internet; accessed February 10, 2005.

18. Lewis, P. R. and Knight, D. P.(1977) *Staining Methods for Sectioned Material, 1st ed.* North-Holland Publishing, New York.

19. Login, G. R. and Giammra, B. (1993) *Rapid Microwave Fixation, Staining and Embedding for Light and Electron Microscopy.* Microscopy Society of America Workshop, Cincinnati, OH.

20. Bancroft, J. D. and Stevens, A. (1982) *Theory and Practice of Histological Techniques.* New York, Churchill Livingstone.

21. Carson, F. L. (1997) *Histotechnology: A Self-Instructional Text, 2nd ed.* ASCP Press, Chicago.

22. Luna, L. G. (1968) *Histologic Staining Methods of the Armed Forces Institute of Pathology, 3rd ed.* McGraw-Hill, New York.

23. Luna, L. G., (1983) Hematoxylin and eosin staining problems and solutions. *J. Histotechnol.* **6,** 16.

24. Naish, S. J. (1989) *Handbook– Immunochemical Staining Methods.* DAKO Corporation, Carpinteria.

25. One Step Pretreatments: DeclereÆ and Trilogy™ (Electric pressure cooker protocol) Cell Marque, Hot Springs, AR.

26. CD117 (c-kit) (Polyclonal) datasheet. Cell Marque, Rev. 2, Hot Spring, AR.

6

Expression of Cell Surface Antigens on Mast Cells

Mast Cell Phenotyping

Alexander W. Hauswirth, Stefan Florian, Gerit-Holger Schernthaner, Maria-Theresa Krauth, Karoline Sonneck, Wolfgang R. Sperr, and Peter Valent

Summary

During the past few decades, a number of functionally important cell surface antigens have been detected on human mast cells (MCs). These antigens include the stem cell factor receptor (SCFR/CD117), the high-affinity immunoglobulin E receptor, adhesion molecules, and activation-linked membrane determinants. Several of these antigens (CD2, CD25, CD35, CD88, CD203c) appear to be upregulated on MCs in patients with systemic mastocytosis and therefore are used as diagnostic markers. Quantitative measurement of these markers on MCs is thus of diagnostic value and is usually performed by multicolor-based flow cytometry techniques utilizing a PE- or APC-labeled antibody against CD117 for MCs detection. This chapter gives an overview about the methods of staining of MC in various tissues with special reference to novel diagnostic markers applied in patients with suspected systemic mastocytosis.

Key Words: Mast cell; mastocytosis; classification; diagnostic criteria; phenotyping; flow cytometry.

1. Introduction

Mast cells (MCs) are multifunctional effector cells of the immune system *(1,2)*. These cells are found in most organs. MCs are derived from multipotent uncommitted CD34[+] hematopoietic progenitor cells *(3–5)*. In contrast to other leukocytes, MCs undergo differentiation and maturation in extramedullary tissues and, as mature cells, are not found in the peripheral blood *(1,2)*. MCs are easily identified in tissue sections by their characteristic granules that stain metachromatic after exposure to basic dyes *(1,2)*. MCs also express a distinct composition of cytoplasmic and cell surface antigens *(2,6)*. The stem cell fac-

From: *Methods in Molecular Biology, vol. 315: Mast Cells: Methods and Protocols*
Edited by: G. Krishnaswamy and D. S. Chi © Humana Press Inc., Totowa, NJ

tor receptor (KIT) is typically expressed on MCs in various organs independently of the maturation stage of MC or cell activation *(6)*. Activation of MCs through cell surface antigens often results in the release of granule-derived proinflammatory and vasoactive mediators, with consecutive clinical symptoms *(7–10)*. The most intriguing example is immunoglobulin E (IgE) receptor-mediated release of histamine in allergic reactions *(7)*.

A number of previous and more recent observations support the concept of MC heterogeneity *(11–14)*. In fact, depending on the environment and other factors, MCs differ from each other in expression of mediators, response to diverse stimuli, and expression of cell surface antigens *(11–14)*. More recently, it also was found that MCs in patients with systemic mastocytosis (SM) clearly differ in their phenotype when compared with normal MCs *(15,16)*. Likewise, in contrast to normal MCs, MCs in patients with SM express CD2 and CD25 *(15–17)*. In addition, MCs in SM express increased amounts of CD63, CD69, CD88, and CD203c *(16–19)*. The organ that usually is analyzed in patients with suspected SM is the bone marrow.

During the past 10 yr, a number of useful techniques for the enumeration and phenotypic analysis of MCs in the bone marrow have been established. Most of these techniques are based on the unique expression of the SCF receptor (KIT/CD117) on these cells *(15,20,21)*. In fact, in the bone marrow, KIT is expressed on MC and CD34+ hematopoietic progenitors but not on other mature hematopoietic cells.

2. Patients and Materials

1. Patients with suspected mastocytosis.
2. Tissue samples (bone marrow aspirate, tissue cell suspensions, blood).
3. FACS-lysing and -fixation solution (Becton Dickinson, San Jose, CA).
4. Monoclonal antibodies (MAbs) from various companies (**Table 1**).
5. Goat F(ab')2 anti-mouse IgG (H+L) FITC (Caltag Lab, Hamburg, Germany).
6. Saponin S-7900 (Sigma-Aldrich, Steinheim, Germany).
7. HEPES buffer (Biomol, Hamburg, Germany).
8. Formaldehyde, 37% (Merck, Darmstadt, Germany).
9. AB-serum (PAA laboratories, Pasching, Austria).
10. Tyrode's buffer, Ca^{2+}-free: 0.2 g/L KCl, 0.05 g/L Na-dihydrogen phosphate, 8 g/L NaCl, and 1 g/L glucose.
11. Collagenase type II (Worthington, Lakewood, NJ).
12. Nytex cloth (Lohmann & Rauscher, Rengsdorf, Germany).
13. RPMI 1640 medium (PAA laboratories).
14. Fetal calf serum (PAA laboratories).
15. Ficoll (Biochrom AG, Berlin, Germany).

3. Methods

3.1. Phenotyping of Bone Marrow MCs

Bone marrow MCs usually are incubated with MAbs in heparinized samples shortly after aspiration without a preceding isolation step or separation from erythrocytes. This procedure has been recommended because bone marrow MCs often are lost in Ficoll separation steps or prior erythrocyte lysis *(15,16,20,21)*. In select cases (patients with high-grade MC diseases, e.g., MC leukemia), MCs also can be enriched by Ficoll isolation without loss of a considerable number of MCs. In low-grade MC disease, however, it is of great importance to provide optimal prestaining conditions and an appropriate protocol for sampling of bone marrow cells *(21)*.

3.1.1. Sampling of Bone Marrow Cells

Correct sampling of bone marrow cells is a first critical step in MC phenotyping in patients with suspected SM *(20,21)*. The selection of patients and pre-invasive steps in the diagnostic work-up in SM have been described in detail elsewhere *(22–24)*. In all patients examined, a bone marrow biopsy is performed *(22–24)*. Usually, the bone marrow is obtained from the posterior iliac crest. Aspiration can be performed with any type of bone marrow-aspiration needle. In recent years several companies have offered biopsy needles through which bone marrow can be aspirated after the biopsy cylinder has been removed (one step procedure and one needle for both the biopsy and aspiration). The quality of the aspirated marrow does not differ from that obtained with conventional aspiration needles (unpublished observation).

In the procedure of aspiration, the goal is to prevent contamination with peripheral blood and to collect as many MCs in the sample as possible (*see* **Note 1**). To reach this goal, aspiration has to be performed firmly and quickly *(21)*. Approximately 1.5–3.0 mL of aspirate should be collected in heparinized tubes or syringes. Harvest of larger aspirate volumes in a single tube will not increase, but rather decrease, the percentage of MCs in the sample *(21)*. After collection, the aspirate is passed through a 25-gage needle to disaggregate bone marrow particles. Quick staining of freshly prepared bone marrow smears with 0.5% toluidine blue may be helpful to determine the content of MCs in the sample *(21)*. In each case, the aspirated cells should be subjected to antibody staining, erythrocyte lysis, and fixation within 6 h *(20,21)*. Sometimes, the technique of staining may also work after 24 h *(21)*. However, the time between aspiration and MC analysis should always be kept to a minimum (*see* **Note 2**).

3.1.2. Incubation of Bone Marrow Samples With Monoclonal Antibodies, Erythrocyte Lysis, and Fixation of Cells

1. After sampling, bone marrow aspirates are incubated with MAbs. Usually, combinations of directly conjugated antibodies (MAbs with different color labels) are co-applied (*15–21*). **Table 1** provides a list of monoclonal antibodies that are recommended to be used in patients with suspected SM. **Table 2** lists proposed antibody combinations that can be applied in suspected SM. Usually, 10^6 nucleated bone marrow cells (determined by counting in a hematocytometer or under a light microscopy) are incubated with MAbs (approx 1 µg of MAb should be applied to 1×10^6 cells) at room temperature for 15 min.
2. After staining with MAbs, erythrocytes are lysed in 2 mL of FACS Lysing Solution containing formaldehyde for cell fixation (*15–21*).
3. Cells are then washed and analyzed on a flow cytometer using an appropriate software (such as Paint-a-gate, Becton Dickinson). Antibody reactions should always be controlled by applying isotype-matched control antibodies (*15–21*).

3.1.3. Antibody Selection and Gating Strategy

The most appropriate marker for identification and enumeration of (normal or neoplastic) MCs in the bone marrow or other tissue is CD117 (*15–21*). However, because CD117 is also expressed on immature hematopoietic progenitor cells and sometimes even on nonhematopoietic cells, additional markers should be applied to define the MCs component by flow cytometry in bone marrow samples: first, to distinguish CD117$^+$ MCs from CD117$^+$ nonhematopoietic cells, staining of MC with a MAb against CD45 is recommended (*15–21*). In addition, we recommend the use of a CD34 MAb to discriminate between MCs and immature myeloid progenitors, which may be of great importance in patients with SM and a co-existing myeloid non-MC lineage neoplasm (*15–21*). By applying these stains and light scatter parameters, MC can easily be identified and discriminated from all other cells in the bone marrow sample (**Fig. 1**), even if their frequency is as low as $1:10^{-4}$ to $1:10^{-5}$ (one MC among 10,000–100,000 cells *[21]*). In patients with suspected SM, several other MC-related markers (such as CD63) can be used, which then reconfirm the identity of MCs (*15–18*). Some of these markers also appear to be upregulated on MCs in SM, so that their investigation is diagnostic (**Table 3** *[15–21]*). The most powerful diagnostic MC markers in suspected SM appear to be CD2 and CD25 (**Fig. 2;** *[15–18,21]; see* **Note 3**). These antigens are usually not expressed on normal MCs or MCs in the reactive bone marrow (**Fig. 2, Table 3**) and therefore have been proposed as diagnostic criteria (*16,22–24*). These two markers should therefore always be applied in flow cytometry analyses in patients with suspected SM (**Table 1** *[21–24]*).

Figure 3 shows abnormal expression of CD203c on MC in SM. The "minimum panel" recommended for the diagnosis of SM should include CD2, CD25, CD34, CD45, and CD117 (*see* **Note 1** *[15,21]*). In addition, a control tube for evaluation

Table 1
Specification of MAbs

Clone	CD	Antigen	Ig class	Source
RPA-2.10	CD2	LFA-2	IgG1	Mouse
M–ΦP9	CD14	LPS-R	IgG1	Mouse
MMA	CD15	3-FAL	IgG1	Mouse
2A3	CD25	IL-2 Rα	IgG1	Mouse
581	CD34	HPCA-1	IgG1	Mouse
E11	CD35	CR1	IgG1	Mouse
2D1	CD45	LCA	IgG1	Mouse
CLB-gran 12	CD63	ME491	IgG1	Mouse
W17/1	CD88	C5aR	IgG1	Mouse
104D2D1	CD117	SCFR,c-kit	IgG1	Mouse
9F5	CD123	IL-3 Rα	IgG1	Mouse
97A6	CD203c	E-NPP3	IgG1	Mouse

IL, interleukin, CR; complement receptor; SCF, stem cell factor.

Table 2
Combination of MAbs Applied in Four-Color
Flow Cytometry Experiments

Tube	FITC	PE	PerCP	APC
1	IgG1	CD34	CD45	CD117
2	CD34	IgG1	CD45	CD117
3	CD2	CD34	CD45	CD117
4	CD34	CD2	CD45	CD117
5	CD25	CD34	CD45	CD117
6	CD11c	CD34	CD45	CD117
7	CD35	CD34	CD45	CD117
8	CD63	CD34	CD45	CD117
9	CD88	CD34	CD45	CD117
10	CD34	CD203c	CD45	CD117
11	CD34	CD123	CD45	CD117

Conjugates: FITC, fluorescein isothiocyanate; PE, phycoerythrin; PerCP, peridinin chlorophyll protein; APC, allophycocyanin.

of baseline autofluorescence levels should always be included in the diagnostic procedure (*21*). With regard to selection of color label, it is of importance to be aware that the expression levels vary among antigens, and that PE and APC provide a more sensitive stain compared to other labels (**Fig. 2** *[18–21]*). Therefore, PE or APC should be used for "relatively weak" antigens such as CD2 (*21*).

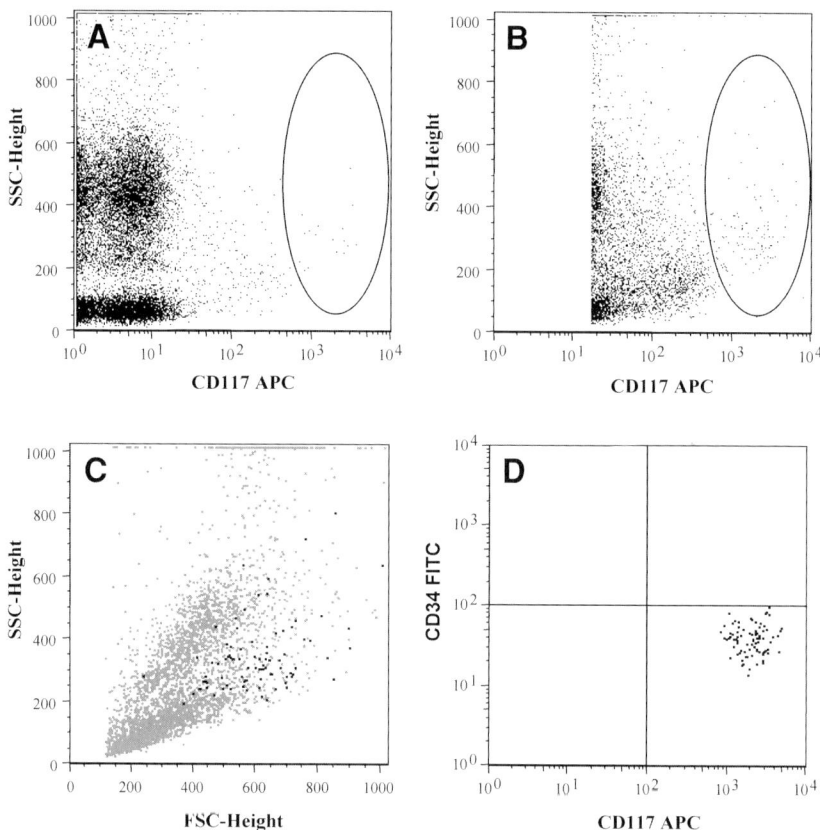

Fig. 1. Gating strategy for the identification of bone marrow mast cells (MCs). Shown is a representative dot plot analysis of bone marrow MCs in a patient with systemic mastocytosis (SM). A total of 50,000 events/tube are acquired and analyzed for expression of CD117 in a stepwise fashion. (**A**) Only a few CD117++ cells are identified in the entire cell population. (**B**) in a next step, an electronic live gate is introduced, resulting in an increased percentage of visible CD117++ cells. (**C**) The forward side scatter diagram shows that the CD117 ++ cells are diffusely distributed suggesting heterogeneity with regard to size and granulation. (**D**) Double staining for CD34 and CD117 confirms that the CD117 ++ cells are indeed (CD34–) MCs.

3.1.4. Data Acquisition and Flow Cytometry

Instrument setup, calibration, and quality control should follow rules identical to those described for the immunophenotyping of other nucleated blood cells (**20,21**). For data acquisition, the use of a double-step procedure is recommended (**20,21**). In a first step, information from a small proportion of cells in the test tube ($2–5 \times 10^4$ events), that is, type of cells and their relative distribu-

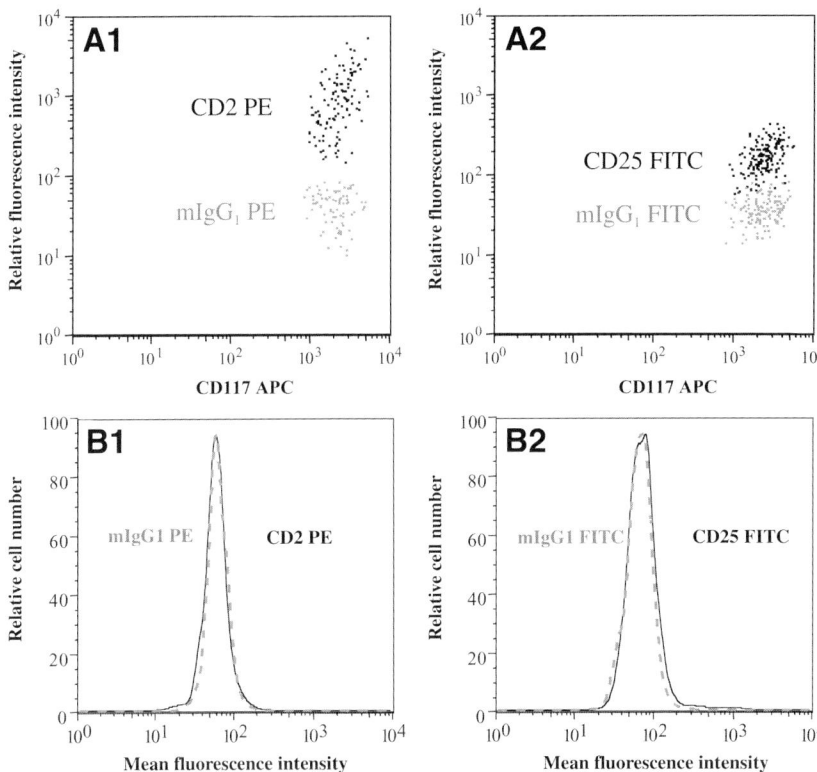

Fig. 2. Surface expression of CD2 and CD25 on bone marrow mast cells (MCs). Expression of CD2 (**A1**) and CD25 (**A2**) on bone marrow MCs in a patient with systemic mastocytosis (SM). MCs were stained with a CD117 APC monoclonal antibodies (MAb) for MC detection, a PE-labeled CD2 MAb, and a FITC-labeled CD25 MAb. Note the difference between labels (PE vs FITC) in sensitivity with regard to detection of surface antigens. Therefore, the isotype-matched control-antibodies (IgG_1) have to be labeled in the same color as the test antibody, in each experiment. Expression of CD2 and CD25 confirms the neoplastic nature of MCs. Normal bone marrow MCs invariably are CD2- (**B1**) and CD25 (**B2**) negative, as exemplified in the histogram shown.

tion in the sample, is obtained. In a second step, information on events acquired through an electronic live gate containing only CD117$^+$ cells is stored (**Fig. 1**). Such data-acquisition procedures have proven to be a reasonable approach in the analysis of rare cells (frequency: <0.01% *[20,21]*). In addition, this approach has overcome the problem related to the acquisition and storage of multiparameter information on large numbers of events (10^6–10^7 per test tube *[20,21]*). Among collected events, a minimum of 10^2–10^3 MCs should be present.

Table 3
Immunophenotype of MCs in Normal Tissues[a]
and Patients With SM

CD	Expression of surface antigens on MCs in	
	Normal tissue[a]	SM
CD2	–	+
CD14	–	–
CD15	–	–
CD25	–	+
CD33	+	+
CD34	–	–
CD35	–	+
CD45	+	+
CD63	+	+[b]
CD69	+	+[b]
CD88	+	+[b]
CD117	+	+
CD123	–	–
CD203c	+	+[b]

[a] In normal internal organs, most of the markers are distributed homogenously on MCs without major subpopulations or organ-dependent heterogeneity.

[b] These antigens are overexpressed on MCs in patients with SM compared with normal MCs. Usually, MCs are obtained from the bone marrow in SM for diagnostic tests.

3.1.5. Alternatives of Immmunophenotyping of Bone Marrow MCs

In a few patients with SM (high-grade disease, i.e., aggressive SM or MC leukemia), reasonable amounts of aspirated MCs can be enriched by Ficoll density gradient centrifugation. In these patients, MCs also can be analyzed phenotypically by single color flow cytometry, immunocytochemistry, or by a combined toluidine blue–immunofluorescence staining technique (*see* **Subheading 3.3.**). In addition, bone marrow MCs can be (and are usually) examined by immunohistochemistry, which is another standard diagnostic approach (*see* **Notes 4** and **5**).

3.2. Phenotyping of MCs in Extramedullary Organs

3.2.1. Other Hematopoietic Organs Analyzed in Patients With Mastocytosis

In almost all patients with suspected SM, the bone marrow is affected and is the primary organ to be analyzed (*22,23*). Other "hematopoietic" organs

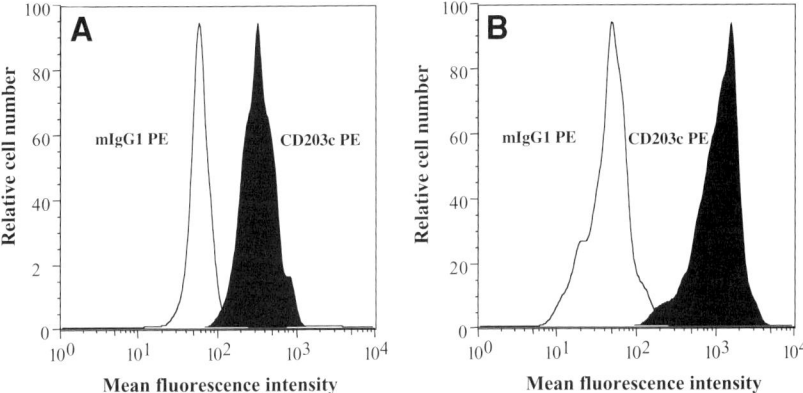

Fig. 3. Expression of CD203c on bone marrow mast cells (MCs). (**A**) Normal bone marrow MCs express low but detectable amounts of CD203c. The graph shows a histogram of MCs stained with the PE-labeled CD203c monoclonal antibody (MAb) 97A6. (**B**) In patients with systemic mastocytosis (SM), the levels of CD203c expressed on bone marrow MCs usually are higher as compared with those found on MCs in the normal bone marrow. A comparison of the two samples analyzed (**A** vs **B**) suggests an approximately fivefold higher expression of CD203c on MCs in a patient with SM (**B**) compared with normal MCs (**A**). Note logarithmic scale of immunofluorescence intensity.

(spleen, liver, lymph nodes, peripheral blood) may also be affected in these patients, and sometimes it may be of importance to know whether these organs contain MC infiltrates (*25,26*). Phenotyping of MCs in these organs usually is performed by immunohistochemistry but not by surface marker studies (*see* **Notes 4** and **5** *[25]*). An exception is blood. Thus, in patients with MC leukemia, circulating MCs can be detected by flow cytometry (*27–29*). In typical MC leukemia, the percentage of MCs in the peripheral blood exceeds 10% of all nucleated white blood cells (*22,30*). However, in some cases (e.g., aleukemic MC leukemia), the percentage of MCs is less than 10% (*22,28*). In these patients, cell surface phenotyping of MCs in the peripheral blood is sometimes helpful to confirm the presence of MCs and to determine their phenotype (*28*).

3.2.2. MC Phenotyping in Extrahematopoietic Tissues

MCs can also be examined phenotypically in nonhematopoietic organs, such as the lung, skin, or gastrointestinal tract (*31–35*). However, cell surface marker analysis on these MC subsets usually cannot be performed in patients with SM but instead has to be performed in surgical specimens obtained from patients who suffer from other neoplastic disorders (*31–35*). Likewise, lung tissue can be obtained at surgery (lobectomy) from patients with bronchiogenic carcinoma. Tissue MCs are isolated as follows:

1. Tissue is chopped into small fragments and washed extensively in Mg^{2+}/Ca^{2+}-free Tyrode's buffer *(31–35)*.
2. Tissue fragments are incubated in collagenase type II (2 mg/mL) at 37°C for 1–3 h *(31–35)*. The additional use of other enzymes may increase the percentage of MC in the final suspension samples. However, many of these enzymes (but not collagenase) are known to degrade various cell surface antigens and, therefore, their use is not recommended for MC isolation.
3. Dispersed cells are separated from the tissue by filtration through Nytex cloth, washed, and recovered in RPMI 1640 medium plus 10% fetal calf serum.

Immunophenotyping of MCs in lung cell suspensions can be performed in the same way as described for cell marker analysis of bone marrow MCs. Again, MCs are detected by CD117 and are delineated from other (CD117+) tissue cells by multicolor flow cytometry *(17,35)*. The MAbs applied are the same as those used to phenotype bone marrow MCs (**Table 2 [17,35]**). Apart from flow cytometry, however, suspended MCs also can be analyzed by combined toluidine blue/immunofluoresence staining technique (*see* **Subheading 3.3.**).

3.3. Combined Toluidine Blue–Immunofluorescence Staining

3.3.1. Indication and Limitations

This technique has been applied in previous years to demonstrate expression of cell-surface antigens on metachromatically stained leukocytes *(31–35)*. The advantage of this technique is that no additional surface markers are required for MC detection and, thus, all metachromatically stained subsets of MCs (including phenotypically distinct subpopulations) are included in the analysis *(31–35)*. The disadvantage of the technique is that it is sometimes impossible to differentiate between MCs and basophils when analyzing very immature cells (leukemic cells, metachromatic blasts) and that completely "agranular" MC progenitors may escape analysis. Another disadvantage is that the technique cannot be performed on samples containing an excess of erythrocytes or samples that were exposed to erythrocyte lysis and fixation buffer.

3.3.2. Technique

1. Cells are incubated with 20% human AB-serum (100 µL per 10^6 cells) for 30 min at 4°C to minimize nonspecific antibody binding *(31–35)*.
2. Cells are incubated with MAbs (1 µg per 10^6 cells) for 30 min at 4°C, washed, and exposed to second-step fluorescein-labeled goat F(ab') 2 anti-mouse IgG (H+L) antibody (30 min, 4°C).
3. Cells are fixed in glutaraldehyde (0.025%) for 1 min *(31–35)*.
4. Cells are washed and incubated with toluidine blue (0.0125%) for approx 8 min *(31–35)*. The exact time of exposure to toluidine blue has to be adjusted in each laboratory and differs significantly when basophils (instead of MC) are analyzed (in the laboratory of the authors, MCs are exposed for 8 min and basophils for 11–12 min).

5. After washing, cells are examined under bright-field and fluorescence light. Isotype matched control antibodies should be examined in parallel in each experiment. With regard to detection of surface antigens on MCs, the combined toluidine blue–immunofluorescence staining technique is equally sensitive compared to multicolor flow cytometry *(35)*.

3.4. Flow Cytometric Evaluation of Cytoplasmic Antigens

Several important MC antigens (signaling molecules, granule-associated antigens, MC tryptase) may be expressed in cytoplasmic compartments but not on the cell surface *(1,2,13,17)*. For these antigens, different immunostaining techniques are available. The traditional approach is immunohistochemistry (*see* **Notes 4** and **5**) or immunocytochemistry *(13,17,25,26)*. More recently, however, flow cytometry-based techniques for detection of cytoplasmic MC antigens like tryptase have been developed *(36–38)*. These techniques have the advantage (over traditional staining techniques) in that MCs can be examined simultaneously for expression of cytoplasmic and cell surface antigens by multicolor staining technique. Another advantage is the possibility to objectively quantify antigen expression in the flow cytometer *(36)*. A number of different protocols are available for detection of cytoplasmic antigens in human leukocytes *(36–38)*. We recommend the use of saponin-based protocols. An example for such protocol using anti-tryptase antibody G3, is given below:

1. Before staining, erythrocytes are lysed in 2 mL of FACS Lysing Solution.
2. Cells are then washed in phosphate buffered saline and permeabilized with 0.1% saponin dissolved in HEPES buffer.
3. Cells are incubated with the anti-tryptase MAb G3 diluted in saponin solution, for 30 min.
4. After washing in saponin, a fluorescein isothiocyanate-conjugated second step antibody (goat anti-mouse) is applied for 30 min.
5. Cells are washed once in saponin solution, once in phosphate-buffered saline, and then are exposed to labeled antibodies against cell surface antigens (for cell detection).
6. Consecutive steps in the procedure and data acquisition are identical to that described for cell-surface antigen phenotyping of MCs (*see* **Subheading 3.1.**).

4. Notes

1. The Spanish Network on Mastocytosis (REMA) has recently provided useful recommendations for the application of immunophenotypic analyses in mastocytosis including cell sampling techniques, antibody selection, and data acquisition *(21)*.
2. Only a few centers and universities in Europe and in the United States offer flow cytometry-based examination of MCs as a routine technique for diagnosis of SM. Some of these centers may also offer examination of referral material. In this case, it is of importance to keep the time of transport of bone marrow samples to an absolute minimum *(21)*.

3. Expression of CD2 and CD25 on bone marrow MCs has been defined as minor criterion of SM in the updated consensus classification of mastocytosis adopted by the WHO in 2001 *(22)*. If at least one major and one minor or at least three minor criteria are fulfilled, the diagnosis SM can be established *(22)*. However, the absence of CD2 or/and CD25 on MC does not exclude the diagnosis SM.

4. Expression of CD2 and CD25 on MC also can be studied by immunohistochemistry (IHC). However, the CD2 IHC-staining protocol is less sensitive compared with flow cytometry. With regard to CD25, however, bone marrow MCs also can be analyzed by IHC, yielding the same results compared with flow cytometry.

5. Only very few patients with SM lack bone marrow infiltrates (= major criterion of SM). These rare patients have splenic mastocytosis or advanced MC sarcoma. In these patients, phenotyping is largely restricted to immunohistochemistry.

References

1. Schwartz, L.B. (1985) The mast cell, in *Allergy, vol 1*, (Kaplan, A. P., ed.), Churchill Livingston, Edinburgh, pp. 53–92.
2. Valent, P., Sillaber, C., and Bettelheim, P. (1991) The growth and differentiation of mast cells. *Prog. Growth Factor Res.* **3**, 27–41.
3. Kitamura, Y., Yokoyama, M., Matsuda, H., Ohno T., and Mori, K. J. (1981) Spleen colony forming cell as common precursor for tissue mast cells and granulocytes. *Nature* **291**, 159–160.
4. Kirschenbaum, A. S., Kessler, S. W., Goff, J. P., and Metcalfe, D. D. (1991) Demonstration of the origin of human mast cells from CD34+ bone marrow progenitor cells. *J. Immunol.* **146**, 1410–1415.
5. Agis, H., Willheim, M., Sperr, W. R., et al. (1993) Monocytes do not make mast cells when cultured in the presence of SCF. Characterization of the circulating mast cell progenitor as a c-kit⁺, CD34⁺, Ly⁻, CD14⁻, CD17⁻, colony forming cell. *J. Immunol.* **151**, 4221–4227.
6. Valent, P. and Bettelheim, P. (1992) Cell surface structures on human basophils and mast cells: biochemical and functional characterization. *Adv. Immunol.* **52**, 333–423.
7. Ishizaka, T. and Ishizaka, K. (1984) Activation of mast cells for mediator release through IgE receptors. *Prog. Allergy* **34**, 188–235.
8. Lewis, R. A. and Austen, K. F. (1981) Mediation of homeostasis and inflammation by leukotrienes and other mast cell dependent compounds. *Nature* **293**, 103–108.
9. Serafin, W. E. and Austen, K. F. (1987) Mediators of immediate hypersensitivity reactions. *N. Engl. J. Med.* **317**, 30–34.
10. Burd, P. R., Rogers, H. W., Gordon, J. R., et al. (1989) Interleukin 3-dependent and -independent mast cells stimulated with IgE and antigen express multiple cytokines. *J. Exp. Med.* **170**, 245–257.
11. Kitamura, Y. (1989) Heterogeneity of mast cells and phenotypic change between subpopulations. *Ann. Rev. Immunol.* **7**, 59–76.
12. Lawrence, I. D., Warner, J. A., Cohan, V. L., Hubbard, W. C., Kagey-Sobotka, A., and Lichtenstein, L. M. (1987) Purification and characterization of human skin mast cells: evidence for human mast cell heterogeneity. *J. Immunol.* **139**, 3062–3069.

13. Irani, A. A., Schechter, N. M., Craig, S. S., DeBlois, G., and Schwartz, L. B. (1986) Two human mast cell subsets with distinct neutral protease composition. *Proc. Natl. Acad. Sci. USA* **83**, 4464–4468.

14. Füreder, W., Agis, H., Willheim, M., et al. (1995) Differential expression of complement receptors on human basophils and mast cells: evidence for mast cell heterogeneity and C5aR/CD88 expression on skin mast cells. *J. Immunol.* **155**, 3152–3160.

15. Escribano, L., Orfao, A., Diaz-Agustin, B., et al. (1998) Indolent systemic mast cell disease in adults: immunophenotypic characterization of bone marrow mast cells and its diagnostic implications. *Blood* **91**, 2731–2736.

16. Escribano, L., Diaz-Agustin, B., Bellas, C., et al. (2001) Utility of flow cytometric analysis of mast cells in the diagnosis and classification of adult mastocytosis. *Leuk. Res.* **25**, 563–270.

17. Schernthaner, G. H., Jordan, J. H., Ghannadan, M., et al. (2001) Expression, epitope analysis, and functional role of the LFA-2 antigen detectable on neoplastic mast cells. *Blood* **98**, 3784–3792.

18. Escribano, L., Orfao, A., Diaz Agustin, B., et al. (1998) Human bone marrow mast cells from indolent systemic mast cell disease constitutively express increased amounts of the CD63 protein on their surface. *Cytometry* **34**, 223–228.

19. Nunez-Lopez, R., Escribano, L., Schernthaner, G. H., et al. (2003) Overexpression of complement receptors and related antigens on the surface of bone marrow mast cells in patients with systemic mastocytosis. *Br. J. Haematol.* **120**, 257–265.

20. Orfao, A., Escribano, L., Villarrubia, J., et al. (1996) Flow cytometric analysis of mast cells from normal and pathological human bone marrow samples. Identification and enumeration. *Am. J. Pathol.* **149**, 1493–1499.

21. Escribano, L., Diaz-Agustin, B., Lopez, A., et al. (2004) Immunophenotypic analysis of mast cells in mastocytosis: when and how to do it. Proposals of the Spanish Network on Mastocytosis (REMA). *Cytometry* **58B**, 1–8.

22. Valent, P., Horny, H. P., Escribano, L., et al. (2001) Diagnostic criteria and classification of mastocytosis: a consensus proposal. *Leuk. Res.* **25**, 603–625.

23. Valent, P., Akin, C., Sperr, W. R., et al. (2003) Diagnosis and treatment of systemic mastocytosis: state of the art. *Br. J. Haematol.* **122**, 695–717.

24. Valent, P., Sperr, W. R., Schwartz, L. B., and Horny, H. P. (2004) Classification of systemic mast cell disorders: delineation from immunologic diseases and non mast cell lineage hematopoietic neoplasms (review). *J. Allergy Clin. Immunol.* **114**, 3–11.

25. Horny, H. P. and Valent, P. (2001) Diagnosis of mastocytosis: general histopathological aspects, morphological criteria, and immunohistochemical findings. *Leuk. Res.* **25**, 543–551.

26. Horny, H. P. and Valent, P. (2002) Histopathological and immunohistochemical aspects of mastocytosis. *Int. Arch. Allergy Immunol.* **127**, 115–117.

27. Dalton, R., Chan, L., Batten, E., and Eridani, S. (1986) Mast cell leukemia: evidence for bone marrow origin of the pathological clone. *Br. J. Haematol.* **64**, 397–406.

28. Baghestanian, M., Bankl, H., Sillaber, C., et al. (1996) A case of malignant mastocytosis with circulating mast cell precursors: biologic and phenotypic characterization of the malignant clone. *Leukemia* **10**, 159–166.

29. Escribano, L., Orfao, A., Villarrubia, J., et al. (1997) Sequential immunopheno-typic analysis of mast cells in a case of systemic mast cell disease evolving to a mast cell leukemia. *Cytometry* **30,** 98–102.

30. Travis, W. D., Li, C. Y., Hoagland, H. C., Travis, L. B., and Banks, P. M. (1986) Mast cell leukemia: report of a case and review of the literature. *Mayo Clin. Proc.* **61,** 957–966.

31. Valent, P., Ashman, L. K., Hinterberger, W., et al. (1989) Mast cell typing: dem-onstration of a distinct hemopoietic cell type and evidence for immunophenotypic relationship to mononuclear phagocytes. *Blood* **73,** 1778–1785.

32. Valent, P., Majdic, O., Maurer, D., Bodger, M., Muhm, M., and Bettelheim P. (1990) Further characterization of surface membrane structures expressed on human basophils and mast cells. *Int. Arch. Allergy Appl. Immunol.* **91,** 198–203.

33. Sperr, W. R., Agis, H., Czerwenka, K., et al. (1992) Differential expression of cell surface integrins on human mast cells and basophils. *Ann. Hematol.* **65,** 10–16.

34. Ghannadan, M., Baghestanian, M., Wimazal, F., et al. (1998) Phenotypic charac-terization of human skin mast cells by combined staining with toluidine blue and CD antibodies. *J. Invest. Dermatol.* **111,** 689–695.

35. Wimazal, F., Ghannadan, M., Müller, M. R., et al. (1999) Expression of homing receptors and related molecules on human mast cells and basophils: a compara-tive analysis using multi-color flow cytometry and toluidine blue/immunofluo-rescence staining techniques. *Tissue Antigens* **54,** 499–507.

36. Sperr, W. R., Jordan, J. H., Baghestanian, M., et al. (2001) Expression of mast cell tryptase by myeloblasts in a group of patients with acute myeloid leukemia. *Blood* **98,** 2200–2209.

37. Knapp, W., Strobl, H., and Majdic, O. (1994) Flow cytometric analysis of cell-surface and intracellular antigens in leukemia diagnosis. *Cytometry* **18,** 187–198.

38. Groeneveld, K., te Marvelde, J. G., van den Beemd, M. W., Hooijkaas, H., and van Dongen, J. J. (1996) Flow cytometric detection of intracellular antigens for immunophenotyping of normal and malignant leukocytes. *Leukemia* **10,** 1383–1389.

7

Identification of Mast Cells in the Cellular Response to Myocardial Infarction

Nikolaos G. Frangogiannis and Mark L. Entman

Summary

Myocardial infarction is associated with an acute inflammatory response, leading to replacement of injured cardiomyocytes with granulation tissue. Mast cells are actively involved in postinfarction inflammation by releasing histamine and tumor necrosis factor-α, triggering a cytokine cascade. During the proliferative phase of healing, mast cells accumulate in the infarct and may regulate fibrous tissue deposition and angiogenesis by releasing growth factors, angiogenic mediators, and proteases. This chapter describes simple and reliable methods used to identify mast cells in control and infarcted canine hearts. Toluidine blue staining, labeling with conjugated avidin, and tryptase histochemistry are useful in the detection of mast cells in canine tissues. In the healing infarct, mast cells are associated with other cell types that are important for granulation tissue formation. We present immunohistochemical methods identifying monocytes, neutrophils, macrophages, endothelial cells, myofibroblasts, and smooth muscle cells in dog infarcts. These techniques are useful tools for pathological studies in canine models.

Key Words: Mast cell; toluidine blue; metachromatic; FITC-avidin; tryptase; histochemistry; pathology; immunohistochemistry; endothelial; macrophage; neutrophil; myofibroblast; smooth muscle cell; wound healing; infarct; myocardial ischemia.

1. Introduction

The presence of mast cells has been established in amphibian, murine, rat, canine, and human heart tissue *(1–3)*. Because of their strategic location, mast cells are likely to play an important role in initiating the inflammatory response through the release of proinflammatory mediators, capable of triggering a cytokine cascade. Gordon and Galli *(4)* identified mouse peritoneal mast cells as an important source of both preformed and immunologically induced tumor necrosis factor (TNF)-α. Additional observations suggested that mast cells are capable of producing multiple cytokines and chemokines, such as interleukin

From: *Methods in Molecular Biology, vol. 315: Mast Cells: Methods and Protocols*
Edited by: G. Krishnaswamy and D. S. Chi © Humana Press Inc., Totowa, NJ

(IL)-4, IL-5, IL-8, Macrophage Inflammatory Protein-1α, Macrophage Inflammatory Protein-1β, Monocyte Chemoattractant Protein-1, and lymphotactin *(5–7)*. Cytokine expression by cardiac mast cells has been recently demonstrated. Mast cells in rupture-prone areas of human coronary atheromas were positive for TNF-α *(8)*. Furthermore, our laboratory *(9)* has demonstrated constitutive expression of TNF-α in canine cardiac mast cells.

A possible role for cardiac mast cells in mediating injury was suggested in a porcine model of C5a-mediated myocardial ischemia *(10)*. Our studies *(9)* indicated a role for mast cell mediators in initiating the cytokine cascade ultimately responsible for intercellular adhesion molecule (ICAM)-1 induction in the reperfused canine myocardium. The constitutive presence of TNF-α in mast cells in control canine hearts led us to postulate that mast cell-derived TNF-α may be released after myocardial ischemia, representing the "upstream" cytokine responsible for initiating the inflammatory cascade (**Fig. 1**).

Our experiments demonstrated a rapid release of histamine and TNF-α bioactivity in the early postischemic cardiac lymph. In addition, histochemical studies indicated mast cell degranulation in ischemic but not in control sections of canine myocardium. These findings suggested rapid mast cell degranulation and mediator release after myocardial ischemia. C5a, adenosine *(11)*, and reactive oxygen may represent the stimuli responsible for initiation of mast cell degranulation. Furthermore, in vitro experiments showed that early postischemic cardiac lymph is capable of inducing IL-6 expression in canine mononuclear cells. Incubation with a neutralizing antibody to TNF-α in part inhibited IL-6 upregulation, suggesting an important role for TNF-α as the upstream cytokine inducer *(9)*. These studies allow us to refine our hypothesis regarding the role of mast cells in myocardial ischemia and reperfusion. Mast cell degranulation appears to be confined in the ischemic area and results in rapid release of TNF-α, inducing IL-6 in infiltrating mononuclear cells. Histamine also may be an important autacoid by stimulating surface expression of P-selectin from Weibel–Palade bodies and inducing leukocyte rolling.

Mast cells also may be involved in regulating fibrous tissue deposition and scar formation in healing infarcts *(12)*. Using labeling with fluorescein-labeled avidin (FITC-avidin), tryptase histochemistry, and toluidine blue staining, we demonstrated a striking accumulation of mast cells in areas of collagen deposition and cell proliferation. The increase in mast cell numbers was first noted after 72 h of reperfusion. After 5–7 d of reperfusion, mast cell numbers in fibrotic areas, in which myocytes were fully replaced by scar, were markedly higher than the numbers from areas of the same section showing intact myocardium. Mast cells are important sources of transforming growth factor (TGF)-β, *(13)* basic fibroblast growth factor *(14)*, and vascular endothelial growth factor *(15)*, factors that can regulate fibroblast growth, modulate extracellular matrix

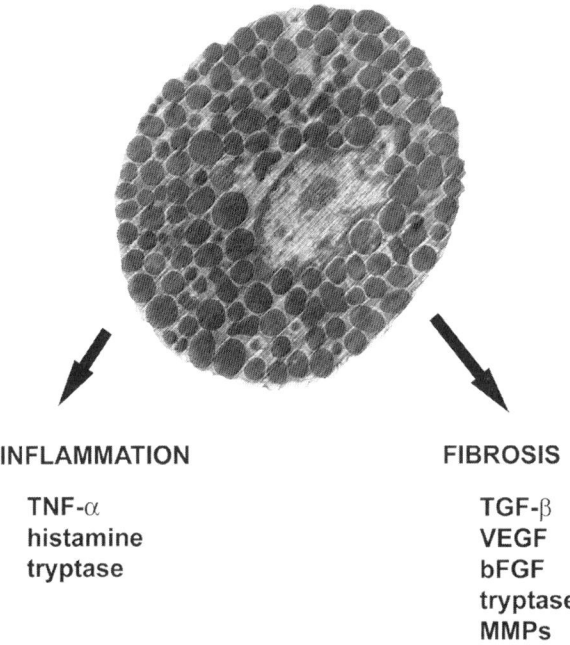

INFLAMMATION

TNF-α
histamine
tryptase

FIBROSIS

TGF-β
VEGF
bFGF
tryptase
MMPs

Fig. 1. Role of the mast cell in myocardial infarction. Mast cells are capable of releasing a wide variety of preformed and newly synthesized mediators important in the proinflammatory (TNF-α, histamine, proteases) and in the proliferative phase of infarct healing (TGF-α, bFGF, VEGF, tryptase, chymase, matrix metalloproteinases [MMPs]).

metabolism, and stimulate angiogenesis *(16)*. Mast cell-derived TGF-β and tryptase may play a significant role in mediating myofibroblast α-smooth muscle actin (α-SMA) expression in the healing scar. Mast cells also may influence healing and tissue remodeling by expressing gelatinases A and B *(17–19)*, which are implicated in extracellular matrix metabolism. Finally, an important role for the chymase pathway in promoting angiotensin II generation and cardiac fibrosis has been suggested *(20)*.

2. Materials

1. Alcohol: 70%.
2. Acetic acid: 10%.
3. Chloroform: 30%.
4. Zinc chloride: 0.6 % in 0.1 % sodium acetate.
5. Sodium acetate: 0.1%.
6. Toluidine blue: 0.5% (w/v) (Sigma, St. Louis).
7. Hydrochloric acid: 0.5 *N*.
8. FITC-avidin.

9. Phosphate-buffered saline (PBS).
10. N-CBZ-GLY-GLY-ARG-β-naphthylamide: 0.54 mM (Sigma).
11. Fast Garnet GBC Salt: 0.22 mM (Sigma).
12. Dimethylformamide: 3.8 % (by volume) in 50 mM Tris-HCl (pH 6.8).
13. Tris-HCl: 50 mM (pH 6.8).
14. Cupric sulfate: 1%.
15. Hydrogen peroxide: 3% (Sigma).
16. Elite Vectastain peroxidase kit (mouse; Vector laboratories, Burlingame CA).
17. Elite Vectastain peroxidase kit (rabbit; Vector Laboratories).
18. Peroxidase substrate kit (Vector).
19. Mouse anti-human macrophage antibody PM-2K (Biogenesis).
20. Mouse anti-human Mac 387 antibody (Dako).
21. Mouse anti-canine neutrophil antibody SG8H6 (kindly donated by Dr. C. W. Smith, Baylor College of Medicine).
22. Mouse anti-human CD31 antibody (Dako).
23. Mouse anti-human α-SMA antibody (Sigma).
24. Rabbit anti-canine chymase antibody (kindly donated by Dr. G. H. Caughey, UCSF).
25. Eosin.
26. Xylene.
27. Aquamount.
28. Cytoseal XYL mounting medium.

3. Methods

The methods described in **Subheadings 3.1.** and **3.2.** outline: (1) the identification and phenotypic characterization of mast cells in the canine heart; and (2) the identification of the cellular content of healing infarcts (macrophages, myofibroblasts, endothelial cells, neutrophils, and monocytes).

3.1. Identification of Canine Cardiac Mast Cells in Paraffin-Embedded Tissue

Mast cells can be identified in paraffin-embedded canine heart using: (1) toluidine blue staining (*see* **Subheading 3.1.1.**); (2) staining with FITC-labeled avidin (**Subheading 3.1.2.**); and (3) tryptase histochemistry (**Subheading 3.1.3.**). Fixation is critical for detection of mast cells in canine tissue (*see* **Note 1**). Tissue samples are collected from the canine heart and fixed in Carnoy's fixative (60% ethanol, 30% chloroform, 10% acetic acid) for 4 h. Fixed tissues are dehydrated in a graded series of alcohols and embedded in paraffin wax. Sections are cut at 5 μ, dewaxed in xylene, rehydrated, and stained.

3.1.1. Toluidine Blue Staining

Sections stained with toluidine blue are rinsed with 0.5 N HCl (pH 0.5) for 5 min, stained with 0.5 % w/v toluidine blue in 0.5 N HCl for 30 min and

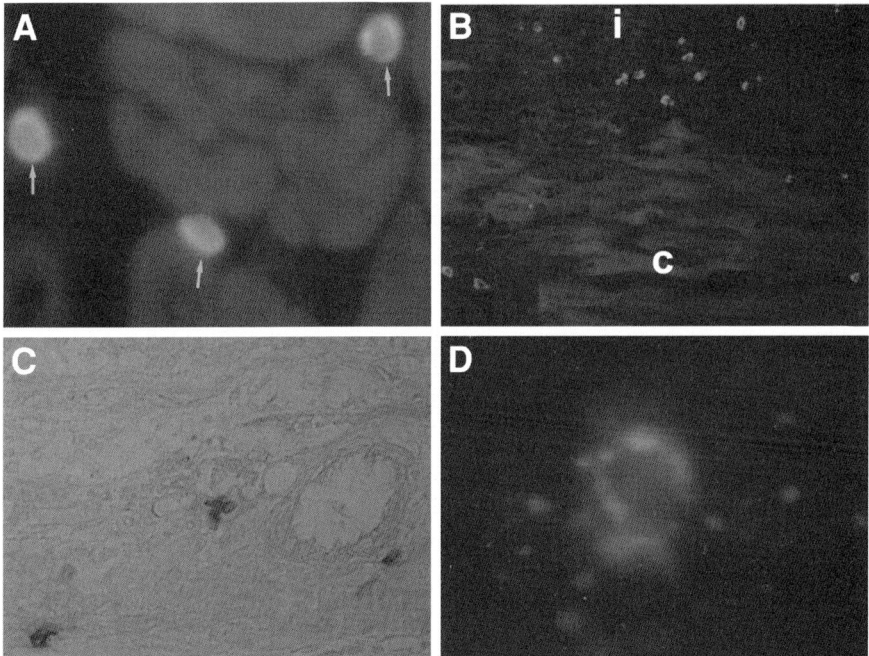

Fig. 2. Identification of mast cells in canine hearts. (**A**) Staining with FITC-conjugated avidin identifies mast cells as intensely fluorescent cells packed with granules. (**B**) In canine infarcts mast cells accumulate in the scar (i) but not in noninfarcted areas (c) (1 h occlusion/7 d reperfusion). (**C**) Tryptase histochemistry identifies mast cells as red/brown granular cells. (**D**) Mast cell degranulation in the infarcted myocardium is demonstrated using FITC-avidin staining.

counterstained for 1 min with fast green. Mast cells are easily identified by the dark violet staining of their granules.

3.1.2 FITC-Avidin Staining

Bergstresser et al. (*21*) described that fluorochrome-conjugated avidin stains rodent and human mast cells. Dewaxed sections are incubated for 60 min at room temperature in FITC-avidin diluted in PBS. The optimal dilution for staining of canine sections fixed in Carnoy's is 1:100. After staining the sections are washed three times for 10 min with PBS and cover slipped with Aquamount without counterstaining. Mast cells are identified as intensely fluorescent granular cells (**Fig. 2A,B**; *see* **Note 2**).

3.1.3 Tryptase Histochemistry

1. To stain for tryptase activity, a reaction mixture is prepared containing 0.54 m*M* *N*-CBZ-GLY-GLY-ARG-β-naphthylamide, 0.22 m*M* Fast Garnet GBC Salt and

3.8% dimethylformamide (by volume) in 50 m*M* Tris-HCl (pH 6.8) as previously described by Caughey et al. *(22)*.

2. After incubation at 30°C in the reaction mixture for 30 min, the slides are immersed in 1% cupric sulfate for 10 min at room temperature, washed in deionized water for 5 min, and cover slipped with Aquamount without counterstaining.
3. Mast cells are easily identified as red-stained granular cells (**Fig. 2C;** *see* **Note 3**).

3.1.4 Identification of Degranulating Mast Cells in Infarcted Canine Hearts

Although electron microscopy is the gold standard for identifying degranulating mast cells, we have used FITC-avidin staining to demonstrate mast cell degranulation in the canine heart *(9)*. Infarcted hearts show a significant number of degranulating mast cells (**Fig. 2D**), whereas the majority of mast cells have normal morphology in noninfarcted myocardium.

3.2. Identification of the Cellular Content of Healing Infarcts

During the proliferative phase of healing, infarcts contain a large number of inflammatory, vascular, and matrix-producing cells. To study the cellular environment in healing infarcts, we developed immunohistochemical methods to identify cell types often associated with mast cells in healing tissues. This section describes immunohistochemical techniques to label neutrophils, macrophages, endothelial cells, fibroblasts, and smooth muscle cells in normal and infarcted canine hearts.

3.2.1 Fixation and Tissue Processing

For optimal staining with the endothelial cell (CD31) and macrophage (PM-2K) markers we use samples fixed in B*5 fixative without formalin (0.6% zinc chloride) as described by Beckstead *(23)*. This fixative combines optimal antigenic survival with good morphological preservation.

3.2.2. Immunohistochemistry

1. Immunohistochemistry is performed using the ELITE mouse kit, which contains all the necessary reagents for the technique except the hydrogen peroxide, PBS, the primary antibodies and the peroxidase substrate kit (diaminobenzidine).
2. 5-μ sections are cut, dewaxed in xylene and graded alcohols, and rehydrated.
3. Sections are pretreated with a solution of 3% hydrogen peroxide to inhibit endogenous peroxidase activity and incubated with 2% horse serum for 1 h to block nonspecific protein binding.
4. Subsequently they are incubated for 2 h at room temperature with the primary antibody diluted in 2% horse serum. The following primary antibodies are used: mouse anti-human macrophage antibody PM-2K (1:200 dilution) to identify mature canine macrophages *(24)*, mouse anti-human Mac 387 antibody (1:1000 dilution) to detect newly recruited myeloid cells (neutrophils and monocytes), mouse anti-canine neutrophil antibody SG8H6 (kindly donated by Dr. C. W. Smith, Baylor

College of Medicine *[25]*), mouse anti-human CD31 antibody (1:100 dilution) to label endothelial cells, and mouse anti-human α-SMA antibody (1:400 dilution) to identify myofibroblasts and smooth muscle cells (*see* **Note 4**).

5. After rinsing with PBS three times, 5 min each slide, the slides are incubated for 30 min with the secondary antibody (0.5% biotinylated anti-mouse IgG) and then again washed in PBS.

6. The biotinylated secondary antibody is detected using the ABC system, a pre-formed macromolecular complex between avidin and biotinylated enzyme. Sections are incubated for 30 min with ABC reagent, which is prepared 30 min before incubation according to the manufacturer's recommendations.

7. After washing with PBS, peroxidase activity is detected using diaminobenzidine (Peroxidase substrate kit).

8. Slides are counterstained with eosin and mounted in Cytoseal XYL mounting medium.

9. Mast cell identification is performed with a rabbit anti-canine antibody to chymase at a 1:500 dilution (kindly donated by Dr. G. H. Caughey, UCSF *[19]*) using the ELITE rabbit kit. The immunohistochemical protocol is similar to the one described previously for the murine antibodies; however a biotinylated anti-rabbit IgG (included in the kit) is used as the secondary antibody.

4. Notes

1. Mast cell heterogeneity was established by the pioneering work of Enerback, who demonstrated a distinctive mucosal mast cell phenotype in the gastrointestinal tract of the rat *(26,27)*. In rodents, the use of modified fixation helps to distinguish mast cell subpopulations: mucosal or "atypical" mast cells are smaller in size, and their granules may become resistant to metachromatic staining after routine fixation with formalin, whereas "typical" or connective tissue mast cells contain large amounts of histamine and stain metachromatically regardless of fixation. In humans, the strict classification into mucosal and connective tissue type mast cells is not possible. However, human mast cell subtypes can also be defined according to staining and fixation properties *(28)*. We have shown that the canine heart contains at least two subpopulations of mast cells, which can be distinguished by their staining properties: approx 40% of the mast cells stained with toluidine blue when the tissue was fixed with formalin (resembling "typical" or "connective tissue" mast cells), whereas the remainder could not be detected unless fixatives such as Carnoy's were used *(2)*.

2. Fluorochrome-conjugated avidin is a simple and reliable technique for detection of mast cells in the canine heart. Avidin binds specifically to individual mast cell granules allowing identification of degranulated mast cells in areas of injury *(29)*. TRITC-avidin and FITC-avidin are equally effective in identifying mast cells. Bergstresser and colleagues suggested that fixation is unimportant for mast cell staining with FITC-avidin *(21)*. However, in our experience, infarcted formalin-fixed canine hearts demonstrated fewer mast cells compared with samples fixed in Carnoy's. The effects of different fixatives on mast cell staining with conjugated avidin have not been systematically studied.

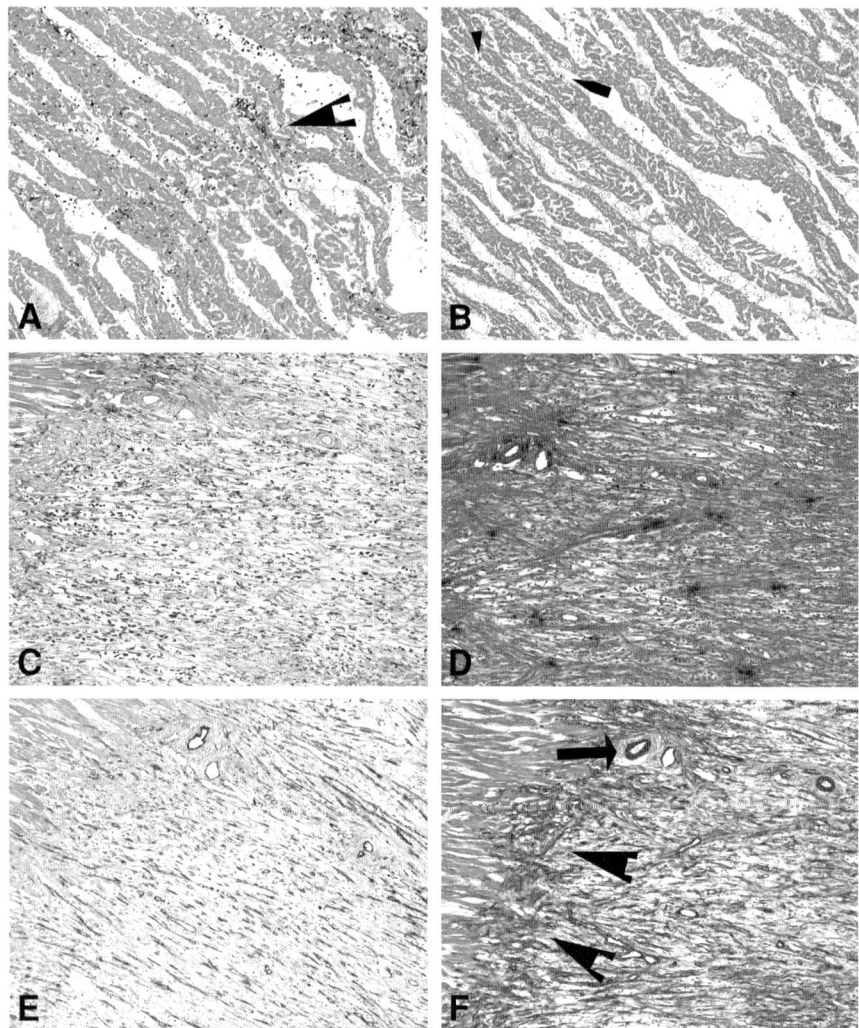

Fig. 3. Identification of the cellular content of canine infarcts (**A** and **B**, 1-h occlu-sion/24-h reperfusion; **C–F,** 1-h occlusion/7-d reperfusion). (**A**) After 24 h of reper-fusion staining with Mac387, an antibody that labels newly recruited myeloid cells (monocytes and neutrophils) identifies a large number of leukocytes in the myocar-dium (**arrowhead**). (**B**) In comparison, at the same time point, staining with PM-2K, a marker for mature macrophages labels a small number of cells (**arrowheads**). (**C**) After 7 d of reperfusion the healing infarct is filled with PM-2K positive mature macrophages. (**D**) Mast cells are identified using immunohistochemistry for chymase. (**E**) CD31 immunohistochemistry labels the vascular endothelium in the healing infarct. (**F**) α-SMA staining identifies myofibroblasts, predominantly localized in the infarct border zone (**arrowheads**) and vascular smooth muscle cells (**arrow**).

3. Tryptase histochemistry has been used to identify mast cells in human, bovine, canine, and murine tissues. Cytochemical reaction mixtures need to be made fresh daily. In addition, the sensitivity of the technique decreases in old histological samples. In our experience, only a small percentage of mast cells can be identified in tissues older than six months. When using fresh samples, however, the method is relatively simple, reliable, and specific for identification of canine mast cells. It is particularly valuable because commercially available antibodies to human tryptase do not crossreact with its canine homologue.

4. Identification of specific cell types in canine tissues requires use of optimal cellular markers (**Fig. 3**). Most anti-human CD68 antibodies do not crossreact with canine species. However, the monoclonal antibodies AM-3K and PM-2K, specific for mature human macrophages, detect canine macrophages in all tissues examined *(24,30)*. Endothelial cell identification requires the use of an anti-CD31 antibody *(31)*. Factor VIII staining labels only arteriolar and venular but not capillary endothelial cells. In addition, lectin histochemistry identified vascular endothelial cells in control hearts, but gave poor results in staining of the infarct vasculature *(31)*. The antibody Mac387 labels myeloid cells, neutrophils and monocytes, but not mature macrophages and serves as a marker of acute inflammatory activity *(30,32)*. In control hearts α-SMA staining labels vascular smooth muscle cells. However in healing infarcts, a large population of phenotypically modulated fibroblasts termed myofibroblasts express α-SMA and are predominantly localized in the border zone of the infarct *(33)*.

Acknowledgments

The authors wish to thank Sharon Malinowski and Connie Mata for editorial assistance with the manuscript. This work was supported by NIH Grant HL-42550, a Grant-in-Aid from the American Heart Association Texas Affiliate, and the DeBakey Heart Center.

References

1. Patella, V., Marino, I., Arbustini, E., et al. (1998) Stem cell factor in mast cells and increased mast cell density in idiopathic and ischemic cardiomyopathy. *Circulation* **97,** 971–978.
2. Frangogiannis, N. G., Burns, A. R., Michael, L. H., and Entman, M. L. (1999) Histochemical and morphological characteristics of canine cardiac mast cells. *Histochem. J.* **31,** 221–229.
3. Gersch, C., Dewald, O., Zoerlein, M., Michael, L. H., Entman, M. L., and Frangogiannis, N. G. (2002) Mast cells and macrophages in normal C57/BL/6 mice. *Histochem. Cell Biol.* **118,** 41–49.
4. Gordon, J. R. and Galli, S. J. (1990) Mast cells as a source of both preformed and immunologically inducible TNF-alpha/cachectin. *Nature* **346,** 274–276.
5. Plaut, M., Pierce, J. H., Watson, C. J., Hanley-Hyde, J., Nordan, R. P., and Paul, W. E. (1989) Mast cell lines produce lymphokines in response to cross-linkage of Fc epsilon RI or to calcium ionophores. *Nature* **339,** 64–67.

6. Baghestanian, M., Hofbauer, R., Kiener, H. P., et al. (1997) The c-kit ligand stem cell factor and anti-IgE promote expression of monocyte chemoattractant protein-1 in human lung mast cells. *Blood* **90,** 4438–4449.

7. Rumsaeng, V., Vliagoftis, H., Oh, C. K., and Metcalfe, D. D. (1997) Lymphotactin gene expression in mast cells following Fc(epsilon) receptor I aggregation: modulation by TGF-beta, IL-4, dexamethasone, and cyclosporin A. *J. Immunol.* **158,** 1353–1360.

8. Kaartinen, M., Penttila, A., and Kovanen, P. T. (1996) Mast cells in rupture-prone areas of human coronary atheromas produce and store TNF-alpha. *Circulation* **94,** 2787–2792.

9. Frangogiannis, N. G., Lindsey, M. L., Michael, L. H., et al. (1998) Resident cardiac mast cells degranulate and release preformed TNF-alpha, initiating the cytokine cascade in experimental canine myocardial ischemia/reperfusion. *Circulation* **98,** 699–710.

10. Ito, B. R., Engler, R. L., and del Balzo, U. (1993) Role of cardiac mast cells in complement C5a-induced myocardial ischemia. *Am. J. Physiol.* **264,** H1346–H1354.

11. Linden, J. (1994) Cloned adenosine A3 receptors: pharmacological properties, species differences and receptor functions. *Trends Pharmacol. Sci.* **15,** 298–306.

12. Frangogiannis, N. G., Smith, C. W., and Entman, M. L. (2002) The inflammatory response in myocardial infarction. *Cardiovasc. Res.* **53,** 31–47.

13. Pennington, D. W., Lopez, A. R., Thomas, P. S., Peck, C., and Gold, W. M. (1992) Dog mastocytoma cells produce transforming growth factor beta 1. *J. Clin. Invest.* **90,** 35–41.

14. Qu, Z., Liebler, J. M., Powers, M. R., et al. (1995) Mast cells are a major source of basic fibroblast growth factor in chronic inflammation and cutaneous hemangioma. *Am. J. Pathol.* **147,** 564–573.

15. Boesiger, J., Tsai, M., Maurer, M., et al. (1998) Mast cells can secrete vascular permeability 3factor/ vascular endothelial cell growth factor and exhibit enhanced release after immunoglobulin E-dependent upregulation of fc epsilon receptor I expression. *J. Exp. Med.* **188,** 1135–1145.

16. Shiota, N., Rysa, J., Kovanen, P. T., Ruskoaho, H., Kokkonen, J. O., and Lindstedt, K. A. (2003) A role for cardiac mast cells in the pathogenesis of hypertensive heart disease. *J. Hypertens.* **21,** 1935–1944.

17. Brower, G. L., Chancey, A. L., Thanigaraj, S., Matsubara, B. B., and Janicki, J. S. (2002) Cause and effect relationship between myocardial mast cell number and matrix metalloproteinase activity. *Am. J. Physiol. Heart Circ. Physiol.* **283,** H518–H525.

18. Chancey, A. L., Brower, G. L., and Janicki, J. S. (2002) Cardiac mast cell-mediated activation of gelatinase and alteration of ventricular diastolic function. *Am. J. Physiol. Heart Circ. Physiol.* **282,** H2152–H2158.

19. Fang, K. C., Wolters, P. J., Steinhoff, M., Bidgol, A., Blount, J. L., and Caughey, G. H. (1999) Mast cell expression of gelatinases A and B is regulated by kit ligand and TGF-beta. *J. Immunol.* **162,** 5528–5535.

20. Matsumoto, T., Wada, A., Tsutamoto, T., Ohnishi, M., Isono, T., and Kinoshita, M. (2003) Chymase inhibition prevents cardiac fibrosis and improves diastolic dysfunction in the progression of heart failure. *Circulation* **107,** 2555–2558.

21. Bergstresser, P. R., Tigelaar, R. E., and Tharp, M. D. (1984) Conjugated avidin identifies cutaneous rodent and human mast cells. *J. Invest. Dermatol.* **83,** 214–218.

22. Caughey, G. H., Viro, N. F., Calonico, L. D., McDonald, D. M., Lazarus, S. C., and Gold, W. M. (1988) Chymase and tryptase in dog mastocytoma cells: asynchronous expression as revealed by enzyme cytochemical staining. *J. Histochem. Cytochem.* **36,** 1053–1060.

23. Beckstead, J. H. (1994) A simple technique for preservation of fixation-sensitive antigens in paraffin-embedded tissues. *J. Histochem. Cytochem.* **42,** 1127–1134.

24. Zeng, L., Takeya, M., Ling, X., Nagasaki, A., and Takahashi, K. (1996) Interspecies reactivities of anti-human macrophage monoclonal antibodies to various animal species. *J. Histochem. Cytochem.* **44,** 845–853.

25. Hawkins, H. K., Entman, M. L., Zhu, J. Y., et al. (1996) Acute inflammatory reaction after myocardial ischemic injury and reperfusion. Development and use of a neutrophil-specific antibody. *Am. J. Pathol.* **148,** 1957–1969.

26. Enerback, L. (1966) Mast cells in rat gastrointestinal mucosa. I. Effects of fixation. *Acta Pathol. Microbiol. Scand.* **66,** 289–302.

27. Enerback, L. (1966) Mast cells in rat gastrointestinal mucosa. 2. Dye-binding and metachromatic properties. *Acta Pathol. Microbiol. Scand.* **66,** 303–312.

28. Miller, J. S. and Schwartz, L. B. (1989) Human mast cell proteases and mast cell heterogeneity. *Curr. Opin. Immunol.* **1,** 637–642.

29. Tharp, M. D., Seelig, L. L., Jr., Tigelaar, R. E., and Bergstresser, P. R. (1985) Conjugated avidin binds to mast cell granules. *J. Histochem. Cytochem.* **33,** 27–32.

30. Frangogiannis, N. G., Mendoza, L. H., Ren, G., et al. (2003) MCSF expression is induced in healing myocardial infarcts and may regulate monocyte and endothelial cell phenotype. *Am. J. Physiol. Heart Circ. Physiol.* **285,** H483–H492.

31. Ren, G., Michael, L. H., Entman, M. L., and Frangogiannis, N. G. (2002) Morphological characteristics of the microvasculature in healing myocardial infarcts. *J. Histochem. Cytochem.* **50,** 71–79.

32. Frangogiannis, N. G., Shimoni, S., Chang, S. M., et al. (2002) Evidence for an active inflammatory process in the hibernating human myocardium. *Am. J. Pathol.* **160,** 1425–1433.

33. Frangogiannis, N. G., Michael, L. H., and Entman, M. L. (2000) Myofibroblasts in reperfused myocardial infarcts express the embryonic form of smooth muscle myosin heavy chain (SMemb). *Cardiovasc. Res.* **48,** 89–100.

III

DEVELOPMENT OF MAST CELLS IN VITRO

8

Growth of Human Mast Cells From Bone Marrow and Peripheral Blood-Derived CD34+ Pluripotent Progenitor Cells

Arnold S. Kirshenbaum and Dean D. Metcalfe

Summary

Human mast cells (HMCs) are derived from a CD34+ pluripotent progenitor cell that is Kit (CD117+), CD13+, FcεRI- and lacks lineage-specific surface markers. Bone marrow and peripheral blood are two tissue sources available for obtaining CD34+ progenitor cells from which to culture HMCs. CD34+ cells can be isolated and enriched by magnetic separation columns and stored under specific conditions until ready for use. Alternatively, enriched CD34+ cells may be immediately cultured in serum-free culture media containing recombinant human stem cell factor (rhSCF), rhIL-6, and rhIL-3 (first week only). Weekly hemidepletions and the removal of adherent cells and/or debris enables the investigator to obtain HMC cultures, identified by Wright–Giemsa and acidic toluidine blue stains, by 8–10 wk.

Key Words: Human mast cells; CD34+ cells; progenitor cells; bone marrow; peripheral blood.

1. Introduction

Human mast cells (HMCs) are derived from a CD34+ pluripotent progenitor cell that is Kit (CD117)+, CD13+, FcεRI- and lacks T-cell (CD2), B-cell (CD19, CD20), macrophage (CD14), and eosinophil lineage surface markers *(1–3)*. In addition to peripheral blood and bone marrow, HMCs have been derived from CD34+ progenitor cells from cord blood *(4–7)*, and fetal liver *(8,9)*; in vitro studies have reported that the mature HMC progeny will differ, depending on the tissue of origin. Furthermore, using rhSCF and rhIL-6, mature FcεRI+/CD117+/CD13+ tryptase+ HMCs require at least 8–10 wk in culture to fully mature. Other lineages that appear in vitro (monocytes) are depleted with weekly passage, and this is believed to prevent competition for growth factors,

From: *Methods in Molecular Biology, vol. 315: Mast Cells: Methods and Protocols*
Edited by: G. Krishnaswamy and D. S. Chi © Humana Press Inc., Totowa, NJ

and release of inhibitory growth factors such as interferon-γ *(10)*, which reduces HMC growth and proliferation.

The use of peripheral blood leukapheresis to collect mononuclear cells, followed by immunomagnetic or affinity column enrichment of CD34+ cells, provides large numbers of CD34+ cells and significantly increases the HMC yield. Laboratory methods are described that detail the isolation of bone marrow and peripheral blood-derived CD34+ cells and growth of HMCs in vitro from these progenitors.

2. Materials

1. MACS High Gradient Magnetic LS Separation Columns (Miltenyi Biotec, Auburn CA).
2. StemPro-34 SFM with nutrient supplement (Invitrogen, Carlsbad, CA).
3. 200 mM (100X) L-glutamine, penicillin-streptomycin (100X; Biofluids, Rockville, MD). Culture concentrations: L-glutamine 2 mM, penicillin 100 IU/mL, streptomycin 50 µg/mL.
4. Ammonium chloride solution (StemCell, Vancouver, BC).
5. RhIL-3, rhIL-6, rhSCF (PeproTech, Rocky Hill, NJ).
6. 75-cm^2 tissue culture flasks (Sarstedt, Newton, NC).
7. 5 mL polystyrene, 15 mL polypropylene, and 50 polypropylene tubes (Becton-Dickinson Labware, Franklin Lakes, NJ).
8. 1X PBS, pH 7.2, containing 0.5% bovine serum albumin (BSA), 2 mM ethylene diamine tetraacetic acid.
9. FITC-conjugated anti-human CD34 (anti-HPCA2, Becton-Dickinson, San Jose, CA).
10. Acidic toluidine blue (pH <1.0).
11. Hematek-2000 Wright–Giemsa slide stainer (Bayer Corporation, Elkhart, IN).
12. Cytospin 3 (Shandon, Pittsburgh, PA).
13. M199 medium 1X with Earles' salts, L-glutamine, sodium bicarbonate, HEPES buffer (Invitrogen).
14. DMSO (Sigma, St. Louis, MO).
15. FBS (Invitrogen).
16. Preservative-free heparin sodium (1000 U/mL; American Pharmaceutical Partners, Schaumburg, IL).
17. Lymphocyte separation media (ICN Biomedicals, Aurora, OH).
18. 30-µm nylon net filter (Millipore, Bedford, MA).
19. Nalgene Cryo 1°C freezing container (Daigger, Vernon Hills, IL).
20. Nunc 1.8-mL SI (377267) cryotubes (Nunc, Roskilde, Denmark).

3. Methods

3.1. Preparation of Bone Marrow or Peripheral Blood for CD34+Selection

CD34+ pluripotent progenitor cells are collected from either bone marrow or peripheral blood. On average, bone marrow contains 1–2% CD34+ cells, and peripheral blood contains 0.01–0.1% CD34+ cells *(11)*, so yields will differ significantly.

1. Preload 10- or 50-mL syringes with 0.5 or 1.0 mL of preservative-free heparin sodium, respectively. Collect aspirated bone marrow in 10-mL syringes. Collect venipuncture-derived peripheral blood into 50-mL syringes. Mix cells and heparin by rotating the syringes for 1 min.
2. Place a maximum of 10 mL of either heparinized bone marrow or peripheral blood into a 50-mL tube and add 25 mL of StemPro serum-free media with nutrient supplement, 2 m*M* L-glutamine, 100 IU/mL penicillin, and 50 µg/mL streptomycin (herein referred to as complete media). Complete media should be kept at 4°C and be remade fresh every 2 mo.
3. Mix cells by gently pipetting and underlayer 14 mL lymphocyte separation media by gently inserting a 10 mL pipet through the mixed bone marrow or peripheral blood, and pipetting 14 mL of separation media slowly into the bottom of the tube (*see* **Note 1**). Centrifuge tubes at 675*g* for 20 min at room temperature. The red cells will collect below the separation media at bottom of the tube. Identify the mononuclear cell layer just above the separation media and pipet off complete media just above the interface.
4. Using a 25-mL pipet, gently skim off and collect the mononuclear cells by back and forth motion (*see* **Note 2**). Discard the remaining red cell pellet and separation media in biohazard waste bags. Add 25 mL of complete media and centrifuge the mononuclear cells at 300*g* for 10 min to remove debris. Remove the supernatant and resuspend the pelleted mononuclear cells in 25 mL of media. Repeat twice.
5. Resuspend mononuclear cells in 5 mL of sterile blocking buffer solution consisting of 1X PBS, pH 7.2, containing 0.5% BSA and 2m*M* ethylene diamine tetraacetic acid. Remove clumps, aggregates, or particles by passing the cell suspension through sterile a 30-µm nylon net filter into a 15-mL tube (*see* **Note 3**). Count cells and record total using a hemocytometer.

3.2. CD34+ Cell Selection and Enrichment (see *Note 4*)

CD34+ purity is important for eliminating unwanted cells from cultures. Magnetic separation columns initially yield a CD34+ cell purity between 65 and 75%. A second CD34+ enrichment using a new column may be necessary to obtain purities of 90–95% CD34+ cells.

1. Resuspend 10^7 mononuclear cells in 100 µL of sterile blocking buffer in a 5-mL tube. Add 10 µL of FITC-conjugated anti-human CD34 and incubate the cells for 30 min at 37°C.
2. Add 2 mL of sterile blocking buffer and centrifuge at 210*g* for 5 min. Decant the supernatant and resuspend the cell pellet in 80 µL of sterile blocking buffer. Add 20 µL of MACS anti-FITC microbeads per 10^7 cells and incubate the cells for 15 min at 6–12°C.

3. Add 2 mL of sterile blocking buffer and centrifuge at 210*g* for 5 min. Decant the supernatant and resuspend the cells at a concentration up to 10^8 cells per 500 µL of sterile blocking buffer.

4. Place the MACS LS column into the magnetic field and run 3 mL of degassed sterile blocking buffer through the column. Pipet the cell suspension onto the column and collect the effluent in a 15-mL tube as the negative fraction. Rinse the column with 1 mL of sterile blocking buffer three times, remove the column from the magnetic cell separator, and place the column on a new 15-mL collection tube. Apply 5 mL of buffer to the LS separation column and flush out magnetically labeled cells by applying the plunger supplied with the column. Count cells and record total using a hemocytometer.

3.3. Cryopreservation of CD34+ Cells

A minimum of 5×10^6 CD34+ cells/mL of cryoprecipitate mixture is recommended for preservation and recovery (*see* **Note 5**). The cryoprecipitate mixture consists of two parts.

1. Part 1: mix M199 media with DMSO in a 4:1 v/v ratio. Aliquot in 15-mL tubes and keep frozen at 20°C until use.

2. Part 2: add 3000 U/mL preservative-free heparin to FBS, aliquot in 15-mL tubes, and keep frozen at 20°C until use.

3. To cryopreserve 5 to 10×10^6 cells, prepare two tubes containing either 0.5 mL of cold (4°C) M199/DMSO or FBS/heparin. Add $2.5–5.0 \times 10^6$ cells into each tube and keep on ice for several minutes. Combine cells into a total of 1 mL and pipet into 1.8-mL cryotubes. Allow cells to equilibrate at 4°C for 30 min. Transfer cells to a Nalgene Cryo 1°C freezing container and place in a –70°C freezer overnight. After 24 h, transfer cryotubes to liquid nitrogen.

4. For recovery, quick thaw cells at 37°C, resuspend in 10 mL of complete media, and centrifuge at 300*g* for 10 min. Suction supernatant completely to remove any DMSO. Resuspend cells in 5–10 mL of complete media, count cells, and record total using a hemocytometer.

3.4. CD34+ and HMC Cultures

Under ideal conditions, 5×10^6 CD34+ cells at 8–10 wk may give rise to $10–20 \times 10^6$ HMCs with less than 5% contamination with other cell types, as determined by Wright–Giemsa and acidic toluidine blue staining.

1. Add 100 ng/mL rhSCF, 100 ng/mL rhIL-6, and 30 ng/mL rhIL-3 (first week only) to complete media and culture $2.5–5.0 \times 10^4$ CD34+ cells/mL in a total volume of 20 mL in 75-cm^2 tissue culture flasks (*see* **Note 6**).

2. Perform hemidepletions weekly by carefully inserting a 5-mL pipet into the back of the flask, remove supernatant, and add back fresh media containing rhSCF and rhIL-6. Check flasks weekly for adherent cells or debris. Monocytes and other cells will proliferate initially and compete for growth factors in suspension, resulting in

Human mast cells derived from CD34+ peripheral blood leukocytes

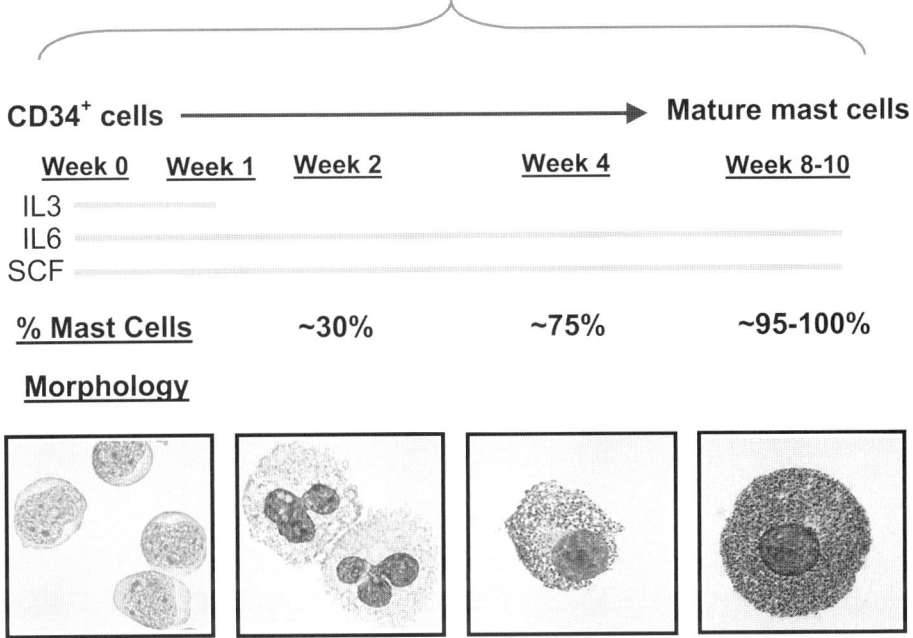

CD34⁺ cells ————————————————→ **Mature mast cells**

Week 0	Week 1	Week 2	Week 4	Week 8-10

IL3
IL6
SCF

% Mast Cells   ~30%   ~75%   ~95-100%

Morphology

Fig. 1. Human mast cells derived from CD34+ peripheral blood leukocytes. (Reproduced with the permission of **ref. *12*.**)

adherent cells or debris from cell death. This extraneous material may have a deleterious effect on HMC yields and must be removed weekly. If adherent cells are present, gently pipet flasks, suction off nonadherent HMCs and move cells and growth media to a new flask. In the event of cell debris, remove nonadherent HMCs and growth media, pipet into a 50-mL tube, and centrifuge at slow speed (150*g*) for 5 min at 22°C. Resuspend the cell pellets in fresh complete media with rhIL-6 and rhSCF, and culture in new flasks (*see* **Note 7**).

3. Check total and HMC counts weekly by staining with Wright-Giemsa and acidic toluidine blue (*see* **Subheading 3.5.**; **Fig. 1** *[12]*).

3.5. HMC Histochemical Stains

HMC numbers are calculated by determining the percentage of acidic toluidine blue positive cells out of total Wright–Giemsa-positive cells. Acidic toluidine blue-positive HMC numbers can be confirmed by tryptase staining.

3.5.1. Wright–Giemsa

1. Count cells directly out of flasks, and concentrate at $210g$ for 5 min to at least 2×10^5 cells/mL, for optimal cytospins.
2. Add 100 µL of cell suspension to cytospin sample chambers and clean slides. Spin slides at $14g$ for 5 min. Let slides air dry and place on an automated Hematek-2000 for Wright–Giemsa stain. Add one to two drops of Permount and cover slip.

3.5.2. Acidic Toluidine Blue

1. Add 0.5 g of toluidine blue to 30 mL of absolute ethanol. Bring the volume to 100 mL with distilled deionized water. Adjust to a pH <1.0 with $1N$ HCl. Store at room temperature.
2. Prepare Mota's fixative in a 100-mL bottle with a magnetic stirrer by adding 4 g of lead acetate (basic) to 50 mL of distilled deionized water. Stir at slow speed and add 2–4 mL of glacial acetic acid to dissolve the lead acetate and make the solution clear. Add 50 mL of absolute ethanol. Keep tightly closed and store at room temperature. Prepare fresh every 1–2 mo.
3. Fix cytospins by adding several drops of Mota's fixative to cover the cells for 10 min. Mota's evaporates quickly, so replenish drops once or twice to prevent crystal formation.
4. Slowly run water down the slides, not directly on cells, to remove fixative, and blot any droplets. Do not disturb the cells.
5. Add two to three drops of acidic toluidine blue to the slide and let stain for 20 min. Run water down the slide to remove the stain, and blot dry. Add one to two drops of Permount and cover slip.

4. Notes

1. It is important not to disturb the bone marrow or peripheral blood when underlaying them with separation media because clots tend to form and make skimming off of mononuclear cells difficult.
2. Before skimming off of mononuclear cells, if clots are noted in the interface or below, suction clots with a 10- or 25-mL pipet placed directly on the clot. The interface is minimally disturbed and clots are avoided in the mononuclear cell suspension.
3. Red blood cells normally contaminate most preparations and will not affect HMC yields if left in culture. For significant red cell contamination, lyse red blood cells by adding ammonium chloride to cells in a 4:1 ratio, incubate cells on ice for 10 min and centrifuge at $300g$ for 5 min at 22°C. Resuspend the mononuclear cell pellet in complete media with growth factors and culture.
4. MACS LS magnetic separation columns have a maximum capacity of 2×10^9 total cells and 10^8 magnetically labeled cells. Use degassed buffer only by applying a vacuum to the buffer at room temperature. Excessive gas in the buffer will form bubbles, and decrease the CD34+ cell yields. Use the column immediately

after filling to avoid formation of air bubbles. Use a maximum cell concentration of 10^8 cells per 500 μL of buffer.

5. CD34+ cells generally survive cryopreservation well, with some variation between procedures. Cell loss attributable to crystallization can occur and can affect overall yields of cells. Viability as measured by trypan blue staining may yield viabilities ranging between 75 and 90%. Remove cell debris from thawed CD34+ cells by centrifuging at 150*g* for at least 5 min. Resuspend CD34+ cells in complete media with growth factors.

6. CD34+ cells may initially proliferate 100 times or more the starting number of cells if rhSCF is combined with rhIL-3 and rhIL-6, so do not culture greater than 5×10^4 cells/mL. Luxurious growth is observed during the first 2–3 wk, although debris will begin to accumulate because of non-HMC lineage cell apoptosis and necrosis. Adherent macrophages also may start increasing in number by 2 wk. Check cultures weekly and separate nonadherent HMC committed progenitors from adherent cells and debris. Gently pipet and remove nonadherent cells to a new flask or centrifuge nonadherent cells and supernatant at 150*g* for 5 min, resuspend cells in complete media with growth factors, and culture in a new flask. The 4-wk time point appears to be a critical juncture, and cultures not properly cared may undergo significant HMC loss. To counteract this, remove and replenish 95% of the media at 4 wk.

7. RhSCF alone will give rise during the course of 8–10 wk to pure HMC cultures; however, HMC numbers are less, and less cell debris is observed at all weeks in culture. IL-3 increases all cell lineages and is a basophil growth factor but will not give rise to significant numbers of basophils if used for the first week only in the presence of rhSCF and rhIL-6. IL-6 helps supports HMC growth and maturation and prevents apoptosis.

Acknowledgments

The authors thank Dr. Alasdair Gilfillan for reviewing the manuscript.

References

1. Kirshenbaum, A. S., Goff, J. P., Semere, T., Foster, B., Scott, L. M., and Metcalfe, D. D. (1999) Demonstration that human mast cells arise from a progenitor cell population that is CD34+, c-*kit*+, and expresses aminopeptidase N (CD13). *Blood* **94**, 2333–2342.
2. Kirshenbaum, A. S., Kessler, S. W., Goff, J. P., and Metcalfe D. D. (1991) Demonstration of the origin of human mast cells from CD34+ bone marrow progenitor cells. *J. Immunol.* **146**, 1410–1415.
3. Rottem, M., Okada T., Goff, J. P., and Metcalfe, D. D. (1994) Mast cells cultured from the peripheral blood of normal donors and patients with mastocytosis originate from a CD34+/FcεRI- cell population. *Blood* **84**, 2489–2496.
4. Toru, H., Eguchi, M., Matsumoto, R., Yanagida, M. Yota, J., and Nakahata, T. (1998) Interleukin-4 promotes the development of tryptase and chymase double-positive human mast cells accompanied by cell maturation. *Blood* **91**, 187–195.

5. Lee, E., Min, H. K., Oskeritzian, C. A., Kambe, N., Schwartz, L. B., and Wook Chang H. (2003) Recombinant human (rh) stem cell factor and rhIL-4 stimulate differentiation and proliferation of CD3+ cells from umbilical cord blood and CD3+ cells enhance FcepsilonR1 expression on fetal liver-derived mast cells in the presence of rhIL-4. *Cell Immunol.* **226,** 30–36.

6. Matsuzawa, S., Sakashita, K., Kinoshita, T., Ito, S., Yamashita, T., and Koike K. (2003) IL-9 enhances the growth of human mast cell progenitors under stimulation with stem cell factor. *J. Immunol.* **170,** 3461–3467.

7. Piliponsky, A. M., Gleich, G. J., Nagler, A., Bar, I., and Levi-Schaffer, F. (2003) Non-IgE-dependent activation of human lung- and cord blood-derived mast cells is induced by eosinophil major basic protein and modulated by the membrane form of stem cell factor. *Blood* **101,** 1898–1904.

8. Kambe, N., Kambe, M., Chang, H. W., et al. (2000) An improved procedure for the development of human mast cells from dispersed fetal liver cells in serum-free culture medium. *J. Immunol. Methods* **240,** 101–110.

9. Kambe, M., Kambe, N., Oskeritzian, C. A., Schechter, N., and Schwartz, L. B. (2001) IL-6 attenuates apoptosis, while neither IL-6 nor IL-10 affect the numbers or protease phenotype of fetal liver-derived human mast cells. *Clin. Exp. Allergy* **31,** 1077–1085.

10. Kirshenbaum, A. S., Worobec, A. S., Davis, T. A., Goff, J. P., Semere, T., and Metcalfe, D. D. (1998) Inhibition of human mast cell growth and differentiation by interferon gamma-1b. *Exp. Hematol.* **26,** 245–251.

11. Lane, T. A., Law, P., Maruyama, M., et al. (1995) Harvesting and enrichment of hematopoietic progenitor cells mobilized into the peripheral blood of normal donors by granulocyte-macrophage colony- stimulating factor (GM-CSF) or G-CSF: potential role in allogeneic marrow transplantation. *Blood* **85,** 275–282.

12. Tkaczyk, C., Okayama, Y., Metcalfe, D. D., and Gilfillan, A. M. (2004) Fcγ receptors on mast cells: activatory and inhibitory regulation of mediator release. *Int. Arch. Allergy Immunol.* **1333,** 305–315. Adapted with permission from S. Karger AG, Basel.

9

Culture of Human Mast Cells
From Hemopoietic Progenitors

Hirohisa Saito

Summary

The survival of hemopoietic stem cells in culture is suppressed by various cytokines and stimuli. The development of human mast cells also is affected by these stem cell-inhibitory mechanisms because it requires a much-longer period as compared with the development of other cell lineages. This chapter introduces the method of forming human mast cell colonies by culturing purified cord blood cells and peripheral blood cells in serum-free methylcellulose supplemented with stem cell factor and interleukin-6 for 6 wk. Mast cells in colonies can be retrieved by dissolving methylcellulose, and can be maintained in liquid medium for more than six months. This method should be useful for obtaining non-neoplasmic functional human mast cells with high methodological reproducibility.

Key Words: Mast cells; cellular differentiation; cord blood-derived cultured mast cells; granulocyte macrophage colony-stimulating factor; hemopoietic stem cell; interleukin-3; interleukin-6; peripheral blood-derived cultured mast cells; stem cell factor.

1. Introduction

A hemopoietic stem cell is capable of dividing into a cell having the identical properties (self-renewal) and into a differentiated cell at the same time. After cell division, differentiated cells (myeloid progenitors) can survive, proliferate, and further differentiate only if the appropriate growth factors, such as granulocyte macrophage colony-stimulating factor (GM-CSF), are present in the microenvironment, whereas the survival of renewed stem cells is supported by the continuous expression of certain transcriptional factors, such as SCL and signal transducers and activators of transcription (STAT)-3 (**Fig. 1**). Stem cell factor (SCF) strongly supports the survival of hemopoietic stem cells by upregulating the basic helix–loop–helix transcriptional factor, SCL,

From: *Methods in Molecular Biology, vol. 315: Mast Cells: Methods and Protocols*
Edited by: G. Krishnaswamy and D. S. Chi © Humana Press Inc., Totowa, NJ

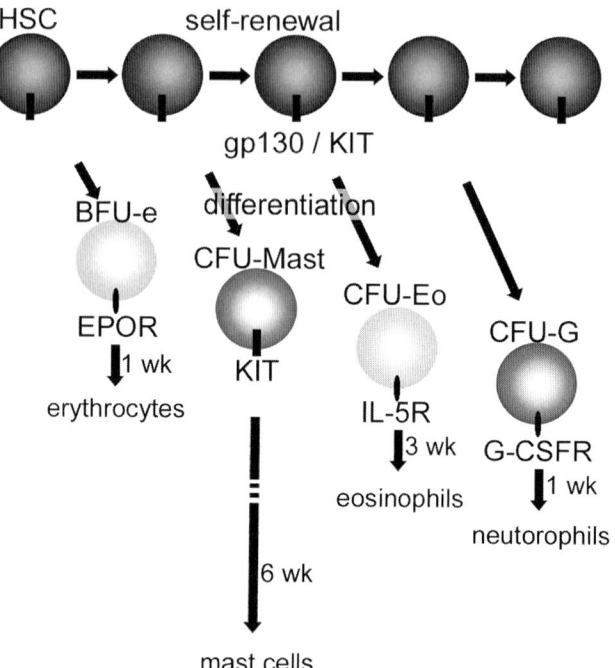

Fig. 1. Differentiation of a mast cell progenitor from a hemopoietic stem cell (HSC). While they are self-renewing, HSCs can differentiate into various types of committed progenitors. Commitment of differentiation is considered to be determined randomly by intrinsic mechanisms. Erythroid progenitors (BFU-e) express erythropoietin receptors (EPOR) and require EPOR for their survival, differentiation, and proliferation. Similarly, mast cell progenitors (CFU-mast), eosinophil progenitors (CFU-Eo), and neutrophil progenitors (CFU-G) can survive, differentiate, and proliferate only when their appropriate growth factors are present. The survival of HSCs in culture is suppressed by various cytokines and stimuli. The development of human mast cells is also downregulated by the HSC-inhibitory mechanisms because it requires a longer period compared with other cell lineages.

whereas GM-CSF supports the proliferation of differentiated myeloid progenitors but suppresses the expression of SCL in hemopoietic stem cells (*1*). IL-6 family cytokines such as IL-11 and leukemia inhibitory factor (LIF) are also capable of supporting the survival of hemopoietic stem cells by upregulating the expression of STAT-3 via gp130 signaling molecule. The IL-6 family-induced expression of STAT-3 is suppressed by suppressor of cytokine signaling (SOCS)-1 (*2*) and SOCS-3 (*3*), which are induced by various cytokines, such as IL-4 and GM-CSF, and pathogen-associated molecular patterns (PAMPs), such as lipopolysaccharide *(4)*. Therefore, the contamination of these cytokines and PAMPs in the culture system, and the culture conditions supporting the production of these cytokines, such as crowding culture with the cytokine-producing cells *(5)*, all suppresses the self-renewing mechanism of hemopoietic stem cells.

SCF also supports the survival and activation of human mast cells. However, mature mast cells do not rapidly proliferate, even in the presence of SCF. However, SCF can support the development and proliferation of mast cells from immature hemopoietic progenitors. Therefore, proliferation of mast cells is mostly caused by the proliferation of immature progenitors. Indeed, human mast cells require a much longer period for their development compared with other cell lineages. It has been previously reported that the combination of SCF and IL-6, the inhibition of the endogenous GM-CSF by prostaglandin E2 *(6)*, the purification of CD34$^+$ hemopoietic cells, and serum-free culture condition *(7)* all support the proliferation of human mast cells from hemopoietic stem cells. However, a good batch of fetal calf serum (FCS) or a good CO_2 incubator (serum-deprived culture is highly sensitive to CO_2 concentration change) is required in these culture conditions and sometimes may limit the reproducibility of these experiments outside in the laboratories.

This chapter introduces the method of forming human mast cell colonies by culturing purified cord blood cells and peripheral blood cells in serum-free methylcellulose supplemented with SCF and IL-6 and by laying the fresh methylcellulose medium every 14 d as has been reported *(8–10)*. Most mast cell progenitors are capable of producing other cell types before 4 wk. However, they become pure colonies consisting only of mast cells after 6 wk of culture. Mast cells can be retrieved by dissolving methylcellulose and transferred into liquid medium.

2. Materials
2.1. Preparation for Methylcellulose Culture

1. Silica (silicon gel; Immuno Biological Laboratories, Fujioka, Japan).
2. Lymphocyte Separation Medium (Organon Teknika Corp. Durham, NC).
3. Magnetic separation column (MACS II, cat. no. 441-01, Miltenyi Biotec, Bergisch Gladbach, Germany).
4. CD4, CD8, CD11b, CD14, and CD19-conjugated MACS beads (Miltenyi Biotec).
5. CD34$^+$ cell isolation kit (Miltenyi Biotec; *see* **Note 1**).
6. Iscove's modified Dulbecco's medium (IMDM; GIBCO, cat. no. 12440-053, Invitrogen Co., Carlsbad, CA).
7. Insulin-Transferrin-Selenium supplement (GIBCO, 41400-045).
8. 2-mercaptoethanol (GIBCO, 21985-023).

9. Penicillin + streptomycin supplement (GIBCO, 15140-122).
10. Bovine serum albumin (BSA; A-8919 Endotoxin-free grade, Sigma, St. Louis, MO).
11. Serum-free Iscove's methylcellulose medium (MethoCult™ SFBIT H4236; Stem Cell Technologies Inc. Vancouver, BC, Canada; *see* **Notes 1** and **2**).
12. 24-well plates (Iwaki Glass, Tokyo, Japan).

2.2. Cytokines

1. SCF (Recombinant Human SCF, PeproTech EC Ltd., London, UK, cat. no. 300-07, size C = 1 mg).
2. IL-6 (Recombinant Human IL-6, PeproTech EC Ltd., cat no. 300-07, size C = 1 mg).
3. IL-3 (Recombinant Human IL-3, R&D Systems, Minneapolis, MN, cat. no. 203-IL-010/CF, carrier-free).
4. GM-CSF (Recombinant Human GM-CSF, R&D Systems, cat. no. 215-GM-005/CF, carrier-free).
5. IL-4 (Recombinant Human IL-4, R&D Systems, cat. no. 204-IL-005/CF, carrier-free).

3. Methods

3.1. Mast Cell Culture in Methylcellulose

1. Umbilical cord blood or peripheral blood was drawn into heparinized syringes and was incubated with 1/10 vol of Silica (silicon gel; Immuno Biological Laboratories) for 30 min at 37°C. Nonphagocytic mononuclear cells (MNCs) were separated by density-gradient centrifugation using lymphocyte separation medium. Because phagocytic monocytes affect the differentiation of hemopoietic stem cells *(2)* by releasing a variety of cytokines and mediators and by adherence, the separation should be finished within 24 h and the samples should be kept at 0°C.
2. Lineage-negative mononuclear cells (lin-MNCs) were selected from the peripheral blood mononuclear cells (*see* **Note 3**) using a magnetic separation column and a mixture of magnetic microbeads-conjugated antibodies against CD4, CD8, CD11b, CD14, and CD19 according to the manufacturer's instructions. CD34$^+$ cells were positively selected from cord blood mononuclear cells using CD34$^+$ cell isolation kit. The frequency of CD34$^+$ cells from peripheral blood is very low (<0.01%). Thus, positive selection of peripheral blood CD34$^+$ cells is not efficient.
3. The lin-MNCs (usually 10^6) obtained from 10 mL of adult peripheral blood or 100 CD34$^+$ cord blood cells were suspended in 0.3 mL of Iscove's modified Dulbecco's medium supplemented with 1% Insulin-Transferrin-Selenium, 5 × 10^{-5}M 2-ME, 1% penicillin + streptomycin and 0.1% BSA. The cells were mixed well with 2.4 mL of serum-free Iscove's methylcellulose medium and 0.3-mL solutions containing adequate concentrations of SCF, IL-6, and IL-3 (*see* **Note 4**). The cell suspension was inoculated at 0.3 mL per well in the 24-well plates at 37°C in 5% CO_2. Every 10–14 d, 0.3 mL of fresh methylcellulose medium containing SCF + IL-6 without cells were layered over the methylcellulose cultures (*see* **Note 5**).

4. After 6 wk of culture, the methylcellulose was dissolved in phosphate-buffered saline and the cells were resuspended and cultured with IMDM containing cytokines with 2% FCS (*see* **Notes 6** and **7**).

3.2. Effect of IL-3 and GM-CSF on Mast Cell Development in the Presence of SCF and IL-6

IL-3 and GM-CSF have strong homology in their amino acid sequences and share the common receptor β-chain CD131. GM-CSF inhibits the mast cell development both in mouse *(11)* and human systems *(6)*, whereas the effect of IL-3 on the human mast cell development is still controversial. IL-3 is not required for the development of cord blood-derived mast cells in the presence of oxygen at a low concentration *(7)*. However, IL-3 enhances the SCF-dependent development of mast cells at low cell densities such as in methylcellulose with normal oxygen concentrations *(8–10)*. In the presence of SCF and IL-6, cord blood CD34$^+$ cells gave rise to pure mast cell colonies after 6 wk of culture **(Fig. 2A)**. The addition of IL-3 or GM-CSF enhanced the mast cell colony formation in a concentration-dependent manner. IL-3 at 1 ng/mL enhanced the mast cell colony growth without inducing granulocyte and macrophage (GM) colonies **(Fig. 2B)**. IL-3 at the concentrations higher than 5 ng/mL and GM-CSF at the concentrations higher than 0.1 ng/ml induced a substantial number of GM colonies **(Fig. 3)**. Macrophages present in culture suppress further mast cell proliferation. Thus, we recommend adding IL-3 at 1 ng/mL only, at the beginning of culture, in addition to SCF and IL-6. Continuous addition of IL-3 at higher concentrations should be avoided because IL-3 may support the growth of other cell lineages and thus suppress further mast cell development.

3.3. Mast Cell Development From Different Progenitor Samples

Using standard conditions, 10^3 human CD34$^+$ cord blood (10^6 cells were usually retrieved from 10 mL of cord blood) progenitors gave rise to 100 mast cell colonies consisting of 15,000 cells per colony on average after 6 wk. Adult peripheral blood contains approx 2–100 mast cell progenitors/mL. A single adult peripheral blood progenitor gives rise to 800 mast cells per colony on average. Adult peripheral progenitor-derived mast cells express far more abundant FcεRI α-chain and release far higher levels of mediators and cytokines after receptor crosslinking compared with neonatal cord blood progenitor-derived mast cells cultured under the same culture conditions *(12)*.

Peripheral blood progenitors derived from the patients with severe allergic diseases can give rise to more eosinophil-basophil colonies **(Fig. 2C)** than those derived from normal donors. However, the number of mast cell colonies is not significantly changed in such allergic patients *(13)*. FcεRI expression and the

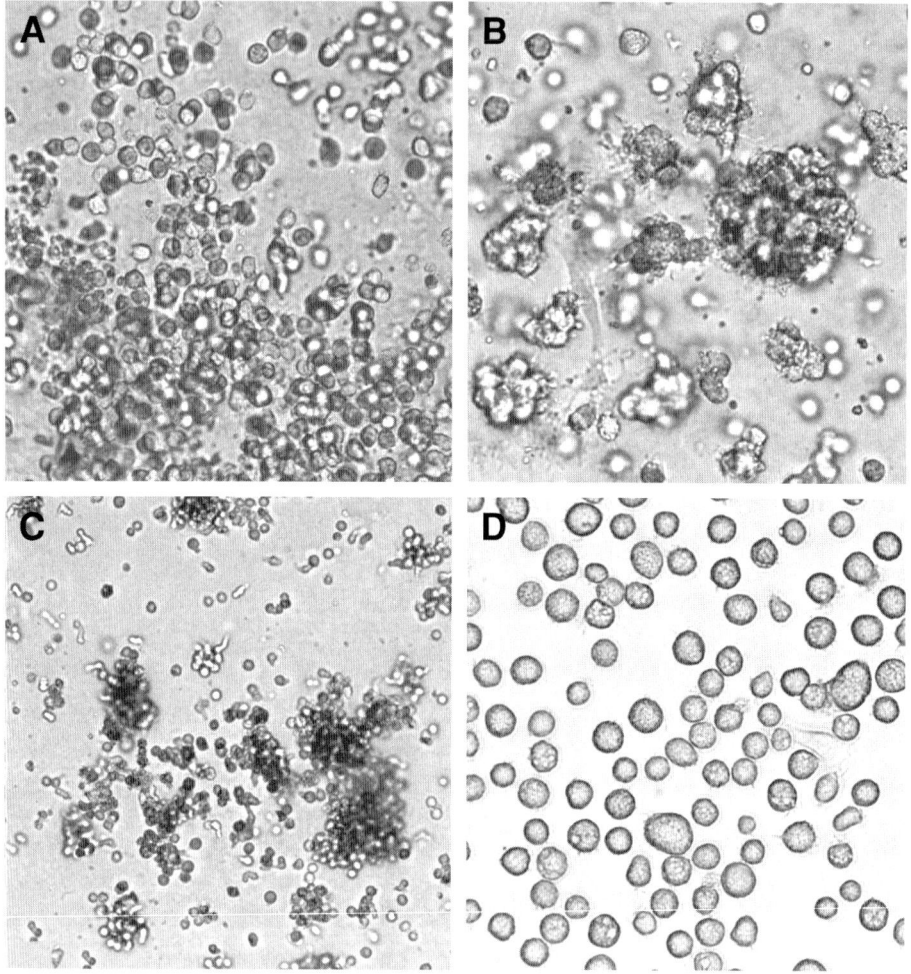

Fig. 2. **(A)** A part of a typical mast cell colony grown at 6 wk of culture from an adult peripheral blood progenitor. Note the retractile nature of round cells. **(B)** A typical GM macrophage colony grown at 4 wk of culture. Note the heterogeneously sized cells with irregular processes. **(C)** A part of a mixed eosinophil basophil colony. Dark compact cell clusters consist of eosinophils, and dispersed long narrow cells are basophils. **(D)** Mast cells in liquid medium at 10 wk of culture. It should be noted these cells were photographed at the same magnification using an objective ×20 lens.

related functions of mast cells derived from the allergic patients were also similar with those from normal volunteers in our study *(13)*. These mast cell functions are profoundly upregulated by the addition of IL-4 into the culture *(14)*.

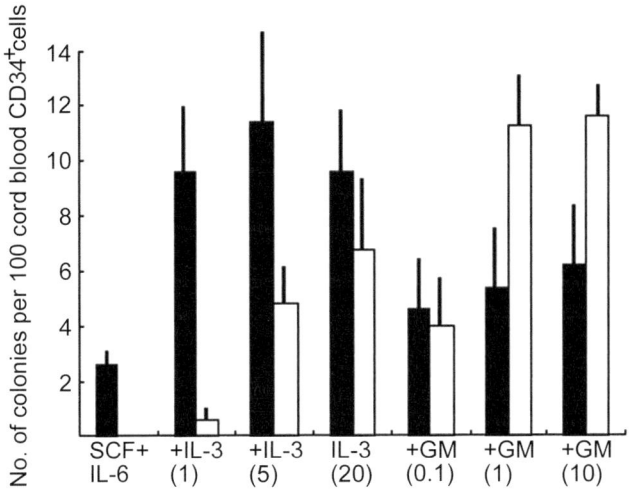

Fig. 3. The number of pure mast cell colonies (closed column and a bar represent the mean +SEM) and mixed mast cell-macrophage colonies (open column and a bar represent the mean +SEM) at 6 wk of culture are shown (when 100 CD34$^+$ cord blood cells were inoculated). (Reproduced with permission from **ref. *10*.**)

Nevertheless, mast cells in colonies can be retrieved by dissolving methylcellulose, and can be maintained in liquid IMDM for more than 6 mo **(Fig. 2D)**. This method is considered to be highly reproducible in every laboratory and should be useful for obtaining non-neoplastic, functional human mast cells.

4. Notes

1. Instead of the CD34$^+$ Isolation kit, the AC133 Isolation kit (Miltenyi Biotech) can be used for the purification of hemopoietic progenitors. Also, instead of IMDM supplemented with insulin, transferring, and selenium, other liquid media, such as Stem Span (Stem Cell Technologies) can be used. There is no reason to use FCS for the expansion of hemopoietic stem cells. However, the addition of FCS may increase the FcεRIα expression on cord blood-derived mast cells.
2. Although they may morphologically look mature **(Fig. 4)**, when cord blood-derived mast cells in serum-free medium almost lack FcεRI expression, the addition of FCS *(15)* or IL-4 *(14)* increases FcεRIα expression but suppresses the proliferation of mast cells derived from progenitors.
3. Peripheral blood progenitors derived from elderly people do not give rise to mast cell colonies, while they give rise to hemopoietic colonies consisting of myeloid and erythroid lineages. Thus, donors for peripheral mast cell progenitors are recommended to be less than 40 yr of age. Progenitors obtained from neonates (cord blood) and infants can create large mast cell colonies *(12,13)*.

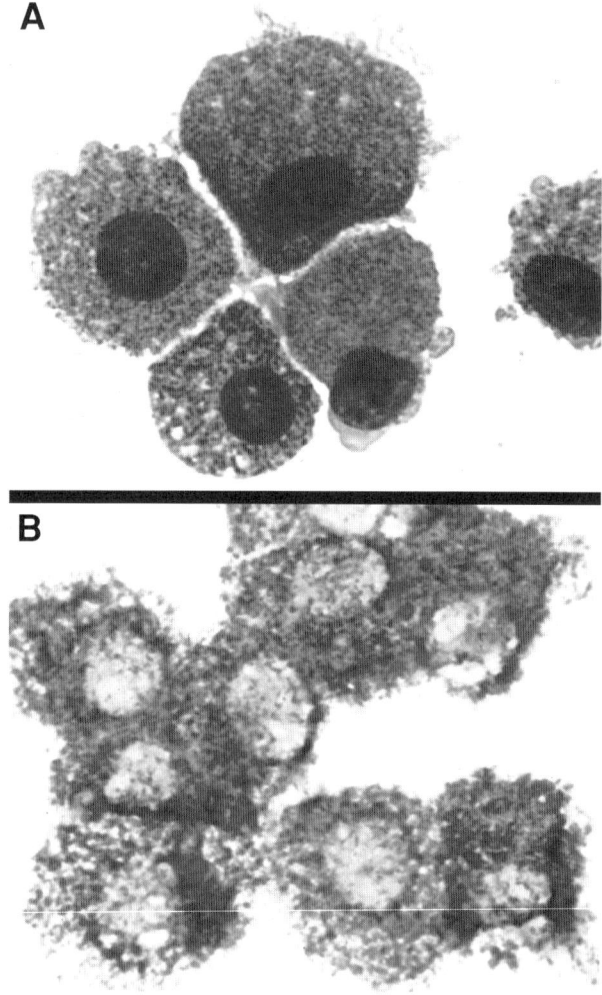

Fig. 4. **(A)** May–Grünwald Giemsa stain and **(B)** antichymase immunostaining of a typical cord blood-derived mast cell colony. Cord blood-derived CD34 ⁺cells were cultured in methylcellulose for 6 wk and further cultured with SCF, IL-6, and IL-4 for 4 wk (magnification ×60)

4. Plating more than 10^3 CD34⁺ cells or 10^6 lin-MNCs per 3 mL of methylcellulose medium at the beginning of culture may result in logarithmic increase in macrophage colonies secreting various cytokines such as GM-CSF in an autocrine manner. It also may result in a profound loss of mast cell colonies.

5. Before 4 wk of culture, agitation of methylcellulose medium may result in profound growth of adherent macrophages on the culture plate bottom and may sup-

press the growth of mast cells. Fresh methylcellulose medium should be softly layered over the old medium.

6. After 15 wk of culture, the addition of FCS or IL-4 do not induce further expression of FcεRIα or chymase messenger ribonucleic acid (mRNA) in cord blood-derived mast cells.

7. After terminal maturation (after 20 wk of culture), mast cells lose some granular compound-related mRNA, such as histidine decarboxylase and chymase. However, they can survive in this state for years without proliferation.

Acknowledgments

This work was supported in part by grants from the RIKEN Yokohama Institute and the Organization for Pharmaceutical Safety and Research of the Ministry of Health, Labour and Welfare (Millennium Genome Project, MPJ-5).

References

1. Caceres-Cortes, J. R., Krosl, G., Tessier, N., Hugo, P., and Hoang, T. (2001) Steel factor sustains SCL expression and the survival of purified CD34+ bone marrow cells in the absence of detectable cell differentiation. *Stem Cells* **19,** 59–70.
2. Magrangeas, F., Boisteau, O., Denis, S., Jacques, Y., and Minvielle, S. (2001) Negative cross-talk between interleukin-3 and interleukin-11 is mediated by suppressor of cytokine signalling-3 (SOCS-3). *Biochem. J.* **353,** 223–230.
3. Schuringa, J. J., van der Schaaf, S., Vellenga, E., Eggen, B. J., and Kruijer, W. (2002) LIF-induced STAT3 signaling in murine versus human embryonal carcinoma (EC) cells. *Exp. Cell Res.* **274,** 119–129.
4. Fujimoto, M. and Naka, T. (2003) Regulation of cytokine signaling by SOCS family molecules. *Trends Immunol.* **24,** 659–666.
5. Metcalf, D., Di Rago, L., and Mifsud, S. (2003) Crowding-dependent production of colony-stimulating factors by cultured syngeneic or allogeneic hematopoietic cells. *Proc. Natl. Acad. Sci. USA* **100,** 1244–1249.
6. Saito, H., Ebisawa, M., Tachimoto, H., et al. (1996) Selective growth of human mast cells induced by Steel factor, interleukin 6 and prostaglandin E$_2$ from cord blood mononuclear cells. *J. Immunol.* **157,** 343–350.
7. Kinoshita, T., Sawai, N., Hidaka, E., Yamashita, T., and Koike, K. (1999) Interleukin-6 directly modulates steel factor-dependent development of human mast cells derived from CD34+ cord blood cells. *Blood* **94,** 496–508.
8. Kempuraj, D., Saito, H., Kaneko, A., et al. (1999) Characterization of mast cell-committed progenitors present in human umbilical cord blood. *Blood* **93,** 3338–3346.
9. Ahn, K., Takai, S., Pawankar, R., et al. (2000) Regulation of chymase production in human mast cell progenitors. *J. Allergy Clin. Immunol.* **106,** 321–328.
10. Saito, H., Kempuraj, D., Tomikawa, M., Tomita, H., Ahn, K., and Iikura, Y. (2001) Human mast cell colony-forming cells in culture. *Int. Arch. Allergy Immunol.* **124,** 301–303.

11. Bressler, R. B., Thompson, H. L., Keffer, J. M., and Metcalfe, D. D. (1989) Inhibition of the growth of IL-3-dependent mast cells from murine bone marrow by recombinant granulocyte macrophage-colony-stimulating factor. *J. Immunol.* **143,** 135–139.

12. Iida, M., Matsumoto, K., Tomita, H., et al. (2001) Selective down-regulation of high-affinity IgE receptor (FcεRI) α-chain messenger RNA among transcriptome in cord blood-derived versus adult peripheral blood-derived cultured human mast cells. *Blood* **97,** 1016–1022.

13. Nomura, I., Katsunuma, T., Matsumoto, K., et al. (2001) Human mast cell progenitors in peripheral blood from atopic subjects with high IgE levels. *Clin. Exp. Allergy* **31,** 1424–1431.

14. Tachimoto, H., Ebisawa, M., Hasegawa, T., et al. (2000) Reciprocal regulation of cultured human mast cell cytokine production by IL-4 and IFN-γ. *J. Allergy Clin. Immunol.* **106,** 141–149.

15. Dahl, C., Saito, H., Nielsen, H. V., and Schiotz, P. O. (2002) The establishment of a combined serum-free and serum-supplemented culture method of obtaining functional cord blood-derived human mast cells. *J. Immunol. Methods* **262,** 137–143.

10

Isolation, Culture, and Characterization of Intestinal Mast Cells

Gernot Sellge and Stephan C. Bischoff

Summary

Mast cells are bone-marrow-derived tissue cells typically located at barrier sites of the body, such as skin, mucosal barriers, or blood barriers, that is, around blood vessels. This location suggests that mast cells might have a function as immunological "gate-keepers" or "watch dogs" and, indeed, some recent functional data support this idea. Mast cells derive from myeloid progenitors, but in contrast to other myeloid cells, they leave the bone marrow in an immature state; therefore, mast cells are not found in the blood under normal conditions. For full maturation, the tissue environment is necessary. Thus, mature mast cells can be only isolated from tissue such as skin or mucosal sites, which makes mast cell isolation rather complicated. Alternatively, mast cell progenitors can be isolated from the bone marrow, peripheral blood, or cord blood, which is easier but requires subsequent in vitro maturation of mast cells as far as possible using cytokines. This chapter describes a rather new technique of mast cell isolation from human intestinal mucosal tissue yielding approx 1–5 million pure and viable human mast cells suitable to perform functional and cell culture experiments.

Key Words: Mast cells; human; intestinal; gut, bowel; innate immunity; isolation; enzymes; mediator release assay; culture; food allergy; inflammatory bowel disease.

1. Introduction

Unlike other immune effector cells, mature mast cells are only found in the tissue, not in the blood. Preferentially, mast cells are located at sites of the host–environment interface, such as the skin and the mucosa of the respiratory, gastrointestinal, and urogenital tract. The normal human gastrointestinal tract contains numerous mast cells. The largest number are found in the lamina propria, where 2–3% of the cells are mast cells. Most of such mast cells belong to the tryptase positive, chymase negative subtype (MC_T), resembling the mucosal

From: *Methods in Molecular Biology, vol. 315: Mast Cells: Methods and Protocols*
Edited by: G. Krishnaswamy and D. S. Chi © Humana Press Inc., Totowa, NJ

mast cell subtype in rodents. In the submucosa, mast cell density is lower compared with the lamina propria (approx 1% of all cells) and, instead, the frequency of the tryptase, chymase double positive mast cell subtype (MC_{TC}), corresponding to the connective tissue mast cells subtype in rodents, is higher than that of the MC_T subtype *(1–3)*. Mast cells originate from immature, bone marrow-derived CD34+ hematopoietic stem cells circulating in the peripheral blood as committed progenitors before homing *(2,4)*. In mice, the crucial role of α4β7 integrin expressed on mast cell precursors and the mucosal address in cell adhesion molecule (MAdCAM)-1 expressed on high endothelial venules in the intestinal lamina propria for the gut homing of mast cell precursors recently have been demonstrated *(5)*. In humans, the regulation of this process and the stage of maturation at which mast cells migrate from the blood into the tissue remain largely unknown. Electron-microscopic studies revealed that mast cell progenitors are not only found in peripheral blood but also in tissue such as the intestine, where they represent 5–15% of total mast cell numbers *(6)*. This suggests that mast cell densities in the intestine are regulated by the influx of early mast cell progenitors and the growth factor-dependent survival and proliferation of late progenitors or even mature mast cells within the tissue. The capacity of mast cells to release proinflammatory and immunoregulatory mediators led to the speculation that they are involved in gastrointestinal pathologies, such as intestinal allergy, celiac disease, and inflammatory bowel disease (IBD). In patients with IBD, the numbers of intestinal mast cell are increased. They account for 60 and 30% of all mucosal cells that were immunoreative for tumor necrosis factor (TNF)-α and interleukin (IL)-5, respectively *(3,7–9)*. In addition, in vitro studies with mast cells isolated from intestinal tissue demonstrated increased release of histamine and eicosanoids in mast cells derived from patients with IBD compared with control patients *(10)*. Such data support the hypothesis that the mast cells were primed or preactivated by the local inflammatory tissue environment.

We have established methods for the isolation, purification, and culture of human intestinal mast cells, providing a unique source of tissue-derived human mast cells. Similar methods have been used by us and by others for the isolation of human mast cell from other organs such as the lung, the skin, or the nasal mucosa *(11–14)*. The following protocols describe the isolation of cells from the human intestinal mucosa by a combination of mechanical fragmentation and enzymatic digestion, the purification of mast cells by magnetic cell sorting, and the culture of mast cells. Using these protocols, as much as 100% of pure tissue mast cells can be obtained *(15,16)*. Furthermore, we describe methods for the characterization of effector functions of human intestinal mast cell with the focus on cytokine production and mediator release.

2. Materials

2.1. Cell Isolation

1. Shaking water bath (37°C).
2. Tyrode buffer: 137 mM NaCl, 2.7 mM KCl, 0.36 mM Na$_2$HPO$_4$, 5.55 mM glucose, adjust to pH 7.4, and store at 4°C.
3. Tissue storage buffer: tyrode buffer, ampicillin 0.5 mg/mL (Ratiopharm), gentamycin 0.2 mg/mL (Gibco), and metronidazol 0.2 mg/mL (Baxter); store at 4°C.
4. TE buffer: Tyrode buffer containing 2 mM ethylene diamine tetraacetic acid (EDTA); store at 4°C.
5. TGMD buffer: tyrode buffer supplemented with gelatin (1 mg/mL, Sigma, cat no. G-9391), 1.23 mM MgCl$_2$, and 15 µg/mL DNAse (Boehringer, cat. no. 1284932); make fresh as required.
6. Enzyme solution PCh: 50 mL of TE buffer, 150 mg of Pronase (Boehringer, cat. no. 1459643), and 21 mg of chymopapain (Sigma, cat. no. S-8526); make fresh as required.
7. Enzyme solution Co: 50 mL of TGMD-buffer, 75 mg of collagenase D (Boehringer, cat. no. 1088882); make fresh as required.
8. RPMI 1640 with phenol red, Glutamax, and 25 mM HEPES (Gibco, cat. no. 32404-014).
9. Culture medium: RPMI 1640 supplemented with 10% (v/v) heat inactivated fetal calf serum (e.g., Biochrom), 100 µg/mL streptomycin, 100 µg/mL gentamycin, 100 U/mL penicillin, and 0.5 µg/mL amphotericin (all antibiotics from Gibco)
10. Trypan blue (Sigma, cat. no. T-8154).
11. May-Grünwald Giemsa stain (Merck, cat. no. 1014250500).
12. Giemsa (Azur-Eosin-Methylenblau; Riedel-de-Haen, cat. no. 32884).
13. Tweezers and scissors, kept in sterile beaker with 70% ethanol.
14. Bottle-top filter (Becton Dickinson, cat. no. 7105).
15. Nylon mesh, pore size 250 and 100 µm (Omnilab, cat. nos. 4-250 and 4-100).
16. 50-mL conical tubes (Falcon, cat. no. 2070).
17. *N*-Acethyl-L-cystein (Sigma, cat. no. A7250).

2.2. Purification of Intestinal Mast Cells

1. 80-cm^2 or 175-cm^2 cell culture flask (e.g., Nunc).
2. Plastic cell scraper (Biochrom, cat. no. 9903).
3. HEPES buffer: 20 mM HEPES (Sigma, cat. no. H-9136), 125 mM NaCl, 5 mM KCl, 0.5 mM glucose, adjust to pH 7.4, store at 4°C.
4. HA buffer: HEPES buffer containing 1 mg/mL bovine serum albumin (Boehringer, cat. no. 775827); make fresh as required.
5. MACS buffer: HA buffer, 2 mM EDTA; make fresh as required.
6. Antihuman CD117 (monoclonal anitbody [MAb] YB5.B8, BD Bioscience, cat. no. 555713) directed against human *c-kit*.

7. Goat anti-mouse IgG antibody coupled to paramagnetic beads (Miltenyi Biotech, cat. no. 130-048-401).
8. MACS LS columns (Miltenyi, cat. no. 130-042-401).
9. MidiMACS Separation Unit (Miltenyi, cat. no. 130-042-302).
10. MACS Multi Stand (Miltenyi, cat. no. 130-042-303).
11. Nylon mesh, pore size 30 μm (Omnilab, cat. no. 4-30).
12. Trypan blue, May-Grünwald stain, Giemsa, Bottle-top filter, 50-mL conical tubes, culture medium (*see* **Subheading 2.1.**).

2.3. Culture of Intestinal Mast Cells

1. CO_2 incubator.
2. Human recombinant stem cell factor (SCF; provided by Amgen).
3. IL-4 (provided by Novartis Research Institute).
4. Other growth factors as required (e.g., IL-3).
5. 6-, 12-, 24-, 48-, or 96-well flat-bottom plates (e.g., Nunc).
6. Trypan blue, May-Grünwald stain, Giemsa, culture medium (*see* **Subheading 2.1.**), plastic cell scraper (*see* **Subheading 2.2.**).

2.4. Mediator Release

1. Shaking water bath (37°C).
2. Sonicater.
3. MAb 22E7 (provided by Hoffmann-La Roche) directed against a non-IgE binding epitope of the high affinity IgE receptor chain.
4. HACM-buffer: HA-buffer (*see* **Subheading 2.1.**), 1 mM $CaCl_2$, 1 mM $MgCl_2$, store at 4°C.
5. Cytokine enzyme-linked immunosorbent assay (ELISA, e.g., R&D, Biosource).
6. Histamine radioimmunoassay (Coulter Immunotech, cat. no. IM2588).
7. Sulfidoleukotriene (sLT) ($LTC_4/D_4/E_4$) RIA (Biotrend, cat. no. 900070).
8. Prostaglandin D_2 (PGD_2) ELISA (Cayman Chemical, cat. no. 512011).
9. HA-buffer (*see* **Subheading 2.3.**).

3. Methods

3.1. Isolation of Cells From the Intestinal Mucosa

For the isolation of cells from the human intestinal mucosa we use the modified four-step enzymatic tissue dispersion method originally described by Schulman et al. *(17)*. Other investigators have succeeded in isolating intestinal cells using simpler methods *(13,18)*. In our hands, the method described here is slightly superior in terms of cell yield, mast cell percentage, and cell integrity.

1. Obtain intestinal tissue from surgical specimens of patients who underwent bowel resection (*see* **Note 1**).
2. Wash specimen with water and remove adherent mesentery and fat from tissue using tweezers and scissors. Place specimen immediately in tissue storage buffer (*see* **Note 2**).

3. Separate mucosa from the submucosa/muscular layer using tweezers and scissors. Discard submucosa/muscularis.

4. Place mucosa in 50-mL Falcon tube containing 30 mL of TE buffer and agitate gently to remove mucus. Transfer mucosa in a 50-mL Falcon tube containing 30–40 mL of TE buffer + 1 mg/mL *N*-acethyl-L-cystein. Incubate for 10 min in a shaking water bath at 37°C. After incubation, agitate tube gently to remove mucus. Repeat **step 4** if mucus is not adequately removed.

5. Transfer mucosa in a 50-mL Falcon tube containing 30–40 mL of Tyrode buffer + 5 m*M* EDTA. Incubate for 20 min in a shaking water bath at 37°C. After incubation, agitate tube gently to remove epithelial cells and residual mucus.

6. Place tissue in a plastic Petri dish containing 20 mL of enzyme solution PCh and cut with scissors into 1-mm^3 pieces.

7. Place tissue suspension on a bottle top filter containing nylon mesh with a pore size of 250 µm. Wash with 50 mL of TE buffer (*see* **Note 3**). Discard filtrate. Close the bottle top filter with the stopper.

8. Suspend tissue in 30 mL of enzyme solution PCh and transfer suspension in a 50-mL Falcon tube. Incubate 30 min in a shaking water bath at 37°C. Filter as in **step 7** and wash with 50 mL of TGMD buffer. Discard filtrate.

9. Suspend tissue in 25 mL of enzyme solution Co and transfer suspension in a 50-mL Falcon tube. Incubate 30 min in a shaking water bath at 37°C. Filter as in **step 7** and wash with 25 mL of TGMD buffer. Centrifuge filtrate (300*g*, 10 min), remove supernatant, resuspend cells in 1–2 mL of cell culture medium, and place at 4°C.

10. Repeat **step 9**.

11. Pool cells collected in **steps 9** and **10**, resuspend in 20 mL of RPMI, and filtrate through a bottle top filter containing nylon mesh with a pore size of 100 µm. Wash with 30 mL of RPMI. Centrifuge (300*g*, 10 min) and resuspend in 10 mL of culture medium.

12. Count the cells after staining with trypan blue. Prepare cytocentrifuge smears and stain with May–Grünwald/Giemsa to perform a differential count (*see* **Note 4, Fig. 1**).

3.2. Enrichment of Intestinal Mast Cells by Positive Selection Using Magnetic Cell Sorting

Enrichment of human intestinal mast cells can be performed by using magnetic cell sorting (MACS). In general, mast cells are 50–75% pure after positive sorting by immunomagnetic labeling of *c-kit* (*15,16*). In some cell preparations, the purity can be greater than 90%. Further purification, as much as 100%, is possible by culture of the cells (*see* **Subheading 3.3.**).

Although this method is a powerful tool for the enrichment of human intestinal mast cells it has also some limitations: (1) recovery of the mast cells is low (30–50%); (2) the positive fraction containing the mast cells frequently are contaminated with high amounts of dead cells and cell debris that

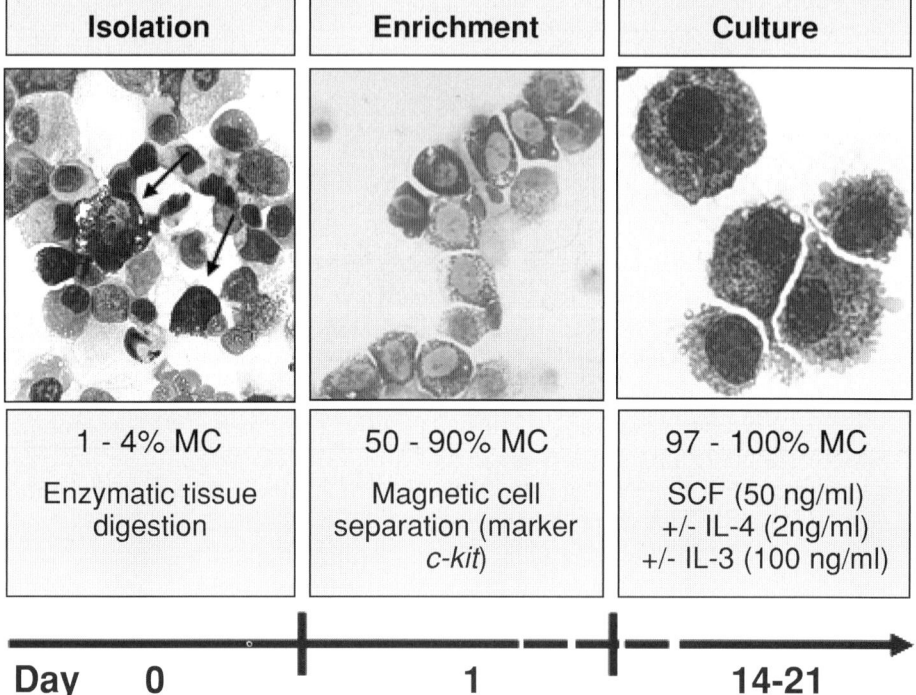

Fig. 1. May–Grünwald/Giemsa stain of cell fractions obtained after cell isolation (arrows, mast cells), MACS enrichment, and culture for 14 d in the presence of SCF (50 ng/mL).

nonspecifically bind to the magnetic beads; and (3) the functional response to physiological activators and the culture sufficiency is diminished directly after MACS purification but can be restored after culture *(15,16)*.

Purification of mast cells can be achieved also by long-term culture of nonenriched cell fractions *(19)*. This approach has the advantage of higher cell numbers and a better culture sufficiency. The disadvantages are that the purity is often poor and the required culture period quite long. This issue will be discussed in detail in the following section.

MACS is the method of choice for the purification of mast cells if long-term culture needs to be avoided.

1. Culture freshly isolated intestinal cells at 4×10^6/mL in culture medium overnight in 75-cm^2 (up to 1.2×10^8 cells) or 150-cm^2 (up to 2.5×10^8 cells) tissue culture flasks (*see* **Note 5**).
2. Harvest cells by gently scraping with a plastic cell scraper (*see* **Note 6**). Count after staining with trypan blue (*see* **Note 7**).

3. To remove clumps, pass cells through a 30-μm filter. Centrifuge cells ($300g$, 10 min, 4°C) and remove supernatant. Keep cells cold during the following steps (use cold solutions, centrifugation at 4°C, and so on).

4. Resuspend cells in MACS buffer ($200 \mu L/10^8$ cells). For fewer cells, use $200 \mu L$. Add MAb YB5.B8 ($1.25 \mu g/10^8$ cells), mix well, and incubate for 15–20 min in a refrigerator at 4–10°C.

5. Wash cells with 10–20 mL of MACS buffer, remove supernatant, and resuspend in MACS buffer ($200 \mu L/10^8$ cells) again. For fewer cells, use $200 \mu L$. Add MAb Goat Anti-Mouse IgG MicroBeads ($1.25 \mu g/10^8$ cells), mix well, and incubate for 15 min at 4–10°C (*see* **Note 8**).

6. Wash cells with 10–20 mL of MACS buffer, remove supernatant, and resuspend in 5 mL of MACS buffer/10^8 cells. For fewer cells, use 5 mL.

7. Place a positive selection column type LS+ in the magnetic field of an appropriate MACS separator (located in a 4°C room). Wash with 5 mL of HA buffer according to the manufacturer's instructions. Discard eluate.

8. Transfer as many as 10^8 cells to the top of the MACS column (*see* **Note 9**). Once the cell suspension has completely entered start washing of the column with at least 10 mL MACS buffer. Collect the effluent in a 50-mL Falcon tube (mast cell-depleted fraction).

9. Remove MACS column from the separator. Fill column with MACS buffer (as much as 7 mL), firmly flush out the positive fraction using the supplied plunger and collect cells in an appropriate tube.

10. Centrifuge cells and resuspend in culture medium. Count the cells after staining with trypan blue. Prepare cytocentrifuge smears and stain with May–Grünwald/ Giemsa to perform a differential count (*see* **Note 10**).

3.3. Culture of Intestinal Mast Cells

In the absence of growth factors, MACS-enriched mast cells die completely within 3–7 d. Mast cell survival is slightly prolonged if nonenriched cell fractions are cultured, which is related to growth factors provided by contaminating cells. Long-term culture of human intestinal mast cells can be achieved in the presence of recombinant SCF preventing mast cell apoptosis and inducing proliferation *(15,19)*. Additional factors such as IL-3 and IL-4 enhance mast cell growth in the presence of SCF by decreasing apoptosis (IL-3) or increasing proliferation (IL-4, **Fig. 2** and **Table 1**). In the absence of SCF, IL-4 has no effect and IL-3 has only a minimal effect on mast cell survival. The addition of IL-3, IL-4 or IL-3 + IL-4 to the culture medium in combination with SCF can enhance mast cell numbers after 2–3 wk of culture approximately two-, three-, or fourfold, respectively, in comparison with mast cells cultured with SCF alone *(16,20)*.

The purity of mast cells largely increases during culture. If mast cells were enriched by MACS before culture, purity is generally 85–95% after 1 wk and 95–100% after 2 wk of culture *(15)*. If nonenriched cell fractions were cultured

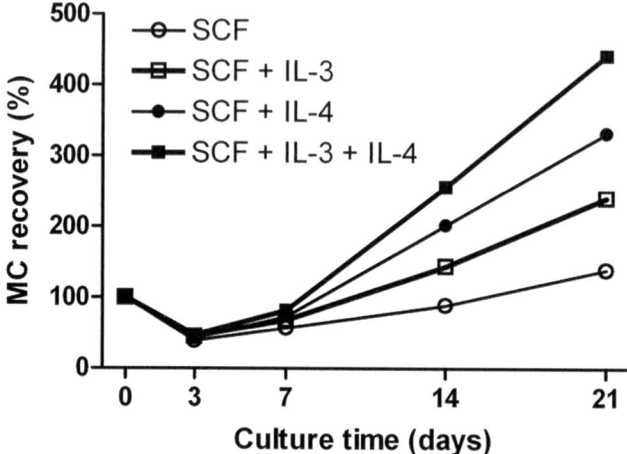

Fig. 2. Mast cell recovery after culture of MACS-enriched human intestinal mast cells. Mast cells were cultured for indicated times in the presence of SCF (50 ng/mL), SCF + IL-3 (100 ng/mL), SCF + IL-4 (2 ng/mL), or SCF + IL-4 + IL-3.

Table 1
Effects of IL-3, IL-4, and TGF-β on Human Intestinal Mast Cells

Cytokine	IL-3	IL-4	TGF-β
Mast cell numbers			
after 21 d of culture[a]	150–250%	200–400%	20–50%
Proliferation[a]	↔	↑	↓
Apoptosis[a]	↓	↔	↑
Histamine[a,b]	↑	↑	↓
$LTC_4/D_4/E_4$[a,b]	↑	↑	↓
PGD_2[a,b]	↔	↔	↑
TNF-α[a,b]	n.t.[d]	↔	↓
IL-6[a,b]	n.t.[d]	↓	n.t.[d]
IL-3, IL-5, IL-13[a,b,c]	n.t.[d]	↑	↓
Ratio of MC_T/MC_{TC}[a]	n.t.[d]	↑	↓

[a] Phenotype of mast cells cultured in the presence of SCF alone is compared with the phenotype of mast cells cultured in the presence of SCF + the indicated cytokine.
[b] Mediator release upon FceRI-crosslinking.
[c] IL-4 induces small amounts of IL-5 even without further stimulation.
[d] Not tested.
PGD_2, prostaglandin D2; LT, leukotrienes; TNF-a, tumor necrosis factor alpha; IL, interleukin; MC, mast cell; T, tryptase; TC, tryptase + chymase; TGF-β, transforming growth factor β.

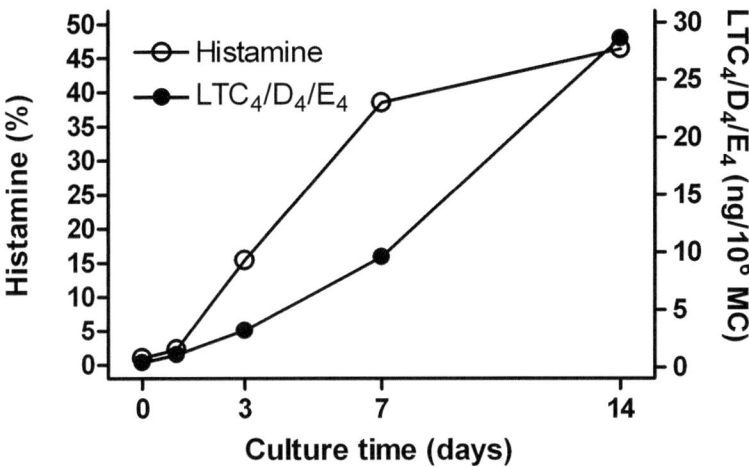

Fig. 3. Influence of culture on histamine and sLT ($LTC_4/D_4/E_4$) release after FcεRI-crosslinking. Mast cells were stimulated with for 30 min with the MAb 22E7 (100 ng/mL) directly after MACS purification or after 3, 7, or 14 d of culture in the presence of SCF (50 ng/mL). Specific histamine release as a percentage of total histamine (determined after cell lysis) is shown.

in the presence with SCF, mast cell survive selectively and highly purified mast cells can be obtained after 4–5 wk of culture. Although 95–100% pure mast cells can be obtained in some cultures, the purity often is poorer because of contaminating fibroblasts. In our hands, IL-4 does not induce the growth of intestinal lymphocytes and improve the purity of mast cells cultures used in combination with SCF (*see* **Notes 11** and **12**).

Cultured mast cells release much higher amounts of mediators in response to Fcε receptor I (FcεRI) crosslinking than freshly isolated mast cells (*see* **Subheading 3.4.** and **Fig. 3**), which is most likely related to the fact that the isolation and purification procedure causes a reversible damage of the cells that reduces their functional capacities. During culture, mast cells regain the full capacity to respond to FcεRI crosslinking. This suggests that cultured mast cells reflect more accurately the phenotype of mast cells in vivo than freshly isolated mast cells *(15,16,19)*.

Human intestinal mast cells also can be maintained in co-culture with human endothelial cells or human fibroblasts. Co-culture with endothelial cells requires direct cell contact. The survival and proliferation of intestinal mast cells are mediated by at least two pathways: (1) the interaction between transmembrane SCF expressed by endothelial cells and c-*kit* on mast cells; and (2) the interaction between the adhesion molecules and very late activation antigen-4, expressed by mast cells and vascular cell adhesion molecule-1 induced on endothelial cells in the presence of mast cells *(21)*. Human intestinal fibroblasts prevent mast cell apoptosis but do not induce proliferation. In contrast to findings with the rodent 3T3-fibroblast cell line, human intestinal fibroblasts mediate mast cell survival independent of SCF by a yet unknown soluble factor *(22)*. Both co-culture systems are useful in studying the interaction of mast cells with the respective cell type; however, they are insufficient techniques if one wishes to obtain high numbers of purified intestinal mast cells.

1. Culture mast cells in culture medium. Adjust the cell concentration to $1–2 \times 10^5$ mast cells/mL for MACS-enriched cells or to 2×10^6 of total cells/mL for unpurified cells. Culture of intestinal mast cells can be performed in 96-, 48-, 24-, 12-, or 6-well flat-bottomed plates in 0.2, 0.5, 1, 2, or 5 mL of cell culture medium, respectively.
2. Add SCF at a concentration of 50 ng/mL. If required add other cytokines (*see* **Table 1** and **Note 12**).
3. Maintain cells in a humidified atmosphere containing 5% CO_2 at 37°C.
4. Change 50% of the culture medium twice during the first week and then once a week thereafter. Add new growth factors each time.
5. Subculture cells if required (*see* **Note 13**).
6. After an appropriate culture period (*see* text above), harvest mast cells using a cell scraper. Count the cells after staining with trypan blue. Prepare cytocentrifuge smears and stain with May–Grünwald/Giemsa to perform a differential count.

We have been using standard assay for the analysis of proliferation (Ki-67, BrdU-, and ^{3}H-thymidin incorporation) and apoptosis (annexin V, caspase assays *[16,20,22]*). These assays are used frequently and they will not be described here. For all assays, use only mast cells that have been cultured for at least 4–7 d. Many mast cells die within the first days of culture because of damage caused by the isolation and MACS procedure (**Fig. 2**). Proliferation starts after approx 4 d *(16)*. Short-term effects can be assayed by using precultured mast cells.

3.4. Mediator Release and Cytokine Production in Human Intestinal Mast Cells

In the gut, mast cells produce histamine, neutral proteases, and eicosanoids mediating various functions such as smooth muscle contraction, leukocyte extravasation, ion and mucus secretion, and degradation of peptides. In addition, intestinal mast cells produce multiple cytokines and growth factors, such as TNF-α, IL-1β, IL-3, IL-5, IL-6, IL-8, IL-13, IL-16, IL-18, transforming growth factor (TGF)-β$_1$, basic fibroblast growth factor, and others *(10,13,18,20, 23)*. These findings emphasize their important role in immunoregulation, tissue homeostasis, host defense against infection, or fibrotic tissue transformation.

Crosslinking of cell surface-bound IgE by antigen or, experimentally, of IgE receptors by anti-IgE receptor antibodies, is the most potent and best characterized stimulus for mast cell activation *(2,10)*. In addition, several IgE-independent triggering agents act on human skin or rodent mast cells, such as C5a, substance P, vasoactive intestinal peptide, morphine, f-Met, compound 48/80, or chemokines *(2,13)*. However, using human intestinal mast cells freshly isolated from surgery specimens or cultured in the presence of SCF, we found no mediator release after challenge with these IgE-independent agonists, thus supporting the concept of MC heterogeneity at distinct anatomical locations and between different species *(10,24)*. So far, only a few IgE-independent triggers causing mediator release in human intestinal mast cells have been identified. SCF triggers histamine release and sLT production under certain conditions *(19)*, and IL-4 induces IL-5 production in mast cells cultured in medium supplemented with SCF *(16,23)*. *Escherichia coli*-producing a-hemolysin causes the release of histamine, sLT, and TNF-α *(9)*. Mediator release after IgE receptor-crosslinking in cultured human intestinal mast cells is altered depending on the presence of cytokines such as IL-4, IL-3, and TGF-β_1 in addition to SCF. IL-4 and IL-3 support the release of histamine and production of sLT but not PGD_2 in intestinal mast cells after activation *(16,20)*. Moreover, IL-4 profoundly alters the cytokine expression pattern in cultured human intestinal mast cells, leading to an increased production of Th2-like cytokines such as IL-3, IL-5, and IL-13 after IgE-dependent activation *(23)*.

For the study of mast cell mediator release and cytokine production in response to FcϵRI crosslinking, we have been using two different protocols. The first protocol describes a method for short time stimulation (up to 60 min) to study degranulation and the production of eicosanoids. The second protocol is useful to investigate the messenger ribonucleic acid (mRNA) transcription and protein production of cytokines and chemokines. The protocols have been optimized to use as small cell numbers as possible.

3.4.1. Short-Term Stimulation Assay for the Study of Degranulation and Eiconsanoid Production

1. Wash mast cells twice in HA buffer (*see* **Note 14**).
2. Resuspend mast cells in HACM buffer (200–1000 µL per condition as required, minimal cell concentration 2×10^4 mast cells/mL) and transfer them into appropriate tubes. Duplicates are recommended.
3. Prepare cell lysates for the detection of total histamine (*see* **Subheading 3.4.2**).
4. Incubate tubes in a shaking water bath at 37°C for 10 min without agonists.
5. Add trigger/agonist of interest (e.g., for FcϵRI crosslinking, MAb 22E7 100 ng/mL). Leave control untreated or add appropriate isotype control.
6. Stop reaction by placing the tubes in ice-cold water at the time point of interest (*see* **Note 15**).

7. Centrifuge cells (300g, 10 min, 4°C) and collect supernatants. Store aliquots at –80°C.
8. Measure mediators of interest in the supernatants (histamine, sLTs, PGD$_2$, cytokines, and so on). Dilution of samples might be required (in particular for histamine). Calculate histamine release as follows: specific histamine release (% of total histamine) = (histamine release induced by the triggering agent – spontaneous release in response to buffer/isotype control)/total histamine in cell lysates.

3.4.2. Preparation of Mast Cell Lysates

1. Place 100 µL of the cell suspension in an appropriate tube and add 100 µL of water.
2. Freeze cell suspension at –80°C.
3. Before determination of histamine, thaw suspension and sonicate for 3–5 min.
4. Centrifuge cell debris down and use supernatant for analysis.

3.4.3. Stimulation Assay for the Study of Cytokine Production

We use this protocol to study cytokine production in mast cells. Histamine and eicosanoid release can be studied with the same protocol. Because of longer incubation time spontaneous histamine release is higher and eicosanoids might be partly degraded using this protocol instead of the protocol described in **Subheading 3.4.1.**

1. Wash mast cells twice in culture medium.
2. Resuspend mast cells in culture medium in the concentration and volume as required. Place cells in a fresh culture plate (*see* **Note 16**).
3. Prepare cell lysates for the detection of total histamine if you wish to study histamine release in parallel (*see* **Subheading 3.4.2.**).
4. Add trigger or agonist of interest (e.g., for FcεRI crosslinking, MAb 22E7 100 ng/ mL). Leave control untreated or add appropriate isotype control.
5. Harvest cells after time of interest and transfer them to a Eppendorf tube free of RNAs (*see* **Note 17**). Centrifuge cells (300g, 10 min, 4°C) and collect supernatants. Store aliquots at –80°C. Resuspend pellet immediately in RLT buffer provided by the RNeasy Mini Kit (Qiagen, cat. no. 74106).
6. Measure mediators of interest in the supernatants by appropriate ELISA. Assay mRNA levels by semiquantitative reverse transcription polymerase chain reaction or real-time reverse transcription polymerase chain reaction.

4. Notes

1. Tissue can be obtained from all parts of the bowel. Most specimens we have obtained have come from patients who underwent resection because of large bowel cancer.
2. Tissue can be stored at 4°C overnight, although immediate processing is preferential. In our hands, numbers and viability of isolated mast cell are only slightly impaired after overnight storage of the tissue specimen.

3. Tissue suspension needs to be stirred using a tweezer or with other appropriate instruments to avoid obstruction of the filter. If residual mucus completely clogs the mesh, transfer tissue suspension to a new bottle top filter.

4. Approximately $1–2.5 \times 10^7$ cells can be obtained from 1 g of mucosal tissue. As much as 10 g can be used in one preparation. If more tissue is available, perform two (or more) preparations in parallel. Normally isolated cells contain 1–4% mast cells, but the percentage can be higher in selected patients. Cell preparations contain 10–40% erythrocytes, which has to be taken in account by calculating mast cell numbers. If required, erythrocytes can be lysed using commercially available solutions (e.g., Sigma, cat. no. R7757).

5. Overnight culture improves the efficiency of MACS purification because *c-kit* expression is low after the isolation procedure and upregulated after overnight culture. Do not add SCF to the culture medium because it downregulates *c-kit* in mast cells and, therefore, diminishes the enrichment efficiency and recovery.

6. Mast cells are semiadherent. Approximately 80–90% of the cells can be harvested by resuspending the cells with the pipet only.

7. Normally, 30–50% of the cells are trypan positive after overnight culture (mast cell survival is generally higher). If more than 60% of the cells are Trypan positive, we do not recommend performing a positive selection by MACS because the enrichment efficiency and mast cell recovery will be very low. We have tried different methods to remove dead cells (density centrifugation and dead cell removal kit from Miltenyi). However, cell loss was always unacceptably high. For example, density gradient centrifugation using Ficoll-Paque is sufficient to remove more than 90% of the dead cells. Unfortunately, only 50% of the mast cells are found in the interface fraction, whereas approx 50% are found in the pellet together with the dead cells.

8. An anti-human *c-kit* Ab directly coupled to magnetic beads will be available soon (Miltenyi).

9. Although it is passed through a 30-μm filter, the cell suspension might obstruct the MACS column, which is related to the high amount of cell clumps and residual mucus. We recommend applying cells in small fractions of 1–2 mL. In the case of obstruction, remove the rest of the cell suspension on the top of the column and replace it with 2 mL of MACS buffer. The obstruction can be overcome by pulling up and down the buffer with a pipet. Continue with this column as recommended in the protocol. For the remaining cells, use a new column.

10. Metachromatic staining of mast cells after MACS is sometimes poor, and exact quantification is difficult. Generally, between 0.5 and 3×10^6 mast cells can be obtained from 5 to 10 g of mucosa.

11. More than the half of the MACS-enriched cell preparation die completely within the first days of culture. This may be related to the damage of the cells acquired during the cell separation. Long-term culture of mast cell succeed in approx 80% if unpurified cell preparations are used and the recovery is higher. If mast cells have passed the critical time period of the first week, no morphological or functional differences can be observed between MACS enriched and nonpurified mast cell cultures *(15)*.

12. To obtain high amounts of pure mast cells, we recommend adding IL-4 at a concentration of 2 ng/mL (in combination with SCF) to the culture. Keep in mind that IL-4 changes the mast cell phenotype (**Table 1**). IL-4 can be added at the beginning of the culture but also later. The "IL-4 phenotype" will be obtained after 1–2 wk.

13. In some cultures mast cells proliferate strongly in particular if IL-4 is added to the culture medium. Proliferation will stop if mast cell numbers exceed $0.5–1 \times 10^6$/mL. Then, split cells in a new culture plate.

14. Washing of cultured mast cell is very important because culture supernatants contain high amounts of histamine.

15. We usually stop the reaction after 30 min in a standard assay for the investigation of degranulation and eicosanoid production in response to FcɛRI crosslinking. For histamine, approx 3–5 min and for sLT, approx 10–15 min are required for maximal release (*11*).

16. For mRNA studies, we use at least 5×10^4 mast cells/condition (preferable is at least 1×10^5). For the measurement of TNF-α or IL-5 protein after FcɛRI crosslinking, cell concentrations of 2×10^5 cells/mL are sufficient. Higher concentrations are recommended if weaker agonists, agonists of unknown efficiency, or other cytokines are studied. We perform experiments in 200–400 µL in a 96- or 48-well plate.

17. For the analysis of mRNA induction for IL-3, IL-5, IL-6, IL-8, IL-9, IL-13, and TNF-α upon FcɛRI crosslinking the optimal time point is 90 min. Upregulation of mRNA is still detectable after 6 h. To measure cytokines in the supernatants, we recommend incubation periods of 6 h or longer.

Acknowledgments

The authors thank all former and current colleagues and in particular C. A. Dahinden, K. Wordelmann, S. Schwengberg, C. Mierke, A. Lorentz, G. Weier, N. Steegmann, T. Gebhardt, and A. Radke, who were involved in establishing the methods described here.

References

1. Weidner, N. and Austen, K. F. (1990) Evidence for morphologic diversity of human mast cells. An ultrastructural study of mast cells from multiple body sites. *Lab. Invest.* **63,** 63–72.

2. Metcalfe, D. D., Baram, D., and Mekori, Y. A. (1997) Mast cells. *Physiol. Rev.* **77,** 1033–1079.

3. Bischoff, S. C., Wedemeyer, J., Herrmann, A., et al. (1996) Quantitative assessment of intestinal eosinophils and mast cells in inflammatory bowel disease. *Histopathology* **28,** 1–13.

4. Bischoff, S. C. and Sellge, G. (2002) Mast cell hyperplasia: role of cytokines. *Int. Arch. Allergy Immunol.* **127,** 118–122.

5. Gurish, M. F., Tao, H., Abonia, J. P., et al. (2001) Intestinal mast cell progenitors require CD49dbeta7 (alpha4beta7 integrin) for tissue-specific homing. *J. Exp. Med.* **194,** 1243–1252.

6. Craig, S. S., Schechter, N. M., and Schwartz, L. B. (1989) Ultrastructural analysis of maturing human T and TC mast cells *in situ. Lab. Invest.* **60,** 147–157.

7. Lorentz, A., Schwengberg, S., Mierke, C., Manns, M. P., and Bischoff, S. C. (1999) Human intestinal mast cells produce IL-5 in vitro upon IgE receptor cross-linking and in vivo in the course of intestinal inflammatory disease. *Eur. J. Immunol.* **29,** 1496–1503.

8. Gelbmann, C. M., Mestermann, S., Gross, V., Kollinger, M., Scholmerich, J., and Falk, W. (1999) Strictures in Crohn's disease are characterised by an accumulation of mast cells colocalised with laminin but not with fibronectin or vitronectin. *Gut* **45,** 210–217.

9. Bischoff, S. C., Lorentz, A., Schwengberg, S., Weier, G., Raab, R., and Manns, M. P. (1999) Mast cells are an important cellular source of tumour necrosis factor alpha in human intestinal tissue. *Gut* **44,** 643–652.

10. Bischoff, S. C., Schwengberg, S., Wordelmann, K., Weimann, A., Raab, R., and Manns, M. P. (1996) Effect of c-kit ligand, stem cell factor, on mediator release by human intestinal mast cells isolated from patients with inflammatory bowel disease and controls. *Gut* **38,** 104–114.

11. Bischoff, S. C. and Dahinden, C. A. (1992) c-kit ligand: a unique potentiator of mediator release by human lung mast cells. *J. Exp. Med.* **175,** 237–244.

12. Gibbs, B. F., Wierecky, J., Welker, P., Henz, B. M., Wolff, H. H., and Grabbe, J. (2001) Human skin mast cells rapidly release preformed and newly generated TNF-alpha and IL-8 following stimulation with anti-IgE and other secretagogues. *Exp. Dermatol.* **10,** 312–320.

13. Lowman, M. A., Rees, P. H., Benyon, R. C., and Church, M. K. (1988) Human mast cell heterogeneity: histamine release from mast cells dispersed from skin, lung, adenoids, tonsils, and colon in response to IgE-dependent and nonimmunologic stimuli. *J. Allergy Clin. Immunol.* **81,** 590–597.

14. Pawankar, R., Okuda, M., Yssel, H., Okumura, K., and Ra, C. (1997) Nasal mast cells in perennial allergic rhinitics exhibit increased expression of the Fc epsilonRI, CD40L, IL-4, and IL-13, and can induce IgE synthesis in B cells. *J. Clin. Invest.* **99,** 1492–1499.

15. Bischoff, S. C., Sellge, G., Schwengberg, S., Lorentz, A., and Manns, M. P. (1999) Stem cell factor-dependent survival, proliferation and enhanced releasability of purified mature mast cells isolated from human intestinal tissue. *Int. Arch. Allergy Immunol.* **118,** 104–107.

16. Bischoff, S. C., Sellge, G., Lorentz, A., Sebald, W., Raab, R., and Manns, M. P. (1999) IL-4 enhances proliferation and mediator release in mature human mast cells. *Proc. Natl. Acad. Sci. USA* **96,** 8080–8085.

17. Schulman, E. S., Macglashan, D. W., Peters, S. P., Schleimer, R. P., Newball, H. H., and Lichtenstein, L. M. (1982) Human lung mast cells: purification and characterization. *J. Immunol.* **129,** 2662–2667.

18. Befus, A. D., Dyck, N., Goodacre, R., and Bienenstock, J. (1987) Mast-cells from the human intestinal lamina propria—isolation, histochemical subtypes, and functional-characterization. *J. Immunol.* **138,** 2604–2610.

19. Bischoff, S. C., Schwengberg, S., Raab, R., and Manns, M. P. (1997) Functional properties of human intestinal mast cells cultured in a new culture system: enhancement of IgE receptor-dependent mediator release and response to stem cell factor. *J. Immunol.* **159,** 5560–5567.

20. Gebhardt, T., Sellge, G., Lorentz, A., Raab, R., Manns, M. P., and Bischoff, S. C. (2002) Cultured human intestinal mast cells express functional IL-3 receptors and respond to IL-3 by enhancing growth and IgE receptor-dependent mediator release *Eur. J. Immunol.* **32,** 2308–2316.

21. Mierke, C. T., Ballmaier, M., Werner, U., Manns, M. P., Welte, K., and Bischoff, S. C. (2000) Human endothelial cells regulate survival and proliferation of human mast cells. *J. Exp. Med.* **192,** 801–811.

22. Sellge, G., Lorentz, A., Gebhardt, T., et al. (2004) Human intestinal fibroblasts prevent apoptosis in human intestinal mast cells by a mechanism independent of stem cell factor, IL-3, IL-4, and nerve growth factor. *J. Immunol.* **172,** 260–267.

23. Lorentz, A., Schwengberg, S., Sellge, G., Manns, M. P., and Bischoff, S. C. (2000) Human intestinal mast cells are capable of producing different cytokine profiles: role of IgE receptor cross-linking and IL-4. *J. Immunol.* **164,** 43–48.

24. Bischoff, S. C., Schwengberg, S., Lorentz, A., et al. (2004) Substance P and other neuropeptides do not induce mediator release in isolated human intestinal mast cells. *Neurogastroenterol. Motil.* **16,** 185–193.

IV

Mast Cell Signaling and Gene Expression

11

Activation of Nuclear Factor-κB

Chuanfu Li, Jim Kelley, and Tuanzhu Ha

Summary

Nuclear factor-κB (NF-κB) is a key transcription factor that regulates the expression of genes involved in immune and inflammatory responses and in cell death and survival. This chapter describes in detail the method for measuring the NF-κB binding activity in the cultured human mast cell line HMC-1 using the electrophoretic mobility shift assay: the activation of NF-κB was illustrated by adding lipopolysaccharide to mast cells, nuclear proteins were isolated, and the NF-κB binding activity was determined. We also demonstrate the specificity of the NF-κB binding activity using a competition and supershift assay with specific antibodies that recognize NF-κB subunits p50 and p65. Lipopolysaccharide caused a rapid and significant increase in NF-κB binding activity.

Key Words: Mast cells; nuclear factor-κB (NF-κB); inflammatory cytokines; signal transduction; Toll-like receptors (TLRs); nuclear proteins; EMSA; HMC-1.

1. Introduction

Mast cells play a critical role in the initiation of the innate and adaptive immune response against various pathogens and represent a potential source of multifunctional cytokines that participates in the recruitment and activation of other cells in the inflammatory microenvironment. Activation of mast cells releases inflammatory cytokines, such as tumor necrosis factor (TNF)-α, interleukin (IL)-1, IL-8, IL-5, IL-10, and IL-13. Nuclear factor-κB (NF-κB) is a key transcription factor that controls the expression of these cytokines (*1–3*). In resting cells, NF-κB exists in an inactive cytoplasmic form, bound to the inhibitory proteins known as I-κBs. Upon cellular stimulation, I-κB proteins are rapidly phosphorylated by I-κB kinases and degraded via the 26S uniquitin–proteasome pathway. The released NF-κB translocates to the nucleus and binds specific deoxyribonucleic acid (DNA) motifs and stimulates the transcription of various genes. These include inflammatory cytokines (TNF-α, IL-1β, IL-2, IL-6, IL-8, interferon-γ), adhesion molecules (i.e., vascular cell adhesion mol-

From: *Methods in Molecular Biology, vol. 315: Mast Cells: Methods and Protocols*
Edited by: G. Krishnaswamy and D. S. Chi © Humana Press Inc., Totowa, NJ

ecule-1 [VCAM-1], intercellular adhesion molecule-1 [ICAM-1], and E-selectin), acute phase response proteins, and other factors that are involved in mediating the immune and inflammatory responses and cell survival and cell death *(1–3)*. We and others have reported that stimulation of mast cells results in activation of NF-κB *(4–7)*. Recent studies have highlighted the Toll-like receptor (TLR)-mediated signaling pathway that directly activates NF-κB *(8)*. Mast cell TLR2 or mast cell TLR4 recognizes the pathogen ligands in a way similar to those of other leukocytes *(9–16)*. TLR2-mediated mast cell activation by peptidogly-can leads to degranulation and IL-4 and IL-5 cytokine production, whereas with TLR4-mediated mast cell activation, TNF-α, IL-1β, IL-6, and IL-13 are the major cytokines produced *(15)*.

Activation of NF-κB in mast cells can be examined using the electrophoretic mobility shift assay (EMSA *[4]*), which is a simple and rapid method for detecting DNA-binding proteins. The principle of the assay is that the migration of protein–DNA complexes through a nondenaturing polyacrylamide gel is slower than that of free DNA fragments or double-stranded oligonucleotides. The procedure of the assay includes: (1) isolation of nuclear proteins from mast cells; (2) labeling the oligonucleotides with ^{32}P-ATP; (3) incubation of nuclear proteins with ^{32}P-labeled oligonucleotides; (4) analysis of protein–DNA interaction by a nondenaturing polyacrylamide gel; (5) drying the gel followed by autoradiography; and (6) determination of the specificity of protein–DNA interaction by addition of excess unlabeled oligonucleotides or unrelated oligonucleotides.

2. Materials

1. Human mast cell line (HMC-1).
2. Mast cell culture medium: 5% heat-inactivated fetal bovine serum, 0.01 M HEPES buffer, 50 μg/mL gentamycin, 0.02 mM 2-mercaptoethanol, 5 μg/mL insulin transferrin sodium selenite, and 2 mM L-glutamine in RPMI 1640 media.
3. Lipopolysaccharide (LPS).
4. Buffer A: 10 mM HEPES, pH 7.9, 10 mM KCl, 0.1 mM ethylene diamine tetraacetic acid (EDTA), 0.1 mM ethylenebis(oxyethylenenitrilo)tetraacetic acid (EGTA), 1 mM dithiothreitol (DTT), 0.5 mM phenylmethyl sulfonyl fluoride (PMSF), 1 μM aprotinin; 14 μM leupeptin, 1 μM pepstatin, 80 μg of benzamidine/ mL, 20 mM p-nitrophenyl phosphate, 40 mM β-glycerol phosphate, 1 mM Na$_3$VO$_4$, 50 mM NaF, and 0.1 mM TPCK.
5. Buffer C: 20 mM HEPES, pH 7.9, 0.4 M NaCl, 1 mM EDTA, 1 mM EGTA, 12 mM DTT, 1 mM PMSF, 1 μM aprotinin; 14 μM leupeptin, 1 μM pepstatin, 80 μg of benzamidine/mL, 20 mM p-nitrophenyl phosphate, 40 mM β-glycerol phosphate, 1 mM Na$_3$VO$_4$, 50 mM NaF, and 0.1 mM TPCK, 25% glycerol.
6. Nonidet P-40 (NP-40).
7. BCA protein assay reagents (Pierce).

8. Transcription factor consensus oligonucleotides: 5'-AGT TGA GGG GAC TTT CCC AGG C-3'.
9. T4 polynucleotide kinase.
10. [γ-^{32}P]ATP (3000 Ci/mmol, 10 mci/mL).
11. TE buffer: 10 mM Tris-HCl, pH 8.0, 1 mM EDTA, pH 8.0.
12. DE 81 filter paper.
13. DNA loading buffer: 0.25% bromophenol blue, 0.25% xylene cyanol FF, and 30% glycerol in water.
14. 5X binding buffer: 2.5 mg/mL of double-stranded poly (dI-dC), 50 mM Tris-HCl (pH 7.5), 250 mM NaCl, 2.5 mM EDTA, 2.5 mM DTT, 5 mM MgCl$_2$, 20% glycerol.
15. Nondenaturing polyacrylamide gel electrophoresis (PAGE) equipment.
16. TBE (5X) buffer: 54 g of Tris base, 27.5 g of boric acid, 20 mL of 0.5 M EDTA (pH 8.0) per liter.
17. Whatman no. 3 filter paper.
18. Gel Drier.
19. X-ray films.

3. Methods

3.1. Preparation of Nuclear Extracts From the Cultured Cells (see Note 1)

1. Culture HMC-1 in mast cell culture media. Subculture the cells as designated groups at 1×10^6.
2. After overnight culture, stimulate the cells with desired stimuli for certain time, for example, stimulate the cells with LPS at 100 ng/mL for 30–60 min. Harvest the cells into a 10-mL culture tube.
3. Centrifuge at 1500g for 5 min to pellet the cells. Discard the supernatant, wash the cells with 10 mL of cold Tris-buffered saline (TBS), resuspend the cells, and obtain a pellet of the cells by centrifugation at 1500g for 5 min at 4°C.
4. Resuspend the cell pellets in 1 mL of TBS, transfer the cells into a 1.5-mL Eppendorf tube, and obtain a pellet of the cells again by centrifugation for 15 s in a microcentrifuge at 10,000g at 4°C.
5. Discard the TBS, add 200 µL of cold buffer A to the cell pellets, and suspend the cells by gentle mixing.
6. Incubate the tube containing the cells on ice for 20 min to swell the cells. Twenty min after incubation, add 12.5 µL of a 10% solution of NP-40 and vortex the tube for 10 s.
7. Centrifuge the homogenate for 1 min at 10,000g in a microcentrifuge at 4°C. Transfer the supernatant, which contains cytoplasmic proteins, to a fresh tube and immediately store at −80°C.
8. Add 1 mL of Buffer A, without NP-40, into the tube to wash the nuclear pellets. After centrifugation in a microcentrifuge at 10,000g for 1 min at 4°C and discard the supernatant.
9. Add 50 µL of ice-cold Buffer C into the nuclear pellets and shake the tube vigorously at 4°C for at least for 20 min using a shaking platform.

10. Centrifuge the nuclear extract for 15 min at 10,000*g* in a microcentrifuge at 4°C, harvest the supernatant, freeze in an liquid nitrogen, and then store at –80°C.
11. Determine the concentration of cytoplasmic and nuclear proteins by the BCA protein assay according to the manufacturer's instruction.

3.2. EMSA for NF-κB Binding Activity

The procedures for the binding reaction include the following: incubate the nuclear extracts with $[\gamma\text{-}^{32}P]$ATP-labeled oligonucleotide probe that contains the specific binding sequence for NF-κB (the binding reaction occurs under specific salt/pH conditions in a binding buffer). Add Poly-dIdC into the binding reaction mixtures to prevent nonspecific binding of proteins to the NF-κB oligonucleotide probe. Determine the subunits of NF-κB binding activity in the nuclear extracts by competition assay and antibody supershift analysis. Separate the binding reaction mixtures on a nondenaturing PAGE gel. Finally, dry the PAGE gel and detect the binding bands by autoradiography *(17–20)*.

3.2.1. Labeling of Consensus Oligonucleotide With $[\gamma\text{-}^{32}P]ATP$ (see **Notes 2** and **3**)

1. Take a sterile 1.5-mL Eppendorf tube and add the items sequentially as shown in **Table 1**.
2. Incubate the reaction mixture at 37°C for 10 min.
3. Stop the reaction by addition of 1 μL of 0.5 *M* EDTA.
4. Add 89 μL of TE buffer and store at –20°C.

3.2.2. Determination of the Percent of $[\gamma\text{-}^{32}P]ATP$ Incorporation Into the Oligonucleotide

1. Take 1 μL of the labeled oligonucleotide and spot onto a DE81 filter paper.
2. Dry the DE81 paper briefly under a heat lamp.
3. Place the DE1 paper into a vial and count cpm in a scintillation counter.
4. After counting, wash the DE81 paper in 50 mL of 0.5 *M* Na$_2$HPO$_4$, twice for 5 min each, to remove the unincorporated $[\gamma\text{-}^{32}P]$ATP. Dry the washed DE81 filter paper under a heat lamp.
5. Place the DE81 paper into a vial and count the cpm in a scintillation counter.
6. Calculate the percent incorporation of $[\gamma\text{-}^{32}P]$ATP into the oligonucleotide.

Percent incorporation = cpm incorporated/total cpm $\times$ 100%

3.2.3. Binding Reaction

1. Take a set of 0.5-mL Eppendorf tubes and mark them with designated numbers using a marker pen.
2. Add each the following items sequentially as shown in **Table 2** into designated 0.5-mL Eppendorf tubes in a total 10 μL of reaction volume (*see* **Note 4**).

Nuclear extracts	x μL (5–10 μg)
5X binding buffer	2 μL

Table 1
Labeling NF-κB Oligonucleotides With [γ-^{32}P]ATP

Items	Volume
NF-κB oligonucleotide (1.75 pmol/μL)	2 mL
T4 polynucleotide kinase 10X buffer	1 mL
[γ-^{32}P]ATP (3,000 Ci/mmol at 10 mCi/mL)	5 mL
dH$_2$O	1 mL
T4 polynucleotide kinase (5–10 U/μL)	1 mL
Total reaction volume	10 mL

Table 2
Binding Reaction Mixtures

Sample No	Nuclear proteins	5X binding Buf	Buf C	^{32}P-oligo probe
Negative control	0	2 μL	7 μL	1 μL
No. 1	(5–10 μg) x μL	2 μL	to 7 μL	1 μL
No. 2	(5–10 μg) x μL	2 μL	to 7 μL	1 μL
No. 3	(5–10 μg) x μL	2 μL	to 7 μL	1 μL

Buffer C	to	7 μL
^{32}P-oligonucleotide probe		1 μL

3. Incubate the reaction mixtures at room temperature for 20 min.
4. Stop the binding reaction by adding 2 μL of DNA loading buffer.
5. Briefly centrifuge a microcentrifuge.
6. Load the samples on 5% nondenatured PAGE gel.

3.2.4. Electrophoresis

1. Set up the polyacrylamide gel casting: take clean plates and the spacers. Tighten them to make the casting module and fit it on the stand with the rubber spacer on bottom.
2. Preparation of 5% nondenaturing polyacrylamide gel (40 mL) as below (*see* **Note 5**).

Components	5% gel
TBE 5X buffer	8.00 mL
30:0.8 (acrylamide:Bis-acrylamide)	6.70 mL
80% glycerol	1.25 mL
dH$_2$O	23.73 mL
TEMED	20 μL
10% Ammonium persulfate	300 μL

3. Use a 20-mL syringe to pour the gel on the side of cast near spacers. Fill the cast from bottom without any air bubbles inside. Take the comb and insert it into the gel without trapping any air bubbles. Polymerize the gel for 0.5 h. Make sure its not leaking when leaving it to polymerize.

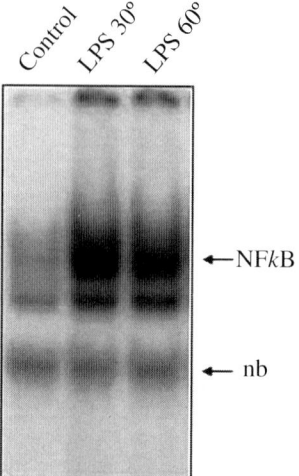

Fig. 1. Lipopolysaccharide (LPS) stimulates nuclear factor-κB (NF-κB) binding activity in mast cells. Mast cells were stimulated with or without LPS at 100 ng/mL for 30 and 60 min, respectively, and nuclear proteins were isolated from the cells. Five micrograms of nuclear proteins from each sample were used for electrophoretic mobility shift assay (EMSA) of NF-κB binding activity. NF-κB binding activity is labeled on the right; nb, nonspecific binding.

4. Prerun the gel for 20 min at 100 V before loading the samples.
5. Load the reaction samples on the gel and run the get at room temperature, in 0.5X TBE buffer at 100 V for approx 2 h or until the bromophenol blue dye is just out of the gel.
6. Collect the gel running buffer into a radioactive liquid waste container. Take the gel cast out and separate the glass plate carefully.
7. Place the gel on a sheet of plastic wrap and cover the gel with Whatman 3MM filter papers and lift the gel. Wrap the gel with plastic wrap and dry with a gel-drier at 80°C for 1 h.
8. Expose the dried gel to X-ray film several hours to overnight at –80°C with an intensifying screen.
9. Develop the film in a dark room (*see* **Note 6**).
10. Scan the gel to determine the relative integrated intensity of the bands. **Fig. 1** shows NF-κB activation in HMC-1 mast cells stimulated with LPS (100 ng/mL) for 30 and 60 min.

3.2.5. Competition and Supershift Assay

To determine the specificity of NF-κB binding activity and the subunits of activated NF-κB, competition with unlabeled oligonucleotides and supershift assay with specific antibodies against subunits of NF-κB are performed as in the next list.

1. Take a set of 0.5-mL Eppendorf tubes and mark them with designated numbers using a marker pen.
2. Add each of the following items sequentially as shown in **Table 3** into designated 0.5-mL Eppendorf tubes in a total 10 μL of reaction volume.

Nuclear extracts	x μL (5–10 μg)
5X binding buffer	2 μL
Buffer C	to 5–7 μL
Unlabeled NF-κB oligonucleotide	2 μL
Other oligonucleotide	2 μL
^{32}P-oligonucleotide probe	1 μL

3. Incubate the binding reaction mixture for 20 min at room temperature.
4. Anti-p50 or anti-p65 2–5 μL.
5. Incubate the binding reaction mixture for 1–2 h at 4°C.
6. Stop the binding reaction by addition of 2 μL of DNA loading buffer.
7. Briefly centrifuge in a microcentrifuge.
8. Load the samples on a 5% nondenatured PAGE gel.

   Figure 2 shows specificity of NF-κB binding activity determined by addition of unlabeled oligonucleotides and by an antibody supershift assay.

4. Notes

1. Isolation of cytoplasmic and nuclear proteins from harvested cells should be performed in ice and proteinase inhibitors should be used.
2. When working with isotope (^{32}P), the regulations for biosafety of radioactivity should be followed. After labeling oligonucleotides with [γ-^{32}P]ATP, it is not necessary to remove unincorporated [γ-^{32}P]ATP from the labeling reaction.
3. After labeling oligonucleotides with [γ-^{32}P]ATP, more than 50% of the radioactivity is typically incorporated in the 5' end-labeling reaction. If the labeling efficiency is low (<30%), the activity of T4 polynucleotide kinase should be checked.
4. For the NF-κB binding assay, 10 μL of a total reaction volume usually is used. If the concentration of nuclear protein preparation is low, 15 μL of a total reaction volume can be used. The volume of nuclear proteins (x μL) plus volume of Buf C = 11 μL. 3 μL of 5X binding buffer will be used.
5. When preparing the nondenaturing polyacrylamide gel, 10% ammonium persulfate should be freshly prepared.
6. If no binding bands are observed, the following should be considered: (1) insufficient amount of nuclear proteins in the assay; (2) low specific activity of ^{32}P-labeled oligonucleotide; (3) inappropriate components in binding buffer; or (4) too much nonspecific competitor DNA or inappropriate type of competitor DNA.

References

1. Baldwin, A. S., Jr. (1996) The NF-kappa B and I-kappa B proteins: new discoveries and insights. *Annu. Rev. Immunol.* **14,** 649–683.
2. Baeuerle, P. A. and Baltimore, D. (1996) NF-κB: ten years after. *Cell* **87,** 13–20.

Table 3
Experimental Design for Competition and Supershift Assay

Sample no.	Nuclear proteins (5–10 mg)	5X binding buffer	Buffer C	Unlabeled NF-κB oligo	Other oligo (APII)	^{32}P-labeled NF-κB oligo	Anti-p50	Anti-p65
No. 1	x µL	2 µL	to 7 µL	2 µL		1 µL	2–5 µL	2–5 µL
No. 1	x µL	2 µL	to 5 µL		2 µL	1 µL	2–5 µL	2–5 µL
No. 2	x µL	2 µL	to 5 µL			1 µL		
No. 3	x µL	2 µL	to 7 µL			1 µL		
No. 4	x µL	2 µL	to 7 µL			1 µL		
No. 5	x µL	2 µL	to 7 µL			1 µL		

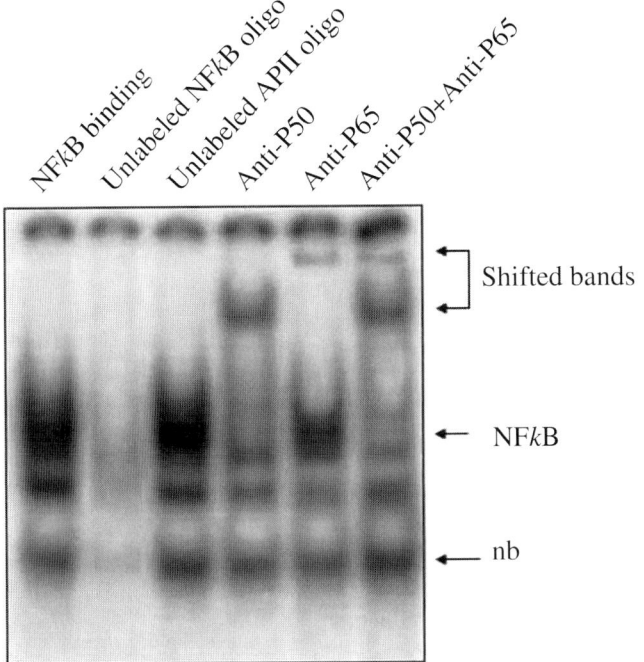

Fig. 2. Specificity of nuclear factor-κB (NF-κB) binding was determined by competition and supershift assays. Nuclear proteins were isolated from mast cells stimulated with lipopolysaccharide (LPS) for 30 min. The binding reaction mixture was added with unlabeled NF-κB oligo, APII oligo, anti-p50, and anti-p65, respectively. The shifted binding bands, NF-κB binding band, and nonspecific binding are labeled on right.

3. May, M. J. and Ghosh, S. (1998) Signal transduction through NF-κB. *Immunol. Today* **19,** 80–88.
4. Krishnaswamy, G., Martin, R., Walker, E., et al. (2003) Moraxella catarrhalis induces mast cell activation and nuclear factor kappa b-dependent cytokine synthesis. *Frontiers Biosci.* **8,** a40–a47.
5. Sarkar, A., Sreenivasan, Y., and Manna, S. K. (2003) α-Melanocyte-stimulating hormone induces cell death in mast cells: involvement of NF-κB. *FEBS Lett.* **549,** 87–93.
6. Coward, W. R., Okayama, Y., Sagara, H., Wilson, S. J., Holgate, S. T., and Church, M. K. (2002) NF-κB and TNF-α: a positive autocrine loop in human lung mast cells? *J. Immunol.* **169,** 5287–5293.
7. Lorentz, A., Klopp, I., Gebhardt, T., Manns, M. P., and Bischoff, S. C. (2003) Role of activator protein 1, nuclear factor-κB, and nuclear factor of activated T cells in IgE receptor-mediated cytokine expression in mature human mast cells. *J. Allergy Clin. Immunol.* **111,** 1062–1068.

8. Medzhitov, R., Preston-Hurlburt, P., and Janeway, Jr. C. A. (1997) A human homologue of the *Drosophila* Toll protein signals activation of adaptive immunity. *Nature* **388,** 394–397.

9. McCurdy, J. D., Olynych, T. J., Maher, L. H., and Marshall, J. S. (2003) Cutting edge: distinct Toll-like receptor 2 activators selectively induce different classes of mediator production from human mast cells. *J. Immunol.* **170,** 1625–1629.

10. Varadaradjalou, S., Feger, F., Thieblemont, N., et al. (2003) Toll-like receptor 2 (TLR2) and TLR4 differentially activate human mast cells. *Eur. J. Immunol.* **33,** 899–906.

11. Applequist, S. E., Wallin, R. P., and Ljunggren, H. G. (2002) Variable expression of Toll-like receptor in murine innate and adaptive immune cell lines. *Int. Immunol.* **14,** 1065–1074.

12. McCurdy, J. D., Lin, T.-J., and Marshall, J. S. (2001) Toll-like receptor 4-mediated activation of murine mast cells. *J. Leukoc. Biol.* **70,** 977–984.

13. Marshall, J. S., McCurdy, J. D., and Olynych, T. (2003) Toll-like receptor-mediated activation of mast cells: implications for allergic disease? *Int. Arch. Allergy Immunol.* **132,** 87–97.

14. Yoshikawa, H. and Tasaka, K. (2003) Caspase-dependent and -independent apoptosis of mast cells induced by withdrawal of IL-3 is prevented by Toll-like receptor 4-mediated lipopolysaccharide stimulation. *Eur. J. Immunol.* **33,** 2149–2159.

15. Supajatura, V., Ushio, H., Nakao, A., et al. (2002) Differential responses of mast cell Toll-like receptors 2 and 4 in allergy and innate immunity. *J. Clin. Invest.* **109,** 1351–1359.

16. Ikeda, T. and Funaba, M. (2003) Altered function of muring mast cells in response to lipopolysaccharide and peptidoglycan. *Immunol. Lett.* **88,** 21–26.

17. Li, C., Browder, W., and Kao, R. L. (1999) Early activation of transcription factor NF-κB during ischemia in perfused rat heart. *Am. J. Physiol.* **276,** H543–H552.

18. Li, C., Ha, T., Liu, L., Browder, W., and Kao, R. L. (2000) Adenosine prevents activation of transcription factor NF-kappa B and enhances activator protein-1 binding activity in ischemic rat heart. *Surgery* **127,** 161–169.

19. Li, C., Kao, R. L., Ha, T., Kelley, J., Browder, I. W., and Williams, D. L. (2001) Early activation of IKKβ during in vivo myocardial ischemia. *Am. J. Physiol. Heart Circ. Physiol.* **280,** H1264–H1271.

20. Li, C., Ha, T., Kelley, J., et al. (2004) Modulating Toll-like receptor mediated signaling by (1→3)-β-D-glucan rapidly induces cardioprotection. *Cardiovasc. Res.* **61,** 538–547.

12

Analysis of Mitogen-Activated Protein Kinase Activation

Stephen C. Armstrong

Summary

The biological functions of mast cells are regulated by several protein kinases, including the tyrosine kinases Fyn, Lyn, Syk, and FAK and the serine/threonine kinases Akt and PKC α/β. The mitogen-activated protein kinases extracellular signal-regulated kinases, JNK, and p38MAPK also play a significant role in the regulation of mast cell biological function. This chapter will detail recent advances in determining mitogen-activated protein kinase activation in single cells. These methods are applicable to studies of signal transduction in mast cells.

Key Words: MAP kinase; ERK; JNK; p38MAPK; immunoblotting; kinase activity assays.

1. Introduction

Mitogen-activated protein (MAP) kinases are classified as: (1) extracellular signal-regulated kinases, (ERK 1/2, 44/42 kDa), which are activated by growth hormone receptors via a Ras/Raf/MEK1/2 pathway; and (2) the stress-activated kinases Jun-NH2-terminal kinases 1/2 (JNK-1/2, 55/46 kDa) and p38MAPK α/β, which are activated via MKK4/MKK7 and MKK3/MKK6 pathways, respectively, by cellular stresses, including reactive oxygen species, heat shock, inflammatory cytokines, and ischemia (*1*). There is also a related MAP kinase that has been termed BMK1 (big MAP kinase) in that it is 115 kDa in size or ERK5 in that it shares extensive homology with ERK 1/2 (*2*). ERK5 is activated by growth factor receptors, G protein-coupled receptors, and osmotic or oxidative stress downstream from MKK5 (*3,4*).

MAP kinases are an important set of protein kinases in the biological functions of mast cells. The neuropeptide substance P rapidly stimulates p38MAPK and JNK phosphorylation in rat peritoneal mast cells. Inhibition of p38MAPK with SB203580 abolishes the production of tumor necrosis factor (TNF)-α by substance P in peritoneal mast cells (*5*). In contrast, the transforming growth

From: *Methods in Molecular Biology, vol. 315: Mast Cells: Methods and Protocols*
Edited by: G. Krishnaswamy and D. S. Chi © Humana Press Inc., Totowa, NJ

factor (TGF)-β1-mediated migration of a human mast cell line (HMC-1) is blocked by ERK 1/2 inhibiton with PD98059, whereas SB203580 does not alter migration *(6)*. JNK and BMK1/ERK5 are activated by FcεRI crosslinking in a murine mast cell line (MC/9) or in embryonic stem cell-derived mast cells. TNF-α expression is dependent upon JNK and BMK1/ERK5 activation *(7,8)*. Permeabilization of mast cells with the virulence factor, streptolysin, activates p38MAPK and JNK. Inhibition of p38 MAPK reduces the streptolysin-mediated production of TNF-α in mast cells *(9)*. Lipopolysaccharide (LPS)-activated JNK and p38MAPK in bone marrow-derived mast cells and inhibition of JNK and p38MAPK suppress the production of interleukin (IL)-5, IL-10, and IL-13 *(10)*. Thus, it can be concluded that the stress kinases JNK and p38MAPK play an important role in the production of cytokines by mast cells, presumably via the transcriptional factors that are downstream substrates of JNK and MAPK.

The MAP kinases share a common Thr-X-Tyr site in the activation loop, and Thr-Tyr phosphorylation initiates kinase activity *(11–13)*. This chapter details the methodologies that have been used to assess activation of the MAP kinases. MAP kinase activity traditionally has been determined by in-gel protein kinase activity assays, in which a cellular sample was separated on an sodium dodecyl sulfate polyacrylamide gel electrophoresis (SDS-PAGE) gel with a specific substrate for a given MAP kinase polymerized into the gel, for example, myelin basic protein, MAPKAPK-2, and Jun substrate for ERK, p38MAPK, and JNK, respectively *(14)*. The gels are renatured and incubated in a protein kinase activity buffer, permitting the protein kinases to express their activity as determined by the incorporation of ^{32}P-ATP into the substrate. The radiolabeling that was associated with a specific MAP kinase was determined by the molecular weight of the radiolabeled band.

This technique has several disadvantages, specifically the use of radioactivity and the lack of specificity. Recently, dual phosphospecific, site-specific antibodies to the MAP kinases have been developed that are directed towards the Thr-X-Tyr activation site, as described previously *(15)*. These phosphospecific antibodies are developed as polyclonal anti-sera that are generated by immunizing rabbits with peptides that contain the dually phosphorylated Thr-X-Tyr site. The anti-sera initially are negatively selected by affinity chromatography with nonphospho peptides, and the eluate is positively selected by dual-phospho peptides. These antibodies permit a simple method to indirectly assess MAP kinase activation. Recently monoclonal antibodies to MAP kinases have been developed. Cellular samples are separated by SDS-PAGE, transferred by Western blotting, and the blots are immunostained with the dual phosphospecific antibodies. My laboratory has extensively used these phospho-specific antibodies to examine MAPK activation during ischemia in isolated adult rabbit cardiomyocytes with a publication on p38MAPK *(16)*, and a manuscript on ERK 1/2 activation is currently in preparation. Dual phospho-specific antibodies can also be used in flow cytometric assays in which the dual phosphorylation and activation of MAP kinases is quantitated on a single cell basis in a large population of cells *(17)*. Finally dual phospho-specific antibodies can be used in immunohistochemistry studies of tissue sections.

Recently, nonradioactive assays have been developed that permit a direct assessment of MAP kinase activity. Cellular samples are immunoprecipitated overnight with an agarose immobilized dual phospho-specific antibody to the Thr-Tyr activation site. The immunoprecipitates are washed and resuspended in a kinase buffer in the presence of a fusion substrate protein and ATP. The incorporation of phosphate into the substrate protein by the immunoprecipitated kinase is determined by immunostaining of blots with a phospho-specific, site-specific antibody to the substrate protein.

The MAP kinases have distinct yet overlapping downstream substrates that mediate their biological functions. These substrates include Elk-1, p90RSK, c-Myc and αB crystallin (ERK1/2); c-Jun (JNK1/2); MAPKAPK-2, MEF2, ATF-2, and CREB (p38MAPK); and p90RSK (ERK5/BMK1). These pathways are outlined in **Fig. 1**.

This chapter will focus on the evaluation of ERK and p38MAPK activation by Western blotting and nonradioactive kinase activity assays. JNK and BMK1/ERK5 dual phosphorylation and kinase activities also can be determined by the protocols described in this chapter. Cardiomyocyte and heart extracts will be used to demonstrate the correspondence of these techniques. The assays described in this chapter can be directly translated to the assessment of MAP kinase activation in mast cells, as described previously *(5–12)*.

2. Materials
2.1. Immunoblotting With Phospho-Specific Antibodies

1. Disruption buffer: Digitonin (0.05%, pH 7.4) diluted in glass distilled water containing 20 mM Tris, 137 mM NaCl, 50 mM sodium fluoride, 5 mM ethylene diamine tetraacetic acid (EDTA), 1 mM [4-(2-aminoethyl) benzenesulfonyl fluoride], 10 mM Na pyrophosphate, 1 mM sodium orthovanadate, and 2 μg/mL leupeptin. Prepare buffer fresh from stock solutions. Sodium fluoride (protein phosphatase inhibitor), AEBSF (serine protease inhibitor), and leupeptin (protease inhibitor) are toxic, and gloves should be worn throughout the preparation and use of this buffer. Digitonin is prepared as a 0.5% (w/v) stock solution in distilled water, heated to 95°C, and cooled to room temperature. AEBSF is less toxic and is a stable water-soluble alternative to PMSF. It is prepared as a 100 mM stock solution in water and is stable for 6 mo with storage at 4°C at pH <7.0. EDTA is prepared as a 0.5 M stock solution that is dissolved by titratation to pH 7.5. Sodium orthovanadate is "activated" by depolymerization of vanadate for maxi-

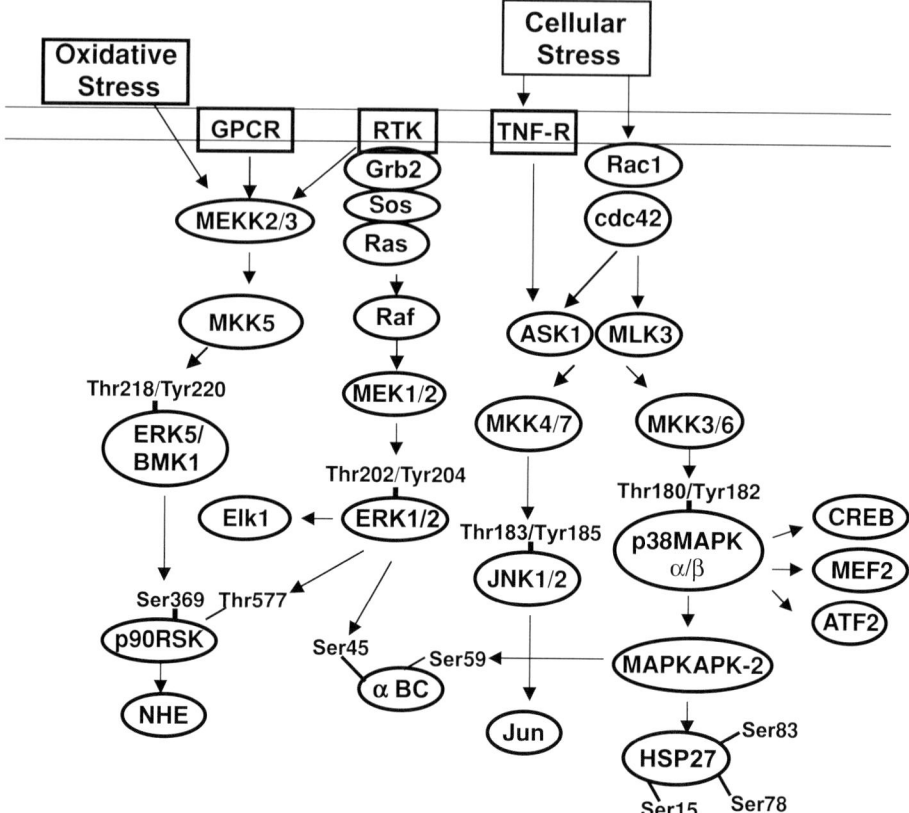

Fig. 1. Diagram of MAP kinase pathways. This diagram details the four types of MAP kinases: ERK1/2 and its homolog, ERK5, and the stress kinases JNK1/2 and p38MAPK α/β. ERK1/2 is activated by growth factor receptors downstream from Ras/ Raf. The stress kinases are activated by cellular stress via the small G proteins, Rac and cdc42. MAP kinase activation is induced by dual phosphorylation of the indicated Thr-X-Tyr motif in the activation loop of each MAP kinase. The downstream substrates of MAP kinases primarily include transcription factors: p90RSK and Elk-1 (ERK); Jun (JNK); and CREB, MEF2 and ATF-2 (p38MAPK). Additionally p38MAPK can initiate the downstream phosphorylation of the small heat shock proteins, heat shock protein 27 (HSP27), and αB crystallin, via its substrate, MAPKAPK-2.

mal inhibition of protein tyrosine phosphatases. A 200 mM solution of sodium orthovanadate is prepared and adjusted to pH 10.0 with sodium hydroxide. This will produce a yellow solution. Incubate the solution at 100°C for 10 min to produce a colorless solution. Repeat the pH adjustment-boiling process till the solution can remain colorless at pH 10.0.
2. Bio-Rad DC protein assay (cat. no. 500-0112, Bio-Rad, Hercules, CA).

3. 1D SDS-PAGE sample buffers (2X): 2% SDS, 2% glycerol, 40 mM dithiothreitol (DTT), 0.1% bromophenol blue, and 250 mM Tris (pH 6.8). 3X sample buffer: 3% SDS, 3% glycerol, 60 mM DTT, 0.15% bromophenol blue, and 375 mM Tris-HCl (pH 6.8). Glycerol is a viscous solution that should be transferred with a large pore pipet.

4. 1D SDS-PAGE separation gel polymerization solution: 30 mL of acrylamide (30%)/bis-acrylamide (0.8%), 18.75 mL of 1.5 M Tris-HCl, pH 8.8; 25.6 mL of glass-distilled water; and 375 µL of 20% SDS. Oxygen is removed from the polymerization solution by vacuum for 10 min. Polymerization is catalyzed by the production of free radicals with 37.5 µL of TEMED and 250 µL of 10% ammonium persulfate.

5. Stacking gel polymerization solution: 28.9 mL of acrylamide (30%)/bis-acrylamide (0.8%); 12.5 mL of 0.5 M Tris, pH 6.8; 28.9 mL of distilled water; and 250 µL of 20% SDS. After 10 min of de-gassing by vacuum, the polymerization is catalyzed by 26 µL of TEMED and 500 µL of 10% ammonium persulfate.

6. Acrylamide and bis-acrylamide (crosslinker) are neurotoxic in the monomer form, and gloves should be worn during routine handling. SDS is an irritant in the powder form and gloves, and face masks should be worn during preparation of stock solutions of SDS, acrylamide and bis-acrylamide. The acrylamide/bis-acrylamide stock solution should be stored at 4°C in brown bottles and is stable for 1 mo.

7. Electrophoresis running buffer: 25 mM Tris, 192 mM glycine, and 10 mM SDS.

8. Kaleidoscope prestained MW standards (cat. no. 161-0324, Bio-Rad).

9. Immunoblotting Transfer Buffer: 25 mM Tris, 192 mM glycine, and 10 mM SDS.

10. Nitrocellulose.

11. Immunostaining blocking buffer: TBS-Tween (TBS-T)-20 mM Tris, pH 7.5; 137 mM NaCl; 0.1% Tween-20; and 5% Carnation nonfat milk powder.

12. Antibody dilution buffer: TBS-Tween with 5% bovine serum albumin, pH 7.5.

13. All polyclonal antibodies are obtained from are obtained from Cell Signaling (Beverly, MA). Phospho-p38MAPK Thr180/Tyr182 (cat. no. 9211); phospho-ERK p44/42 Thr202/Tyr204 (cat. no. 9101); total p38 MAPK (cat. no. 9212); and total ERK p44/42 (cat. no. 9102).

14. Anti-rabbit horseradish peroxidase-conjugate (Sigma).

15. LumiGlo substrate solution (Kirkegaard and Perry, Gaithersburg, MD).

16. Kodak X-Omat LS MAT X-ray film.

17. GBX developer and fixer.

18. Colloidal Gold Total Protein Stain (cat. no. 170-6527, Bio-Rad).

2.2. Nonradioative Kinase Activity Assay

1. Kits for the nonradioactive assay of p38MAPK and ERK kinase activites (cat. no. 9820 and 9800, respectively) are obtained from Cell Signaling (Beverly, MA)

2. Lysis buffer: 1% Triton X-100 with 20 mM Tris, pH 7.5, 150 mM NaCl, 1 mM β-glycerolphosphate, 1 mM EDTA, 1 mM ethylenebis(oxyethylenenitrilo)tetraacetic acid, 1 mM phenylmethyl sulfonyl fluoride (PMSF), 2.5 mM Na pyrophosphate, 1 mM sodium orthovanadate, and 1 µg/mL leupeptin.

3. Kinase buffer: 25 m*M* Tris-HCl, pH 7.5, 5 m*M* β-glycerolphosphate, 2 m*M* DTT, 10 m*M* MgCl$_2$, 1 m*M* PMSF, 2.5 m*M* Na pyrophosphate, and 0.1 m*M* sodium orthovanadate. These components are provided as two separate 10X concentrates in the non-radioactive kinase activity assay kits (with the exception of PMSF or as an alternative, AEBSF, as described previously).
4. Immobilized phospho-p38 MAPK or phospho-ERK 1/2 polyclonal antibodies (Cell Signaling; cat. no. 9219 and 9109, respectively).
5. 10 m*M* ATP (Cell Signaling; cat. no. 9804).
6. Fusion substrate proteins: ATF-2 or Elk-1 for p38MAPK and ERK 1/2 (Cell Signaling; cat. no. 9224 and 9184), respectively.
7. Phosphospecific antibodies for substrate proteins: anti-ATF-2 (Thr71) or anti-Elk-1 (Ser383) for p38MAPK and ERK 1/2 (Cell Signaling; cat. no. 9221 and 9181), respectively.
8. Active p44 and p42 MAP kinase (cat. no. 14-439 and 14-173, respectively, Upstate; Charlottesville, VA).
9. Active p38MAPK α (cat. no. 14-210, Upstate).

3. Methods

The methods described in **Subheadings 3.1.** and **3.2.** outline: (1) the use of phosphospecific MAP kinase antibodies to determine MAP kinase activation by Western blotting; and (2) the use of phospho-specific antibodies to assay kinase activity in a nonradioactive mode.

3.1. Determination of MAPK Activation With Phospho-Specific Antibodies

3.1.1. In Vitro Ischemia Model

1. Cardiomyocytes are isolated by the collagenase digestion of a heart perfused with calcium-free Krebs-Henseleit buffer.
2. An aliquot of isolated cardiomyocytes is placed in a series of microcentrifuge tubes and centrifuged into a pellet. Excess supernatant is removed to leave a fluid layer above the pelleted cells of approximately one third the volume of the pellet.
3. After nitrogenation of the tube, the cell pellets are incubated for 0–90 min without agitation at 37°C. At the indicated time interval, a tube is removed, and the cells are briefly resuspended in ice cold TBS/vandate and collected by rapid centrifugation for snap freezing in liquid nitrogen.
4. For the myocardial studies, a rabbit heart is placed in ice-cold HEPES–Krebs–Henseleit buffer and the ventricular tissue is dissected and sectioned into four pieces. A section is immediately snap frozen with liquid nitrogen as the oxygenated control. In vitro ischemia is induced by incubating the ventricular tissue on a sterile gauze, moistened with saline, for 0–75 min. A section is removed at the indicated time interval and snap frozen with liquid nitrogen.

3.1.2. Cell Fractionation

1. Cardiomyocytes (or activated mast cells) are fractionated by lysing frozen cells for 5 min in 300 µL of ice-cold disruption buffer and centrifuged for 5 min at 10,000*g*.

2. The supernatant containing the cytosolic fraction is transferred to another microcentrifuge tube. Aliquots of cytosolic fractions are diluted with equal volumes of 2X sample buffer and stored at −20°C.

3. Myocardial tissue is homogenized in 4 mL of disruption buffer, and the lysate is processed as described for cardiomyocytes. The concentration of protein in the cellular samples is determined by using the Bio-Rad DC protein assay kit, a Lowry that has been modified to accommodate the presence of a variety of detergents.

3.1.3. One-Dimensional SDS-PAGE

1. One-dimensional gel electrophoresis is run with 4.25% stack gels and 12% separating gels (16 cm in width and 12 cm in height).

2. Cytosolic fractions are incubated at 100°C for 5 min, loaded at 50 µg/lane, and resolved with electrophoresis buffer at a constant current of 50 mA before immunoblotting.

3. Kaleidoscope prestained molecular weight standards in which proteins (7–195 kDa) are labeled with separate dyes, are used at 10 µL per bracketing lanes to: (1) assess protein separation during electrophoresis; (2) assess the transfer of proteins during immunoblotting; and (3) to provide an estimate of the molecular weights of immunostained bands.

3.1.4. Western Blotting and Immunostaining

1. Polyacrylamide gels are transferred by a Genie blotting apparatus to nitrocellulose paper for 90 min in transfer buffer.

2. The blots are incubated in blocking buffer for 1 h at room temperature to prevent nonspecific binding of antibody protein.

3. The blocked blots are incubated (overnight at 4°C, with rotation) with primary polyclonal antibodies diluted in antibody dilution buffer.

4. Blots are washed separately (to prevent cross-contamination of primary antibody) with TBS-T three times, 5 min each time, to remove excess primary antibody.

5. Blots are then incubated with antirabbit peroxidase conjugate (1:2500), incubated for 1 h at room temperature, followed by three 5-min rinses in TBS-T (*see* **Note 1**).

6. Blots are incubated in Lumi-Glo substrate solution for 1 min, drained by contacting an edge to filter paper (do not dry), wrapped in plastic film (Saran wrap), and immediately exposed to X-ray film in an exposure cassette for 1–30 min, depending on signal intensity (*see* **Note 2**).

7. Films are developed with GBX developer and fixer and analyzed by densitometry using Bio-Rad Quantity One software.

8. After immunostaining and exposure to film the blots are stained for total protein to assess the transfer of protein and the equivalency of protein loading in each lane.

9. Several alternatives exist for this procedure, including Sypro Ruby Protein Blot stain or Amido Black. My laboratory uses Colloidal Gold Total Protein Stain. The blots must be thoroughly washed with glass-distilled water to remove chloride ions that would interfere with the staining procedure. Stain for 15–60 min depending on protein load and background staining.

The primary advantage of the Western blotting method is that it is a relatively rapid assay that is not technically challenging. Whole cell lysates can be obtained by solubilization with 2% SDS (at 100°C) and dispersion with a 26-gage needle to shear DNA. However, our studies use fractionation of cardiomyocytes into cytosolic, membrane, and cytoskeletal/nuclear fractions by solubilization with digitonin, Triton X-100, and SDS, respectively. The cytosolic fractions are primarily used for our studies of MAP kinases. The translocation of MAP kinases to the nucleus has been reported (18,19). However, MAP kinase nuclear translocation is not pursued in our current studies.

The activation of ERK and p38MAPK in oxygenated and in vitro ischemic isolated adult rabbit cardiomyocytes was determined by immunoblotting with dual phospho-specific antibodies. In isolated cardiomyocytes, MAP kinase phosphorylation is clearly observed by well-defined bands **(Fig. 2A)**. ERK and p38MAPK dual phosphorylation is observed at high and low levels, respectively, in oxygenated cardiomyocytes. ERK and p38MAPK dual phosphorylation is significantly decreased and increased by 30 min of in vitro ischemia, respectively **(Fig. 2B)**, indicating a reciprocal relationship between the activation of these MAP kinases, as previously described in other systems (20). A subsequent loss of p38MAPK dual phosphorylation is observed after 60 min of in vitro ischemia.

3.2. Nonradioactive Assay of MAP Kinase Activity

1. Nonradioactive kits are used to directly determine p38MAPK and ERK1/2 activity in the cytosolic fractions of cardiomyocytes.
2. All materials (microcentrifuge, buffers, and micro-tubes) are kept ice cold throughout the procedure. An aliquot of the cytosolic fraction (200 μg in 200 μL of lysis buffer) is immunoprecipitated with 20 μL of immobilized phospho-p38MAPK or immobilized phospho-p44/p42 MAPK, overnight at 4°C.
3. Incubate immobilized antibodies on ice for 15 min before resuspension, repeated inversion, or gentle vortexing. In the ERK1/2 kit, purified active ERK2 is provided as a positive control. A control tube with 20 ng of active ERK2 in 200 μL of lysis buffer is immunoprecipitated as described previously.
4. The immunoprecipitates are collected after 30 s of centrifugation (10,000*g*) and washed twice in lysis buffer and twice in kinase buffer.
5. The immunoprecipitates are resuspended in 50 μL of kinase buffer in the presence of 200 μ*M* ATP and 2 μg of substrate protein: ATF-2 and ElK-1 fusion proteins for p38MAPK and ERK activity assays, respectively (*see* **Note 3**). The reaction mixture is incubated for 30 min at 30°C, and the reaction is terminated with 25 μL of 3X sample buffer.
6. The reaction mixture is incubated at 100°C for 5 min and briefly vortexed before centrifugation at 10,000*g* for 2 min.
7. The supernatant (30 μL) is loaded onto 12% 1D-SDS PAGE gels, electrophoresed and subjected to Western blotting, as described previously.

A

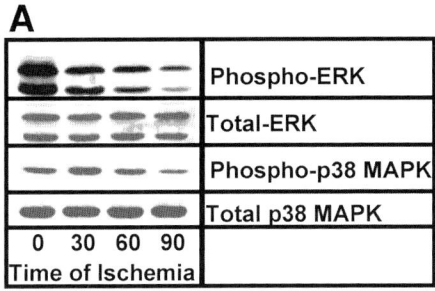

B

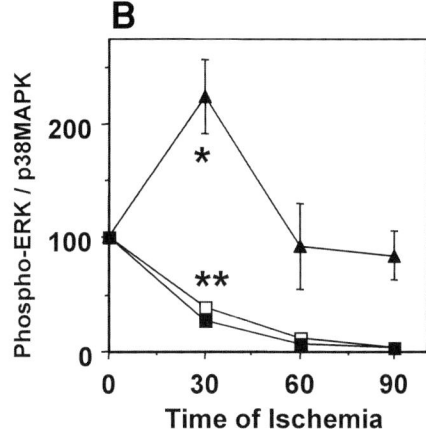

Fig. 2. MAP kinase dual phosphorylation in isolated cardiomyocytes. (**A**) Phosphorylation of ERK 1/2 and p38MAPK is observed at high and low levels, respectively, in oxygenated cardiomyocytes. (**B**) Ischemia significantly decreased ERK p44 and p42, (■ and □, $*p < 0.0001$ vs 0 min control, respectively, $n = 10$). Ischemia increased p38MAPK (closed triangle, $**p < 0.01$ vs 0 min control, $n = 4$). Ischemia did not induce the loss of total ERK1/2 or p38MAPK.

8. The blots are immunostained with phospho-specific antibodies to the substrate proteins: phospho-ATF2 (Thr71) or phospho-Elk1 (Ser383) for p38MAPK or ERK 1/2 activity assays, respectively, as described previously.

These assays use phospho-specific antibodies to determine the ability of an immunoprecipitated MAP kinase to phosphorylate a downstream substrate. The use of immunoblotting with phospho-specific antibodies to determine MAP kinase activation presumes that phosphorylation of the Thr-X-Tyr activation site directly relates kinase activity. However, it is conceivable that phosphorylation of negative regulatory sites on MAP kinases or the crossinhibition of MAP kinases by other signal transduction pathways (*20*) could modulate MAP kinase activity, independent of Thr-X-Tyr phosphorylation. Thus the basic presumption of the immunoblotting assay needs to be validated by kinase activity assays. The non-radioactive assays offer a convenient, specific, and nonhazardous method to determine MAP kinase activity.

3.2.1. Nonradioactive Assay of MAP Kinase Activity in Tissue

Adult rabbit myocardium was sectioned and subjected to various time intervals of in vitro ischemia. Myocardial sections were fractionated by homogenization in the digitonin buffer described above to produce a cytosolic fraction. The myocardial cytosolic fractions were immunoprecipitated and subjected to the nonradioactive kinase activity assay. The bands that were observed subsequent to immunostaining blots with phospho-specific or total MAP kinase antibodies were not as distinct and clear as observed with isolated cardiomyocytes, reflecting increased background and cellular heterogeneity in myocardial tissue (**Fig. 3A**). However, the resolution was sufficient to permit the quantitation of ERK or p38MAPK dual phosphorylation.

The results of the dual phosphorylation studies were compared with the kinase activities of myocardial ERK and p38MAPK as determined by nonradioactive assays (**Fig. 3B,C**). These comparisons demonstrate a correlation between the dual phosphorylation and kinase activities of myocardial ERK1/2 (**Fig. 3B**). In contrast to the dual phosphorylation of ERK1/2 in oxygenated cardiomyocytes (**Fig. 2B**), the dual phosphorylation and kinase activities of myocardial ERK1/2 was low in oxygenated myocardium and increased by 15 min of ischemia, with a subsequent decrease by 30–75 min. The explanation for this discrepancy will be resolved by future studies. The variance in the myocardial ERK1/2 kinase activity results during early ischemia was greater than that observed with the myocardial ERK1/2 and p38MAPK dual phosphorylation studies. The dual phosphorylation and kinase activities of myocardial p38MAPK were directly correlated in that the peak of dual phosphorylation and kinase activity peaked at 15 min of in vitro myocardial in vitro ischemia with a decrease by 30 min of ischemia (**Fig. 3C**).

In conclusion, immunoblotting studies with dual phospho-specific MAP kinase antibodies offer a convenient method to determine MAP kinase activation. The results of these studies can be verified by the nonradioactive kinase activity assays that are now available. These techniques will afford a clearer understanding of the role of MAP kinases in mast cell signal transduction and biological function.

4. Notes

1. The avidity of the phospho-specific antibodies is not as strong as polyclonal antibodies to the total protein. Thus it is important to minimize the washes to the 5-min, three times method described in **Subheading 3.1.4.** This is also the reason that bovine serum albumin is used in the antibody dilution buffer and the incubation period with the primary phospho-specific antibody is overnight at 4°C. This does not increase the background if blots are blocked with nonfat milk for only 1 h at room temperature. The background also is decreased by using nitrocellulose for Western blotting, although polyvinyldiene fluoride is a possible substitute.

2. It is important to expose the blots to X-ray film immediately after incubation in the Lumi-Glo buffer. The peroxidase conjugated secondary antibody catalyzes the breakdown of hydrogen peroxide (Reagent B) to free radicals that excites Luminol (Reagent A), producing light. This production of light peaks at 5 min after incubation and declines by 1–2 h.

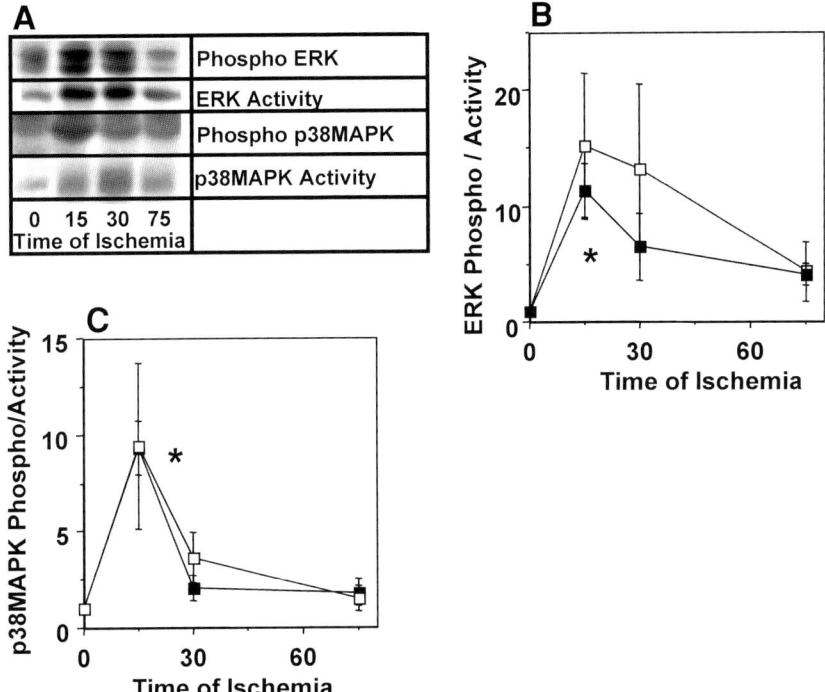

Fig. 3. MAP kinase dual phosphorylation and kinase activities in myocardial extracts. (A) A direct correlation between the dual phosphorylation and kinase activities of ERK1/2 and p38MAPK is observed in immunoblots of myocardial extracts. (B) The dual phosphorylation of ERK p44 was significantly increased by 15 min of ischemia (n, $p < 0.004$ vs 0 min control, $n = 5$). This increase in dual phosphorylation directly correlated to the increase in ERK kinase activity ($\square$, $n = 3$) as determined by a nonradioactive kinase activity assay. (C) The dual phosphorylation of p38MAPK was significantly increased by 15 min of ischemia ($\blacksquare$, $p < 0.03$ vs 0 min control, $n = 3$). This increase in dual phosphorylation directly correlated to the increase in p38MAPK kinase activity ($\square$, $n = 4$), as determined by a nonradioactive kinase activity assay.

3. In the nonradioactive kinase activity assay, it is critical that all components are ice cold. The immobilized anti-phospho MAPK antibody must be fully resuspended (gently vortex if necessary) and added with a large bore pipet tip (cut off the tip) inserted only to the top of the bead slurry. It is also essential to conduct the immunoprecipitation step overnight at 4°C. During the washings the pelleted immunoprecipitate must be fully visualized to verify the complete removal of wash buffer without disturbing the pellet. This step is particularly important after the last wash, before the addition of the reaction kinase buffer, ATP and substrate protein.

References

1. Raingeaud, J., Gupta, S., Rogers, J. S., et al. (1995) Pro-inflammatory cytokines and environmental stress cause p38 mitogen-activated protein kinase activation by dual phosphorylation on tyrosine and threonine. *J. Biol. Chem.* **270,** 7420–7426.

2. Lee, J. D., Ulevitch, R. J., and Han, J. (1995) Primary structure of BMK1: a new mammalian map kinase. *Biochem. Biophys. Res. Commun.* **213,** 715–724.

3. Abe, J., Kusuhara, M., Ulevitch, R. J., Berk, B. C., and Lee, J. D. (1996) Big mitogen-activated protein kinase 1 (BMK1) is a redox-sensitive kinase. *J. Biol. Chem.* **271,** 16,586–16,590.

4. Kato, Y., Tapping, R. I., Huang, S., Watson, M. H., Ulevitch, R. J., and Lee, J. D. (1998) Bmk1/Erk5 is required for cell proliferation induced by epidermal growth factor. *Nature* **395,** 713–716.

5. Azzolina, A., Guarneri, P., and Lampiasi, N. (2002) Involvement of p38 and JNK MAPKs pathways in Substance P-induced production of TNF-alpha by peritoneal mast cells. *Cytokine* **18,** 72–80.

6. Olsson, N., Piek, E., Sundstrom, M., ten Dijke, P., and Nilsson, G. (2001) Transforming growth factor-beta-mediated mast cell migration depends on mitogen-activated protein kinase activity. *Cell. Signal* **13,** 483–490.

7. Chayama, K., Papst, P. J., Garrington, T. P., et al. (2001) Role of MEKK2-MEK5 in the regulation of TNF-alpha gene expression and MEKK2-MKK7 in the activation of c-Jun N-terminal kinase in mast cells. *Proc. Natl. Acad. Sci. USA* **98,** 4599–4604.

8. Garrington, T. P., Ishizuka, T., Papst, P. J., et al. (2000) MEKK2 gene disruption causes loss of cytokine production in response to IgE and c-Kit ligand stimulation of ES cell-derived mast cells. *EMBO J.* **19,** 5387–5395.

9. Stassen, M., Muller, C., Richter, C., et al. (2003) The streptococcal exotoxin streptolysin O activates mast cells to produce tumor necrosis factor alpha by p38 mitogen-activated protein kinase- and protein kinase C-dependent pathways. *Infect. Immun.* **71,** 6171–6177.

10. Masuda, A., Yoshikai, Y., Aiba, K., and Matsuguchi, T. (2002) Th2 cytokine production from mast cells is directly induced by lipopolysaccharide and distinctly regulated by c-Jun N-terminal kinase and p38 pathways. *J. Immunol.* **169,** 3801–3810.

11. Zhou, B. and Zhang, Z. Y. (2002) The activity of the extracellular signal-regulated kinase 2 is regulated by differential phosphorylation in the activation loop. *J. Biol. Chem.* **277,** 13,889–13,899.

12. Jiang, Y., Li, Z., Schwarz, E. M., et al. (1997) Structure-function studies of p38 mitogen-activated protein kinase. Loop 12 influences substrate specificity and autophosphorylation, but not upstream kinase selection. *J. Biol. Chem.* **272,** 11,096–11,102.

13. Burack, W. R. and Sturgill, T. W. (1997) The activating dual phosphorylation of MAPK by MEK is nonprocessive. *Biochemistry* **36,** 5929–5933.

14. Boyevitch, M. A., Gillespie-Brown, J., Ketterman, A. J., et al. (1996) Stimulation of stress-activated mitogen-activated protein kinase subfamilies in perfused heart.

p38/RK mitogen-activated protein kinases and c-Jun N-terminal kinases are activated by ischemia/reperfusion. *Circ. Res.* **79,** 162–173.

15. Yung, Y., Dolginov, Y., Yao, Z., et al. (1997) Detection of ERK activation by a novel monoclonal antibody. *FEBS Lett.* **408,** 292–296.
16. Armstrong, S. C., Delacey, M., and Ganote, C. E. (1999) Phosphorylation state of hsp27 and p38 MAPK during preconditioning and protein phosphatase inhibitor protection of rabbit cardiomyocytes. *J. Mol. Cell. Cardiol.* **31,** 555–567.
17. Bou, G., Villasis-Keever, A., and Paya, C. V. (2003) Detection of JNK and p38 activation by flow cytometry analysis. *Anal. Biochem.* **317,** 147–155.
18. Mizukami, Y., Yoshioka, K., Morimoto, S., and Yoshida, K. (1997) A novel mechanism of JNK1 activation. Nuclear translocation and activation of JNK1 during ischemia and reperfusion. *J. Biol. Chem.* **272,** 16,657–16,662.
19. Raviv, Z., Kalie, E., and Seger, R. (2004) MEK5 and ERK5 are localized in the nuclei of resting as well as stimulated cells, while MEKK2 translocates from the cytosol to the nucleus upon stimulation. *J. Cell. Sci.* **117,** 1773–1784.
20. Zhang, H., Shi, X., Hampong, M., Blanis, L., and Pelech, S. (2001) Stress-induced inhibition of ERK1 and ERK2 by direct interaction with p38 MAP kinase. *J. Biol. Chem.* **276,** 6905–6908.

13

Microarray and Gene-Clustering Analysis

Tsung-Hsien Tsai, Denise M. Milhorn, and Shau-Ku Huang

Summary

Human mast cells are capable of secreting a plethora of inflammatory mediators and cytokines that may play a pivotal role in innate immune and inflammatory responses. Activation of mast cells by antigen and immunoglobulin E (IgE) results in signaling, gene expression, and expression of inflammatory mediators. Although a variety of techniques have been used to evaluate mast cell biology, recent advances in molecular techniques have provided unprecedented tools to study these cells. The complimentary deoxyribonucleic acid (DNA) oligonucleotide microarray, or DNA-chip technology, allows simultaneous monitoring of gene expression, provides a format for identifying genes as well as changes in their activity on a whole genome scale, and potentially offers a global view of pathophysiologic changes. This chapter reviews the use of DNA-chip technology in studying the expression of genes (transcriptional profiling) in activated human mast cells obtained from cultured cord blood-derived mononuclear cells and comments on the use of bioinformatics on analysis of gene expression. The most powerful applications of transcriptional profiling involve identification of the common patterns of gene expression across many experiments using various gene-clustering analyses. Several techniques have been used for the analysis of gene-expression data including hierarchical clustering and self-organizing maps. In this chapter, a general laboratory protocol for array analysis currently being used in our laboratory and the use of bioinformatics is discussed. Although the focus is on Affymetrix oligonucleotide arrays, the techniques described are generally applicable to expression data generated using other array formats.

Key Words: Mast cells; inflammation; oligonucleotide array sequence analysis; computational biology; cytokines; chemokines.

1. Introduction

Accumulated evidence has indicated that highly interactive molecular networks are involved in mast cell function. The regulation of mast cell function involves gene expression for components of receptors, signal transduction pathways, and modulators of transcription and translation. Thus, the identification

From: *Methods in Molecular Biology, vol. 315: Mast Cells: Methods and Protocols*
Edited by: G. Krishnaswamy and D. S. Chi © Humana Press Inc., Totowa, NJ

of genes associated with mast cell activation and characterization of their expression patterns across the whole genome will be significant in our understanding of the role of mast cells in normal physiology and in disease. Recently, new approaches, as a form of functional genomics, have been developed that allow for the analyses of gene expression patterns and their functions on a genome-wide scale. These include complementary deoxyribonucleic acid (cDNA) and oligonucleotide arrays *(1,2)*, a method involving serial analysis of gene expression (SAGE *[3]*), and differential display *(4)*. The cDNA oligonucleotide microarray or DNA-chip technology allows the simultaneous monitoring of gene expression, provides a format for identifying genes as well as changes in their activity on a whole genome scale, and potentially offers a global view of pathophysiologic changes. Two recent studies have been informative in categorizing genes in a rat mast cell line *(5)*, RBL, and in an interleukin (IL)-3-dependent human mast cell line *(6)*. Furthermore, human primary mast cells only recently have been studied for profiling gene expression in unstimulated mast cells using microarray analyses *(7)* and SAGE *(8)*, with an effort towards construction of mast cell transcriptome *(9)*.

Gene microarray analysis typically has been used to identify differential gene expression using a postnormalization cut-off and hybridization signal ratios to search for those that are consistently either up- or downregulated, usually following a simple statistical analysis of gene-expression levels. The most powerful applications of transcriptional profiling involve identification of the common patterns of gene expression across many experiments using various gene-clustering analyses *(10)*. Several techniques have been used for the analysis of gene-expression data, including hierarchical clustering *(11)* and self-organizing maps (SOM *[12]*). The premise of these clustering techniques is based on current understanding of cellular processes, in which genes belonging to a particular pathway tend to be coregulated and consequently show similar patterns of expression. Thus, identifying patterns of gene expression and grouping genes into expression classes might provide much greater insight into their biological function and relevance.

During the past few years we have performed experiments to demonstrate the utility of this technology in profiling differential gene expression using human T cells *(13)* and mast cells. Additionally, using Affymetrix array, we have performed studies of differential gene expression in the bronchial alveolar lavages of asthmatic subjects and in the peripheral blood mononuclear cells of subjects after allergen immunotherapy. In our experience, a successful analysis of gene expression requires the use of various laboratory protocols and access to relevant database and software tools to provide efficient data collection and analysis. Although several detailed laboratory protocols have been published *(14,15)*, the computational tools necessary to analyze the data are evolving and no clear consensus exists as to the best method for revealing patterns of gene expression. The purpose of this chapter is to provide a general laboratory protocol for microarray analysis that is currently being used in our laboratory. Although the focus is on Affymetrix oligonucleotide arrays, the techniques described are generally applicable to expression data generated using other array formats.

2. Materials

1. M-MLV reverse transcriptase (M-MLV RT; 200 U/μL).
2. T7-oligo (dT)$_{24}$ promoter primer 10 μ*M*.
3. DNA polymerase I, DNA ligase, T4 DNA polymerase.
4. T7 RNA polymerase.
5. Biotin-11-CTP, biotin-16-UTP.
6. 5X fragmentation buffer: 200 m*M* Tris-acetate, pH 8.1, 500 m*M* potassium acetate, 150 m*M* magnesium acetate.
7. Herring sperm DNA (10 mg/mL).
8. Acetylated BSA (50 mg/mL).
9. 20X eukaryotic hybridization control.

3. Methods

3.1. RNA Amplification of Human Mast Cells

Human mast cells are generated from umbilical cord mononuclear cells (*see* **Note 1**) and ribonucleic acid (RNA) is isolated. In most of our study samples, only a small amount of total RNA (*see* **Note 2**) from each sample is available, and very often the array analysis requires a large amount (10–20 μg) of good-quality total RNA per hybridization experiment. To increase the yield of total RNA, we usually began with 1–5 μg of total RNA for the first-strand cDNA synthesis. The cDNA synthesized from each preparation is used as a template to make a biotinylated RNA probe through in vitro transcription (T7 Megascript System or MessageAmp™ aRNA kit, Ambion). The unincorporated nucleotides are removed, and biotin-labeled cRNA is fragmented into 35–200 bases in size. The oligonucleotide-based Affymetrix GeneChip array is then used for analysis of gene expression, which currently allows analysis of 38,500 genes and ESTs (Affymetrix Human genome U133 Plus 2.0). For the differential gene expression analysis, the methods provided by the manufacturer (Affymetrix, Santa Clara, CA) for the preparation of cRNA and subsequent steps leading to the hybridization and scanning of GeneChip arrays are used.

3.1.1. Synthesis of First-Strand cDNA (ss-cDNA)

1. Place up to 5 μg of total RNA in a tube.
2. Add 1 μL of 10 μ*M* oligo-dT primer containing a T7 promoter sequence.
3. Add nuclease-free water to bring the final volume of 12 μL.
4. Mix briefly and quick spin.
5. Heat mixture for 10 min at 70°C.

6. Centrifuge briefly and quick chill on ice. Add: 2 μL 10X First-strand buffer; 1 μL of ribonuclease inhibitor (10 U/μL); 4 μL of dNTP mix; 1 μL of M-MLV RT.
7. Incubate mixture for 2 h at 42°C.

3.1.2. Synthesis of Second-Strand cDNA (ds-cDNA)

1. Centrifuge briefly the first-strand cDNA sample and put on ice. Add: 63 μL of nuclease-free water; 10 μL of 10X Second-Strand Buffer; 4 μL of dNTP Mix; 2 μL of DNA polymerase; 1 μL of RNase H.
2. Incubate mixture for 2 h at 16°C.

3.1.3. cDNA Cleanup

1. Place a filter cartridge in a 2-mL microcentrifuge tube, add 50 μL of cDNA binding buffer, and incubate at room temperature for 5 min.
2. Add 250 μL of cDNA binding buffer to each DNA sample, mix thoroughly by repeated pipetting, and apply mixture to an equilibrated cDNA filter cartridge.
3. Centrifuge for 1 min at 10,000g.
4. Discard the flow through and replace the filter cartridge into the tube.
5. Apply 500 μL of cDNA wash buffer to each filter cartridge and centrifuge 1 min at 10,000g.
6. Discard flow through and spin an additional minute.
7. Transfer filter cartridge to a fresh elute tube.
8. Add 10 μL of preheated nuclease free water to the center of the filter and let stand at room temperature for 2 min.
9. Centrifuge for 1.5 min at 10,000g.
10. Repeat **steps 8** and **9**.

3.2. Generation of Hybridization Probes

3.2.1. Prepare Biotin Labeling Antisense RNA (aRNA)

1. Add 7.5 μL of 10 μM biotin-11-CTP and 7.5 μL of 10 μM biotin-16-UTP to the eluted dscDNA.
2. Concentrate the mixture in a vacuum centrifuge concentrator until the volume is reduced to 18 μL.
3. Set up the following 40-μL reaction mixture at room temperature by adding the following reagents: 4 μL of 75 mM T7 ATP and T7 GTP solution; 3 μL of 75 mM T7 CTP and T7 UTP solution; 4 μμL of T7 10X reaction buffer; 4 μL of T7 enzyme mix.
4. Incubate the reaction for 6–14 h at 37°C.
5. Add 2 μL of DNase I (2 U/μL) to each reaction, mix, and incubate for 30 min at 37°C.

3.2.2. Clean Up Biotin-Labeling aRNA

1. Add 60 μL of aRNA elution buffer to each aRNA sample and mix thoroughly.
2. Add 350 μL of aRNA binding buffer to each aRNA sample and mix thoroughly.
3. Add 250 μL of 100% ethanol, mix thoroughly, and apply to the center of an equilibrated aRNA filter cartridge.
4. Centrifuge for 1 min at 10,000g.

5. Discard the flow through and replace the filter cartridge into the tube.
6. Add 650 μL of aRNA wash buffer to each filter cartridge and centrifuge for 1 min at 10,000*g*.
7. Discard the flow through and spin an additional minute at 10,000*g*.
8. Transfer the filter cartridge to a fresh 2-mL microcentrifuge tube.
9. Apply 50 mL of preheated nuclease-free water to the center of the filter, let stand at room temperature for 2 min.
10. Centrifuge for 1 min at 10,000*g*.
11. Repeat **steps 9** and **10**.
12. Quantify aRNA concentration by UV absorbance.

3.2.3. Fragmenting the aRNA for Target Preparation

1. Add 20 μg of aRNA (volume from 1 to 32 μL).
2. Add 8 μL of 5X fragmentation buffer.
3. Add nuclease-free water to bring the final volume 40 μL.
4. Mix thoroughly and incubate the mixture for 35 min at 94°C.
5. Quick spin and place on ice.
6. Run 2 μL of the reaction mixture on 1.5% agarose gel for checking fragmentation efficiency.

3.3. aRNA Hybridization

1. Add 15 μg of fragmented aRNA to a tube.
2. Add 5 μL of control oligonucleotide B2 (3 n*M*).
3. Heat 20X eukaryotic controls to 65°C and add 15 μL of dissolved 20X eukaryotic controls (bioB, bioC, bioD, cre).
4. Add 3 μL of Herring sperm DNA (10 mg/mL).
5. Add 3 μL of acetylated BSA (50 mg/mL).
6. Add 150 μL of 2X hybridization buffer.
7. Add water to a final volume of 300 μL.
8. Heat at 99°C for 5 min.
9. Lower temperature to 45°C and incubate for an additional 5 min.
10. Spin at maximal speed for 5 min.
11. Store the reaction cocktail at −20°C until ready for hybridization.

3.4. Preparation of Affymetrix Gene Chip and Hybridization

1. Remove the Affymetrix chip from 4°C and bring it to room temperature for 10 min.
2. Add 1X hybridization buffer to wet the chip.
3. Put the chip into the hybridization oven and rotate at 0.2358*g* for 5 min.
4. Remove the chip from the hybridization oven.
5. Add 250 μL of hybridization mixture to the chip.
6. Place chip to rotisserie box in 45°C and rotate at 0.2358*g* for 16 h to hybridize.
7. After hybridization, wash the probe array 10 times with a non-stringent buffer at 25°C, followed by four washes with a stringent buffer at 50°C (following Affymetrix protocol program of the fluidics station).

8. After the washes, the hybridization array is stained with 6 µL of streptavidin-phycoerythrin (10 µg/mL) for 30 min at 25°C, and then washed 10 times with a nonstringent buffer at 25°C.

3.5. Data Analysis

3.5.1. Data Collection and Normalization

1. The probe arrays are scanned using a confocal scanner with a 560-nm long-pass filter supplied with the Affymetrix system.
2. The array images are analyzed to identify the arrayed spots and to measure the relative intensities for each element (*see* **Note 3**).The data from each hybridization experiment are processed using Affymetrix GENECHIP 5.0 software, provided by the manufacturer. Most commercially available array scanner manufacturers provide image-processing software.
3. After processing the image, it is necessary to normalize the relative hybridization intensities. Normalization adjusts for differences in labeling and detection efficiencies for the probes and differences in the quantity of initial RNA from the samples examined in the assay (*see* **Note 4**).

3.5.2. Comparing Expression Data

1. Before data analysis, the normalized intensity requires adjustment for subsequent analysis. First, for relatively stringent criteria to exclude artifacts near background range, all genes with a signal less than threefold over the background are eliminated. This step is arbitrary, and there is no absolute cut-off point for background adjustment.
2. Fulfilling these criteria, genes are then selected and subjected to statistical analysis. To distinguish gene expression patterns, genes that are differentially regulated are selected based on the analysis of the paired *t* test to calculate statistical significance.
3. After normalization and adjustment for the background, the data for each gene are typically reported as an expression ratio (generally with log transformation). Most published studies have used a post-normalization cut-off of twofold increase or decrease to define differential expression. Although there is no firm theoretical basis for selecting this level as significant, this threshold is determined by the limits of the current technology and represents a reproducible and reliable a cut-off point for selecting genes whose expression can be validated by other techniques (e.g., real-time PCR).

3.5.3. Clustering Analysis

1. Although the expression ratios often reveal some expression patterns in the data, they remove all information about the absolute gene-expression level. The true power of microarray analysis comes from the analysis of many hybridizations to identify common patterns of gene expression. It is assumed that genes belonging to a particular pathway tend to be co-regulated, and consequently, show similar

patterns of expression. To accomplish this type of analysis, there has been development of several algorithms and methods, generally referred to as "Cluster analysis." Two commonly used are "Hierarchical clustering" and "Self-organizing maps" (*see* **Note 5**).

2. In some microarray experiments, an additional adjustment or re-scaling is needed to control for the significant variability in the intensity value among different genes, some of which may dominate and obscure the difference. One method to circumvent this problem is to re-scale the intensity of each gene, so that the average expression of each gene is zero. In this process, the basal expression level of a gene is subtracted from each measurement, thereby enhancing the variation of the expression pattern of each gene across experiments without regard to whether the gene is up- or downregulated. This is particularly useful for the analysis of time-course experiments (*see* **Note 6**).

4. Notes

1. Human mast cells were generated from umbilical cord mononuclear cells by established techniques *(16)*. Cord blood-derived mast cells (CBDMCs) were generated from freshly isolated cord blood collected with patient consent and institutional review board approval. The blood was diluted 1:1 with phosphate-buffered saline (PBS), layered over Lymphoprep, centrifuged, and washed with PBS. The cells were then grown in DMEM F12 media supplemented with 20% fetal bovine serum (Atlanta Biologicals, Atlanta, GA); $5 \times 10^{-5} M$ 2-mercapto-ethanol (Fisher, Pittsburgh, PA); 0.5 mL of insulin-transferin-sodium selenite solution (Sigma-Aldrich, St. Louis, MO); 25 mM HEPES (Gibco, Carlsbad, CA); 300 nM prostaglandin E_2 (Cayman, Ann Arbor, MI); 100 ng/mL recombinant human IL-6 (kindly provided by Amgen, Thousand Oaks, CA); and 80 ng/mL stem cell factor (kindly provided by Amgen) for about 16 wk or until mature. We observed the maturity of the CBDMCs by using anti-chymase and anti-tryptase antibody staining. Crosslinking of FcεRI on the surfaces of CBDMCs was performed using myeloma IgE at 1 µg/mL and anti-IgE at 1.5 µg/mL. IgE was added overnight at 37°C before the addition of anti-IgE.

2. For isolating total RNA, we commonly use a Qiagen kit, RNeasy, which in our experience generally yields a relatively high quality of RNA and is compatible with the subsequent array analysis. The RNA is quantified by spectrophotometry and stored at –70°C. The integrity and accuracy of quantification of DNase I-treated RNA is assessed by ethidium bromide-formamide gel electrophoresis and observance of the 28s and 18s ribosomal RNA bands. In our experience, further purification of mRNA is not necessary because the use of a RNA-amplification strategy (see below) has proven to successfully enrich, linearly, the amount of mRNA from the original total RNA pools.

3. Each gene on the chip is assayed by measuring intensity resulting from hybridization to 11 oligonucleotide probe pairs; each pair consists of a perfect-match complement and a one-base mismatched variant to a gene-specific sequence. GeneChip software generates a mean intensity for each gene by first calculating

the difference between each of the perfect and mismatcyhed probe pairs and then averaging these differences across the gene-specific probe set, yielding an average intensity value for each gene. To ensure that the estimate of expression was not based on the biased representation of a few probe pairs, we only included genes that have seven or more positive probe pairs as a conservative limit. This approach assures positive intensity measures for all genes which we can accurately assess expression, and it eliminates those genes for which the chip does not provide reliable data. Intensity values are averaged across all good probe sets to provide a single measure for each gene.

4. There are three commonly used techniques that can be used to normalize gene-expression data from the array hybridization: (1) total intensity normalization: this is used based on the assumption that the quantity of the input mRNA is the same for the samples under comparison. It is also assumed that for the thousands of genes in the array, the changes should balance out so that the total quantity of RNA hybridizing to the array from each sample is the same; (2) normalization to housekeeping genes; and (3) normalization to an exogenous control that has been 'spiked' into the RNA before labeling. In addition to these methods, normalization using regression techniques *(17)* and ratio statistics *(18)* has been used, although this is not very common. The normalization factor is then used to adjust the data to compensate for experimental variability from the two samples under comparison.

5. Clustering algorithms sort the data and group genes together on the basis of their relative levels (normalized) of expression. Several clustering techniques have been applied to the identification of patterns in gene-expression data, most of which are hierarchical, and the classification has an increasing number of nested classes resembling a phylogenetic classification. The two most commonly used techniques are: (1) Hierarchical clustering; Hierarchical clustering is relatively simple and the result can be easily visualized, therefore, it has been widely used for the analysis of gene-expression data. Hierarchical clustering is an agglomerative approach to sort the expression profiles into different groups, which are further sorted into various subgroups until the process has been completed, forming a single hierarchical tree. (2) SOM; SOM is a neural network-based clustering approach, which assigns genes to a series of partitions on the basis of the similarity of their expression levels to user defined reference levels for each partition. In general, while these are powerful techniques, they are still subjective depending on the use of different algorithms and normalizations, which will yield different clusters. These techniques are still evolving, and at present the ultimate confirmation still rely upon the functional tests using molecular biologic means.

6. Microarray analysis offers a great opportunity to identify differential gene expression and the patterns of gene expression across different experimental conditions and on a genome-wide scale. Consequently, the use of this technique should be informative for the biological interpretation of genes and their functions. Although the technical aspects of this analysis, including the array design and format, have

been relatively well established, the analytical tools, such as clustering techniques, have not reached their maturity. The successful use of gene clustering techniques and various algorithms are still dependent on the particular methods used, the way in which the data are normalized, and the manner in which the similarity in gene expression is measured. Therefore, at present there is no single correct classification, and the application of more than one technique often is needed. It is expected that many new algorithms and software that are under development will provide much-needed bioinformatics tools for increasing the accuracy and efficiency of gene expression analysis. Finally, a standardized reporting format (the Minimum Information About a Microarray Experiment, or MIAME) *(19)*, involving sample collection, array hybridization, and data analysis, has been developed as a requirement for reporting array data in the literature, which has greatly facilitated data sharing and verification.

References

1. Lockhart, D. J., Dong, H., Byrne, M. C., et al. (1996) Expression monitoring by hybridization to high-density oligonucleotide arrays. *Nat. Biotechnol.* **14,** 1675–1680.
2. Schena, M., Shalon, D., Davis, R. W., and Brown, P. O. (1995) Quantitative monitoring of gene expression patterns with complementary DNA microarray. *Science* **270,** 467–470.
3. Velculescu, V. E., Zhang, L., Vogelstein, B., and Kinzler, K. W. (1995) Serial analysis of gene expression. *Science* **270,** 484–487.
4. Liang, P. and Pardee, A. B. (1992) Differential display of eukaryotic messenger RNA by means of the polymerase chain reaction. *Science* **257,** 967–971.
5. Cho, J. J., Vliagoftis H., Rumsaeng V., Metcalfe, D. D., and Oh, C. K. (1998) Identification and categorization of inducible mast cell genes in a subtraction library. *Biochem. Biophys. Res. Commun.* **242,** 226–230.
6. Chen, H., Centola, M., Altschul, S. F., and Metzger, H. (1998) Characterization of gene expression in resting and activated mast cells. *J. Exp. Med.* **188,** 1657–1668.
7. Nakajima, T., Matsumoto, K., Suto, H., et al. (2001) Gene expression screening of human mast cells and eosinophils using high-density oligonucleotide probe arrays: abundant expression of major basic protein in mast cells. *Blood* **98,** 1127–1134.
8. Kuramasu, A., Kubota, Y., Matsumoto, K., et al. (2001) Identification of novel mast cell genes by serial analysis of gene expression in cord blood-derived mast cells. *FEBS Lett.* **498,** 37–41.
9. Saito, H., Nakajima, T., and Matsumoto, K. (2001) Human mast cell transcriptome project. *Int. Arch. Allergy Immunol.* **125,** 1–8.
10. Quackenbush, J. (2001) Computational analysis of microarray data. *Nat. Rev. Genet.* **2,** 418–427.
11. Eisen, M. B., Spellman, P. T., Brown, P. O., and Botstein, D. (1998) Cluster analysis and display of genome-wide expression patterns. *Proc. Natl. Acad. Sci. USA* **95,** 14,863–14,868.

12. Tamayo, P., Slonim, D., Mesirov, J., et al. (1999) Interpreting patterns of gene expression with self-organizing maps: methods and application to hematopoietic differentiation. *Proc. Natl. Acad. Sci. USA* **96,** 2907–2912.
13. Li, X. D., Essayan, D. M., Liu, M. C., Beaty, T. H., and Huang, S. K. (1998) Profiling of differential gene expression in activated, allergen-specific human Th2 cells. *Genes Immunol.* **2,** 88–98.
14 Eisen, M. B. and Brown, P. O. (1999) DNA arrays for analysis of gene expression. *Methods Enzymol.* **303,** 179–205.
15. Hegde, P., Qi, R., Abernathy, K., et al. (2000) A concise guide to cDNA microarray analysis. *Biotechniques* **29,** 548–560.
16. Krishnaswamy, G., Hall, K., Youngberg, G., et al. (2002) Regulation of eosinophil-active cytokine production from human cord blood-derived mast cells. *J. Interferon Cytokine Res.* **22,** 379–388.
17. Hedenfalk, I., Duggan, D., Chen, Y., et al. (2001) Gene-expression profiles in hereditary breast cancer. *N. Engl. J. Med.* **344,** 539–548.
18. Chen, Y., Dougherty, E. R., and Bittner, M. (1997) Ratio-based decisions and the quantitative analysis of cDNA microarray images. *J. Biomed. Opt.* **2,** 364–374.
19. Brazma, A., Hingamp, P., Quackenbush, J., et al. (2001) Minimum information about a microarray experiment (MIAME)-toward standards for microarray data. *Nat. Genet.* **29,** 365–371.

14

Techniques to Study FcεRI Signaling

Yuko Kawakami, Jiro Kitaura, and Toshiaki Kawakami

Summary

Mast cells are the crucial effector cells for allergic reactions. They are activated through the aggregation of the high-affinity immunoglobulin E (IgE) receptor (FcεRI) with allergen and allergen-specific IgE. Tyrosine phosphorylation of FcεRI subunits and various signaling proteins is an initial triggering event, leading to the activation of several signaling pathways in mast cells. Much has been learned from analysis of mast cells derived from gene-targeted mice. Therefore, in this chapter we will first describe how to generate mast cells from mouse bone marrow cells and how to correct the genetic defect by retroviral transduction. Then, we will describe how to assess early activation events by measuring several protein–tyrosine kinases and serine/threonine kinases such as protein kinase B (= Akt), protein kinase C, and JNK. As signal transduction is highly dependent on protein–protein interactions, we will describe experimental details of co-immunoprecipitation methods that are used to confirm such interactions.

Key Words: Mast cell; FcεRI; Lyn; Fyn; Src; Syk; Btk; JNK; PKC; Akt; co-immunoprecipitation; retroviral transduction; in vitro kinase assay.

1. Introduction

Despite a recent flurry of articles indicating roles for mast cells in innate immunity, autoimmune disease models, angiogenesis, and chronic cardiac failure, immediate hypersensitivity and allergic diseases remain the most important focus in mast cell research (*1*). Because allergic reactions in these diseases are largely dependent on allergen and allergen-specific immunoglobulin E (IgE), the study of the effector cells that are activated by these allergy-triggering agents is central to our understanding of allergy. Mast cells (and basophils) are considered to be the major effector cell type. IgE is bound to the high-affinity IgE receptor, FcεRI, on the surface of mast cells, and IgE-bound FcεRI molecules are aggregated with multivalent allergen. The FcεRI expressed on mast cells consists of IgE-binding α subunit, a signal-amplifying β subunit, and two disulfide-bonded γ subunits with a signal-initiating capability (*2*).

From: *Methods in Molecular Biology, vol. 315: Mast Cells: Methods and Protocols*
Edited by: G. Krishnaswamy and D. S. Chi © Humana Press Inc., Totowa, NJ

Upon receptor aggregation, receptor-bound Src family protein tyrosine kinases (PTKs), such as Lyn and Fyn, are activated. Activated Src PTKs phosphorylate tyrosine residues in the immunoreceptor tyrosine-based activation motifs (ITAMs) in the β and γ subunits. Phosphorylation of ITAMs in the β and γ subunits creates the binding sites for Lyn and Syk (another PTK with two tandem SH2 domains upstream of its catalytic domain), respectively. These PTKs are activated and phosphorylate a variety of substrates, including adaptor proteins, enzymes (kinases, phosphatases, phospholipases), transcription factors, and cytoskeletal proteins. These phosphorylations eventually lead to the activation of several signaling pathways, such as phospholipase C/Ca^{2+}, Ras/mitogen-activated protein kinase, nuclear factor-κB, AP1, and NF-AT. Finally, coordinate activation of these pathways results in degranulation, synthesis and release of lipid mediators, and synthesis and secretion of cytokines and chemokines *(3,4)*.

Much of signaling networks has been figured out by analysis of mast cells derived from gene-targeted mice. Therefore, this chapter will begin with a description of how to generate mast cells from bone marrow cells *(5)*. Biological and biochemical phenotypes found in mast cells derived from gene-targeted mice can most definitively be ascribed to the lack of the gene by reconstituting the mutant cells with wild-type gene or complimentary deoxyribonucleic acid (cDNA). The current standard method of gene transduction in mast cells is retroviral transduction *(6)*. Therefore, we will describe our standard procedures for retroviral transduction. Although the research in FcεRI signaling deals with many classes of molecules, our description here will be focused on early activation events, that is, activation of PTKs of the Src, Syk, and Tec families and several serine/threonine kinases (PS/TKs). Because signal transduction often depends on protein–protein interactions, experimental details in co-immunoprecipitation will be depicted as well.

2. Materials

2.1. The Generation of Bone Marrow-Derived Mast Cells (see Note 1)

1. BMMC medium (600 mL): 500 mL RPMI1640 (GIBCO, Carlsbad, CA), 10% FCS (60 mL, not heat-inactivated, GIBCO), 40 mL D11* (~7%, IL-3), 2 m*M* L-Glutamine (6 mL of 200 m*M* solution, Calbiochem, La Jolla, CA), 0.1 m*M* nonessential amino acids (6 mL of 10 m*M* solution, GIBCO), 50 μg/mL Gentamycin sulfate (0.6 mL of 50 mg/mL solution, Calbiochem), 50 μ*M* 2-mercaptoethanol (0.6 mL of 50 m*M* solution, Sigma, St. Louis, MO).

2.2. Retroviral Transduction

1. sBMMC medium (600 mL): 438 mL RPMI1640, 15% FCS (90 mL, not heat-inactivated), 60 mL D11*, 2 m*M* L-Glutamine, 0.1 m*M* nonessential amino acids, 50 μg/mL Gentamycin sulfate, 50 μ*M* 2-mercaptoethanol, 50 ng/mL recombinant mouse stem cell factor (SCF).

2.3. FcεRI Stimulation

1. Tyrode's buffer: 112 mM NaCl, 2.7 mM KCl, 0.4 mM NaH$_2$PO$_4$, 1.6 mM CaCl$_2$, 1 mM MgCl$_2$, 10 mM HEPES, pH 7.94, 0.05% gelatin, and 0.1% glucose.
2. Anti-DNP IgE.
3. DNP$_{23}$-HSA.

2.4. Kinase Assays

1. Lysis buffer: 1% Nonidet-P40 (NP-40) lysis buffer: 1% Igepal CA-630 (Sigma; *see* **Note 2**), 20 mM Tris-HCl, pH 7.5, 0.15 M NaCl, and 0.1% NaN$_3$.
2. Inhibitors (all from Sigma): add inhibitors to the lysis buffer right before use. 1 mM Na$_3$VO$_4$, 1 mM phenylmethyl sulfonyl fluoride, 1 µg/mL aprotinin, 1 µg/ mL leupeptin, 1 µM pepstatin, 25 µM *p*-nitrophenyl *p*'-guanidinobenzoate, 2 mM NaF.
3. 5X sodium dodecyl sulfate-polyacrylamide gel electrophoresis (SDS–PAGE) sample buffer: 0.5 M dithiothreitol (DTT), 10% SDS, 0.4 M Tris-HCl, pH 6.8, and 50% glycerol.
4. PTK kinase buffer:
   a. –ATP buffer: 20 mM HEPES, pH 7.5, 10 mM MgCl$_2$, and 10 mM MnCl$_2$.
   b. +ATP buffer (for autophosphorylation): –ATP buffer, 0.1 mM cold ATP, and 10 µCi [γ-^{32}P] ATP (ICN; Irvine, CA)/reaction.
   c. +ATP buffer with substrate: the above buffer + 2 mg enolase/reaction.
5. Preparation of acid-denatured enolase:
   a. Thaw 100 µL aliquot of frozen enolase (2 mg/mL in H$_2$O; keep at –20°C).
   b. Add 100 µL of 50 mM acetic acid.
   c. Incubate at room temperature for 5 min.
   d. Add 50 µL of 1 M HEPES, pH 7.0.
   e. Keep at room temperature until use.
6. Akt kinase buffer:
   a. –ATP buffer: 20 mM Tris-HCl, pH 7.5, 50 mM MgCl$_2$, 1 mM DTT, 25 mM ethylene glycol-bis(2-aminoethylether)-*N,N,N'N'*-tetraacetic acid (EGTA), 5 mM Na-o-vanadate, and 1 mg/mL mycrocystin.
   b. +ATP buffer: –ATP buffer, 2 µg of crosstide (Upstate, Charlottesville, VA)/ reaction, 50 µM cold ATP, 10 µCi [γ-^{32}P]ATP/reaction.

2.5. Immunoprecipitation

1. Antibodies:
   - Anti-Lyn: Lyn (44)
   - Anti-Btk: Btk (M138)
   - Anti-Akt: Akt1 (C-20)
   - Anti-JNK1: JNK1 (C-17)
   - Anti-PKCα: PKCα (C-20)
   - Anti-PKCβI: PKCβI (C-16)
   - Anti-PKCβII: PKCβII (C-18)

(All antibodies are from Santa Cruz Biotechnology, Santa Cruz, CA).

2. Pansorbin (Calbiochem; La Jolla, CA).
3. Protein G PLUS-Agarose (Santa Cruz Biotechnology).
4. High salt wash buffer for coimmunoprecipitation: 1 M NaCl, 1% Triton X-100, and 10 mM Tris-HCl, pH 7.2.

2.6. Equipment

1. Culture flasks and tubes; all from BD Falcon.
2. Dissection kit: forceps, scissors, 10-mL syringes, and 26-gauge needles.
3. SDS-PAGE apparatus (Biometra/Labrepco, Horsham, PA).
4. Gel transfer apparatus (Amersham; Piscataway, NJ).
5. Liquid scintillation counter (Beckmann).

3. Methods

The methods described in **Subheading 3.1.–3.4.** will outline; (1) the generation of BMMCS from mouse bone marrow cells; (2) the genetic manipulation of BMMCS by retroviral transduction; (3) the measurement of PTKs and PS/TKs; and (4) a detailed procedure to detect protein–protein interactions by co-immunoprecipitation.

3.1. Generation of BMMCS

Here we describe our standard procedures for BMMC generation, which usually takes 4–6 wk (*see* **Note 1**). After this period, mast cells constitute more than 95% of live cells, as assessed by flow cytometry for positive expression of FcεRI and c-Kit. With this high percentage, the cells are ready for biological (e.g., assays for degranulation, leukotriene, and cytokine secretion), biochemical (e.g., kinase assays, phosphatase assays, GTPase measurement, and so on), genetic (e.g., cDNA transfection, siRNA, and so on), and pharmacological (e.g., inhibitors and activators) experimentations.

3.1.1. Day-by-Day Procedures

Day 1

1. Euthanize a mouse with carbon dioxide (CO_2). Drench the mouse in 70% alcohol to sterilize it.
2. Strip off the skin from one leg.
3. Holding the femur with the forceps, cut away as much of the quadriceps muscle as possible. Then cut the muscles behind the knee joint.
4. Bend the knee joint in the "unnatural" or "incorrect" direction to dislocate it. Cut off the lower leg at the broken knee joint.
5. Snip off a small amount of bone from each end to expose the bone marrow.
6. While holding the femur above the open small flasks (25 cm^2), take a syringe (with a 26-gauge needle containing 10 mL of BMMC media) and insert the tip of the needle into the exposed bone marrow.

7. Push the full l0 mL of media through the femur slowly and into the flask to wash out the cells and collect the drops in the flask.
8. Repeat **steps 2–7** with the other leg.
9. Store the flasks in a 37°C, 5% CO_2 incubator for 2 d.

DAY 3

1. Transfer each 10-mL culture from the small flask to a medium flask (75 cm²) containing 40 mL of BMDMC medium.

DAY 8

1. Transfer the cultures to 50-mL tubes.
2. Centrifuge the cells at 300g for 5 min and aspirate supernatant.
3. Resuspend the cells in an optimum volume of BMMC medium and transfer to a new flask (*see* **Note 3**).
4. Store the flasks in the incubator for 1 wk.

DAY 15 (1 WK LATER)

1. Change the media and flasks again.
2. Store the flasks in the incubator for 1 wk.

DAY 22

1. Change the media and flasks again.
2. Store the flasks in the incubator for 1 wk.

DAY 29

1. Change the media and flasks again.
2. The cells are now ready to use. At this point, BMMCs can be used for approx 2–3 more weeks.

3.2. Retroviral Transduction of BMMCS

This section can be divided into: (1) the construction of retroviral expression vector; (2) the generation of recombinant retrovirus; and (3) the infection of replicating mast cells with recombinant retrovirus (*see* **Note 4**).

3.2.1. Construction of Retroviral Vector

A Moloney murine leukemia virus-based vector, pMX-puro (*8,9*), has been extensively used for transfection of mouse BMMC. As almost all gene-targeted mice have a "neo" gene cassette in their genome, the retroviral vector must have a different drug-resistance gene, such as the puromycin resistance gene or another way of selection, for example, a green fluorescent protein gene in the bicistronic gene expression allele. The expression of the latter can be detected by flow cytometry or fluorescent microscopy. The most popular vector, pMX-puro (**Fig. 1**), can accommodate a gene or cDNA in the region

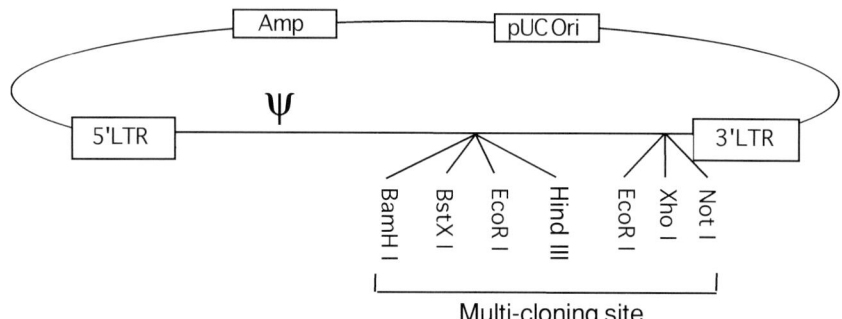

Fig. 1. The most popular vector, pMX-puro (the original figure was kindly provided by Dr. Toshio Kitamura of the University of Tokyo), can accommodate a gene or cDNA in the region between the BamHI (nucleotide 1884) and NotI (nucleotide 3161) sites.

between the Bam HI (nucleotide 1884) and Not I (nucleotide 3161) sites. Standard molecular biological techniques are used to construct recombinant vectors.

3.2.2. Generation of Recombinant Retrovirus

Recombinant retroviral vectors can be transfected into a packaging cell line to generate infectious virus particles. There are several packaging cell lines available for this purpose: for example, BOSC 23 *(10)*, Phoenix *(11)*, and Plat-E *(12)*. Our experience indicates that all of these packaging cell lines yield titers of viruses high enough to produce transfected BMMC in a scale of 5 to 20×10^7 cells after puromycin selection. These numbers of transfectants allow for most of biological and some biochemical analyses. In this section, we will describe our standard protocol using BOSC 23 cells.

3.2.3. Infection of Mast Cells and Selection of Transgene-Expressing Cells

Retroviral genomes can integrate into a host genome only when host cells are replicating. Although IL-3 usually is used as a growth factor to generate BMMC, IL-3 alone is not strong enough to induce vigorous cell cycling for efficient retroviral transduction in BMMC. For this purpose we and others feed bone marrow cells in IL-3 and SCF to generate BMMC that are ready for retroviral infection (hereafter abbreviated as sBMMC).

3.2.4. Day-by-Day Procedures

APPROXIMATELY 10 DAYS BEFORE TRANSFECTION

1. Reconstitute a vial of frozen BOSC 23 cells in DMEM/10% FCS/Gln.

2 Days Later

1. Change medium to GPT selection medium. GPT selection medium: Dulbecco's modified Eagle's medium (DMEM), 10% FCS/Gln, and GPT Selection Reagent (the kit contains 500X mycophenolic acid and 100X aminopterin solution; Specialty Media, Phillisburg, NJ).

BOSC 23 Cells Passage

1. After BOSC 23 cells become confluent, passage every 3 or 4 days by three- to fivefold dilution.
2. Aspirate medium very carefully with Pasteur pipet and wash once with 5 mL of PBS.
3. Add 1 mL of trypsin–EDTA and incubate at room temperature for 1–2 min.
4. Add 3 mL of DMEM and pipet well to separate individual cells. It is very important to prevent cells from making cramps.
5. Centrifuge the cells.
6. Suspend in 8 mL of GPT medium per 100-mm dish.
7. Plate BOSC 23 cells homogenously. Pipet BOSC 23 cells well to prevent them from making cramps.

2 Days Before Transfection

1. Remove GPT selection medium from BOSC 23 cells 48 h before transfection and add DMEM/10% FCS/Gln.

1 Day Before Transfection

1. Plate $5.5–6.5 \times 10^6$ cells per 100-mm dish or 2×10^6 cells per 60-mm dish. For each transfection, prepare three plates/cell densities of 5.5×10^6, 6×10^6, and 6.5×10^6.

Day 1

1. Make DNA/Lipofectamine mixtures:
   a. Mix 10 µg of DNA with 0.75 mL of OPTI-MEM (Gibco) in a Falcon 2059 tube. Add 20 µL of Plus Reagent (Invitrogen) and incubate at room temperature (RT) for 15 min.
   b. Mix 30 µL of Lipofectamine reagent (Invitrogen) with 0.75 mL of OPTI-MEM (Lipofectamine cocktail).
   c. Transfer Lipofectamine cocktail to the DNA tube, mix, and incubate at room temperature for 15 min.
2. Add 4.5 mL of OPTI-MEM (final total volume: 6 mL/transfection).
3. Pick up BOSC cell plates of the best condition (~60% confluent).
4. Rinse BOSC cells once with 5 mL of OPTI-MEM and overlay the above described DNA-Lipofectamine complex solution (6 mL) onto the rinsed BOSC cells.
5. Incubate at 37°C for 5 h in a CO_2 incubator.
6. Add 6 mL of DMEM/20% FCS/Gln.

DAY 2

1. Replace the medium with 9 mL (per 100-mm dish) of fresh complete medium (DMEM/10% FCS/Gln) at 24 h after transfection.

DAY 3

1. At 48 h after transfection, collect the supernatant of BOSC cells and centrifuge for 5 min at 350g at 4°C to remove living cells.
2. Infection cocktail (10 mL): Supernatant of BOSC cells (8 mL), D11 (1 mL), FCS (1 mL), 0.15 mg/mL SCF (3.3 µL), and 4 mg/mL polybrene (freshly prepared; 25 µL).
3. Centrifuge 1×10^7 cells/tube sBMMC, remove supernatant, and suspend the cells in the 10 mL of infection cocktail.
4. Plate sBMMC cells into a 100-mm dish. After 8 h, add 10 mL of fresh sBMMC medium with 10 µg/mL polybrene.
5. Incubate 16 h in 5% CO_2 incubator.

DAY 4

1. At 24 h after infection, wash the cells, suspend in 25 mL of fresh sBMMC medium, and culture them in a 75-cm^2 flask (Falcon cat. no. 3111).

DAY 5

1. At 48 h after infection, start to select the cells with puromycin. Add 10 mL of puromycin-containing sBMMC medium to 25 mL of cell culture fluid (final puromycin concentration: 1.5 µg/mL).

DAY 8

1. At 3 d after selection, add 15 mL of sBMMC medium.

DAY 15

1. At 10 d after selection, remove 15–20 mL of supernatant and add 15–20 mL of fresh medium, including puromycin.

DAY 19

1. After 14–16 d of selection, the cells usually start to grow well, then select living cells using Ficoll as follows.
2. Collect the cells in a 50-mL tube. Spin down at 300g for 5 min.
3. Resuspend the cells in 6 mL of BMMC medium.
4. Overlay the cell suspension in a 15-mL tube containing 6 mL of Ficoll (Roche).
5. Spin at 300g for 15 min.
6. Save the live cells packed between Ficoll and medium and transfer to a 50-mL tube.
7. Wash the cells twice with 30 mL of BMMC medium.
8. Transfer the cells to a 75-cm^2 flask. Keep incubate for several more days in the selection medium.

2 Days Before Using the Cells for Experiment

1. Wash the cells twice with BMMC medium and remove puromycin.
2. Suspend the cells in sBMMC medium, and keep incubating until the day the experiment is performed.

The Day of Experiment

1. Wash the cells twice with BMMC medium to remove SCF from medium.
2. Incubate the cells in BMMC medium with or without IgE for 6–8 h (*see* **Note 5**).
3. Stimulate cells with antigen as described in **Subheading 3.3.2.**

3.3. FcεRI Stimulation in BMMC

3.3.1. Sensitization

1. Count mast cell numbers.
2. Transfer the cells to 200-mL centrifuge tubes or 50-mL tubes.
3. Spin down the cells at 300*g* for 5 min.
4. Resuspend the cells in BMMC medium to a density of 2×10^6/mL.
5. Add IgE to a final concentration of 0.5 µg/mL.
6. Incubate overnight in a CO_2 incubator.

3.3.2. Stimulation

1. Spin down the cells in a 50-mL tube for 5 min at 300*g*.
2. Wash once in Tyrode's buffer.
3. Resuspend the cells in Tyrode's buffer to 2×10^7 cells/mL.
4. Make 1-mL aliquots.
5. Add antigen (DNP-HSA) to a final concentration of 10–100 ng/mL.
6. Incubate at 37°C for predetermined periods (depending on the purpose of the experiment).
7. Spin down the cells and aspirate sup.
8. If you continue experiment, add an appropriate buffer to the pellet. Otherwise, freeze down the cells in dry ice and keep frozen at −80°C until use.

3.4. In Vitro Kinase Assays

Two representative methods will be described here: one is an assay on Btk, in which reaction products are analyzed by SDS-PAGE and followed by blotting, and the other is an assay on Akt, in which reaction products are blotted onto phosphocellulose filters followed by counting the radioactivity. Both methods can be adapted for other PTKs and PS/TKs using proper substrates and kinase reaction conditions (*see* **Note 6**). These methods are also easy to be adapted when different sources of enzyme, for example, purified or recombinant kinases, can be used in place of cell lysates.

3.4.1. Cell Lysis

1. Add 200 µL of lysis buffer (+ inhibitors) to the tube containing 2×10^7 cells (*see* **Note 7**).

2. Incubate on ice with occasional vortexing for 10 min.
3. Spin down the cells at 4°C for 12 min at 15,000g and save sup.

3.4.2. Measurement of Protein Concentration

1. Measure the protein concentration of cleared cell lysate using a Bio-Rad Dc Protein Assay kit following the manufacturer's protocol.
2. Calculate the protein concentration.
3. Make 0.2–1 mg (depends on the protein you want to immunoprecipitate) aliquots at 200–500 µL (make up with lysis buffer as needed).

3.4.3. Btk Kinase Assay

3.4.3.1. IMMUNOPRECIPITATION

1. To 1 mg of the lysate, add 4 µg of anti-Btk (M138) antibody.
2. Let sit on ice for 1.5 h.
3. Add 20 µL of Pansorbin to each tube and vortex at 4°C for 30 min.
4. Wash Pansorbin 4X with 1 mL of lysis buffer and 1X with 1 mL of Btk kinase buffer (–ATP).
5. Remove all sup using Pipetman.

3.4.3.2. KINASE REACTION

1. Add 20 µL of kinase buffer (–ATP) to the Pansorbin, mix well.
2. Let sit on ice.
3. Add 20 µL of kinase buffer (+ATP) and mix well by tapping.
4. Incubate at 30°C for 10 min.
5. Stop reaction by adding 10 µL of 5X SDS/DTT Sample buffer.

3.4.3.3. SDS-PAGE AND BLOTTING

1. Boil sample and load onto 8% SDS–polyacrylamide gel.
2. Run the gel overnight at approx 40 V.
3. Transfer the proteins to PVDF membrane (Millipore), dry the membrane, and then detect the kinase activity by autoradiography.

3.4.4. Akt Kinase Assay

3.4.4.1. IMMUNOPRECIPITATION

1. To 0.5 mg of the lysate, add 2 µg of anti Akt1 (C-20).
2. Let sit on ice for 1.5 h.
3. Add 20 µL of Protein G PLUS agarose and shake at 4°C for 30 min.
4. Wash the agarose 4X with 1 mL lysis buffer and 1Xwith 1 mL Akt kinase buffer (–ATP).
5. Remove the buffer exhaustively using 1-mL syringe with 30-gauge needle.

3.4.4.2. KINASE REACTION (SEE **NOTE 8**)

1. Add 15 µL of kinase buffer (– ATP) to the agarose, carefully mix by swirling the tube using tip of Pipetman (see **Note 9**).
2. Let sit on ice.

3. Add 10 μL of kinase buffer (+ ATP).
4. Incubate at 30°C for 10 min.
5. Stop reaction by adding 45 μL of ice-cold 10% trichloroacetic acid.
6. Spin at 8000*g* for 2 min.
7. Spot one third of the volume of the total reaction (23.3 μL) of sup to P81 phospho-cellulose filter squares (Upstate cell signaling solutions; 11.6 μL to each square, and use 2 squares/rxn).
8. Wash filters with 100 mL of cold 0.5% phosphoric acid for 5 min.
9. Repeat washes four times.
10. Wash once with 100 mL of acetone at room temperature.
11. Dry the filters at room temperature.
12. Put filters in a scintillation vial and measure Cerenkov counts.

3.5. Co-Immunoprecipitation

Protein–protein interactions can be studied by a variety of methods: the yeast two hybrid experiment has been used to identify a novel binding partner for many years. With the advent of proteomics techniques, a more recently invented method termed tandem affinity purification is used more often. Structural requirements for interactions between a given protein and its partner have been studied using "pull-down" methods with a precipitable affinity ligand incubated with cell lysates that express the binding partner or a purified, recombinant, or in vitro translated binding protein. A wide selection of affinity ligands, such as glutathione *S*-transferase (GST), hexahistidine, and maltose-binding protein, are available. However, interactions between endogenous cellular proteins are usually confirmed by co-immunoprecipitation of interacting proteins: a protein will be immunoprecipitated by a specific antibody, and immune complexes are analyzed by SDS-PAGE and followed by immunoblotting with an antibody to the interacting partner (*see* **Note 10**). What follows is the protocol used in our previous study *(13)*.

3.5.1. Co-immunoprecipitation of Btk and PKCβI

1. The cells are sensitized and stimulated as shown in **Subheading 3.3.**
2. Add 500 μL of 1% NP-40 lysis buffer containing inhibitors to 4–5 × 10⁷ cells. Incubate on ice with occasional vortexing for 10 min, centrifuge at 15,000*g* for 12 min, and save the sup.
3. Measure the protein concentration using Bio-Rad Dc Protein Assay kit following the manufacturer's protocol.
4. Preclear the lysate with Pansorbin. Add 20 μL of Pansorbin/1 mg of lysate and incubate at 4°C for 30 min on the shaker.
5. Spin down at 15,000*g* for 5 min and save the sup.
6. Add 5 μg of anti-Btk (raised in rabbit against mouse Btk carboxyl terminal peptide) or 5 μg of normal rabbit IgG to 2 mg of the precleared lysate, let sit on ice for 1.5 h. Use 5 μg of anti-PKCβI (C-16) for the protein kinase C (PKC) immunoprecipitation.

7. Add 25 µL of bovine serum albumin (BSA)-coated Pansorbin and shake at 4°C for 30 min (*see* **Note 11**).
8. Wash once with 1% NP-40 lysis buffer, once with high salt wash buffer, then twice with 1% NP-40 lysis buffer.
9. Remove all the washing buffer using Pipetman, then add 40 µL of SDS/DTT sample buffer.
10. Boil at 95°C for 3 min and load onto 8% polyacrylamide/Tris-SDS gel.
11. Transfer the protein onto PVDF membrane and blot against anti-PKC (C-16) or anti-Btk (C-20).

4. Notes

1. The number of BMMC obtained by our protocol widely varies from 5×10^6 to 4×10^8 cells per mouse, mainly as the result of the mouse strain: C57BL/6 and BALB/c mice tend to give lower numbers of BMMC whereas 129/SvJ mice give larger numbers. Mice with a mixed background of C57BL/6 and 129/SvJ give the greatest numbers of BMMC in our experience. Knockout of some genes might also affect mast cell generation. Although we use mouse IL-3 gene-transfected fibroblasts (D11) as a source of IL-3 for an economic reason, one can use recombinant IL-3 instead. Some laboratories use WEHI-3 culture supernatants as a source of IL-3. Previous optimization for IL-3 sources is required by culturing bone marrow cells. Similarly, a large amount of fetal bovine serum should be tested using bone marrow cells or IL-3-dependent mouse mast cell lines such as PT-18 or MC/9. The heterogeneity of mast cells generated in vitro as well as those in tissues has been well known *(14)*. BMMC generated in our standard protocol are "immature" mast cells with similarities to mucosal mast cells. When bone marrow cells or BMMC that have been generated in IL-3 are exposed to SCF for some time, the resultant mast cells become more "mature," with similarities to connective-tissue mast cells. Therefore, it will not be so surprising to note differences in phenotypes between BMMC and sBMMC. One should carefully assess whether an observed difference is the result of an effect of differentiation or genetic difference or simply a result of c-Kit (SCF receptor) signaling. One should also be cautious in interpreting data using RBL-2H3 rat mast cells because these cells have an activating mutation in c-Kit. *D11 is culture supernatant of IL-3 gene-transfected cells S15 72F-D11 *(7)*. Optimal amounts of D11 supernatant must be titrated by culturing IL-3-dependent mast cells, such as BMMC, PT-18, or MC/9.
2. NP-40 is not commercially available. Igepal CA-630 is recommended as the substitute for NP-40 by Sigma, and we have been using this without any problem.
3. The optimum cell concentration is approx 3×10^5 cells/mL.
4. Retroviral transduction of a transgene results in its integration into the host (sBMMC) genome. Although the integration event is thought to be a nonsequence-specific phenomenon, the randomness of integration may not be absolute. Regardless of the extent of randomness, the positional effect associated with transgene insertion is an inherent problem with retroviral transduction (be reminded of the recent leukemia/lymphoma complications in patients who received a gene

therapy). One way to avoid this problem is to use other vectors that do not involve transgene integration. Unfortunately, no systematic application of such vectors has been attempted with mast cells. However, a practical solution is to study mass populations of retrovirally transduced cells. Even using such populations of mast cells, one has to keep it in mind that the resultant cells might be skewed to have a growth advantage in SCF-containing media. We usually perform three or more transduction experiments before we draw a conclusion on the effect of gene knockout on a mast cell phenotype.

5. This sensitization protocol is different from the one described next. Because sBMMC begin to die from apoptosis 10–24 h after SCF depletion, one needs to shorten the sensitization time.

6. Most PTKs have an autophosphorylating capacity. Autophosphorylating activity is usually more robust in in vitro kinase assays than the activity to phosphorylate an exogenous substrate. It is generally assumed that autophosphorylating activity is correlated with endogenous substrate-phosphorylating activity. Traditionally, acid-denatured enolase has been used as an exogenous substrate for Src family PTKs. Enolase is also a substrate for Btk. Although several other substrates such as poly-(Glu-Tyr) and band III have been used for the same purpose, it is not known whether phosphorylation of these substrates in vitro faithfully reflects the activity of the tested kinase *in situ*. This question can be addressed by immunoblotting cell lysates by a phospho-specific antibody that detects an activated kinase (or an antibody that detects an inactivated kinase) and by confocal microscopic analysis of cells stained by a phospho-specific antibody. Synthetic peptides have been extensively used as a substrate for a variety of kinases, particularly PS/TKs. Phosphorylation of synthetic peptides can be quantified by SDS–PAGE and autoradiography or by counting the radioactivity of filter papers that are spotted with reaction mixtures. Unlike the latter method, SDS–PAGE analysis gives a higher level of confidence for results because the detected radioactive band can make sure the identity of the substrate. However, short peptides (<10 residues) cannot be analyzed by this method. Another potential problem is that some peptides contain more than one phosphorylatable residue. This could be particularly problematic when an enzyme source comes from a complex mixture of proteins such as cell lysates. Fortuitous co-precipitation of an unintended kinase might phosphorylate the peptide at an unintended residue.

7. 2×10^7 cells make approx 1 mg of lysate when lysed in 1% NP-40 lysis buffer.

8. Make samples in triplicate. To reduce the background, perform kinase assays without crosstide, and subtract the count from the one with crosstide.

9. Do not vortex or tap hard. The agarose beads will jump up and stick on the wall.

10. To perform a proper negative control precipitation is critical, given that non-specific bands are usually seen by immunoblotting total cell lysates even with preimmune sera. Our experience also indicates that antibody-precipitating media, such as Pansorbin, protein A agarose, and protein G agarose, precipitate from cell lysates numerous proteins that be detected by staining SDS-PAGE gels. Therefore, it is imperative to show negative control data. We believe such data are essential even when time course studies are carried out. Remember that some

proteins, such as PKC, are very sticky. How can you reduce the chance of fortuitous precipitations of your protein? Because of its unpredictable nature, there is no fixed way to solve this problem. Once you are faced with it, you can try several tricks: (1) change the precipitating media; (2) coat the precipitating media with BSA or gelatin; (3) change the lysis buffer from a mild detergent to a harsher detergent; (4) wash the precipitate with high salt buffer; or (5) a combination of these changes. These changes were all tried before we could generate the clean co-immunoprecipitation data on Btk–PKC interactions *(13)*.

11. Pansorbin usually is incubated with 1 mg/mL BSA during the preparation, but to reduce the nonspecific PKC binding, one needs to incubate Pansorbin with 10 mg/mL BSA in PBS for 30 min right before use, and wash 3X with PBS followed by washing with 1% NP40 lysis buffer.

References

1. Galli, S. J. and Lantz, C. S. (1999) Allergy, in *Fundamental Immunology* (Paul, W. E., ed.), Lippincott-Raven Press, Philadelphia, PA, pp. 1137–1184.
2. Kinet, J. P. (1999) The high-affinity IgE receptor (Fc epsilon RI): from physiology to pathology. *Annu. Rev. Immunol.* **17,** 931–972.
3. Turner, H. and Kinet, J. P. (1999) Signalling through the high-affinity IgE receptor Fc epsilonRI. *Nature* **402,** B24–B30.
4. Kawakami, T. and Galli, S. J. (2002) Regulation of mast-cell and basophil function and survival by IgE. *Nat. Rev. Immunol.* **2,** 773–786.
5. Kawakami, T., Inagaki, N., Takei, M., et al. (1992) Tyrosine phosphorylation is required for mast cell activation by Fc epsilon RI cross-linking. *J. Immunol.* **148,** 3513–3519.
6. Hata, D., Kawakami, Y., Inagaki, N., et al. (1998) Involvement of Bruton's tyrosine kinase in FcepsilonRI-dependent mast cell degranulation and cytokine production. *J. Exp. Med.* **187,** 1235–1247.
7. Yokota, T., Lee, F., Arai, N., et al. (1986) Strategies for cloning mouse and human lymphokine genes using mammalian cDNA expression vector. *Lymphokines* **13,** 1–19.
8. Onishi, M., Kinoshita, S., Morikawa, Y., et al. (1996) Applications of retrovirus-mediated expression cloning. *Exp. Hematol.* **24,** 324–329.
9. Kawakami, Y., Miura, T., Bissonnette, R., et al. (1997) Bruton's tyrosine kinase regulates apoptosis and JNK/SAPK kinase activity. *Proc. Natl. Acad. Sci. USA* **94,** 3938–3942.
10. Pear, W. S., Nolan, G. P., Scott, M. L., and Baltimore, D. (1993) Production of high-titer helper-free retroviruses by transient transfection. *Proc. Natl. Acad. Sci. USA* **90,** 8392–8396.
11. Grignani, F., Kinsella, T., Mencarelli, A., et al. (1998) High-efficiency gene transfer and selection of human hematopoietic progenitor cells with a hybrid EBV/retroviral vector expressing the green fluorescence protein. *Cancer Res.* **58,** 14–19.
12. Morita, S., Kojima, T., and Kitamura, T. (2000) Plat-E: an efficient and stable system for transient packaging of retroviruses. *Gene Ther.* **7,** 1063–1066.

13. Yao, L., Kawakami, Y., and Kawakami, T. (1994) The pleckstrin homology domain of Bruton tyrosine kinase interacts with protein kinase C. *Proc. Natl. Acad. Sci. USA* **91,** 9175–9179.
14. Wong, G. W., Friend, D. S., and Stevens, R. L. (1998) Mouse and rat models of mast cell development, in *Signal Transduction in Mast Cells and Basophils*, (Razin, E., and Rivera, J., eds.), Springer-Verlag, New York, NY, pp. 39–53.

V

MAST CELL EXPRESSION AND RELEASE
OF INFLAMMATORY MEDIATORS

15

Human Mast Cell Proteases

Activity Assays Using Thiobenzyl Ester Substrates

David A. Johnson

Summary

Human mast cells contain proteases that are important functional components and serve as markers of mast cell activation or degranulation. Although tryptase is the best recognized mast cell protease, chymase and Cathepsin G also are found in some human mast cells. Methods for measuring the activities of these enzymes using sensitive synthetic peptide thiobenzyl ester substrates are described in this chapter. Using a visible plate reader with kinetic software femtomole quantities of these proteases can be measured. These methods are demonstrated in assays of tryptase and chymase in cell-free extracts of the HMC-1 and 5C6 human mast cell lines, as well as in extracts of cord blood derived mast cells.

Key Words: Protease; tryptase; chymase; cathepsin G; activity assays; thiobenzyl ester substrate.

1. Introduction

Human mast cells contain three serine proteases in their granules that are released upon degranulation. Most, if not all, mast cells contain tryptase, and some mast cells also contain chymase (*1*). Additionally, cathepsin G, which is normally thought of as a component of neutrophils, also has been shown to be present in mast cells (*2,3*). The activities of these proteolytic enzymes add additional functions to the mast cell. Consequently, the measurement of these enzyme activities is critical to studying mast cell function. Both chymase and CatG are chymotrypsin-like enzymes and distinguishing between their activities is difficult. Although tryptase is the only trypsin-like protease in mast cells, CatG also cleaves synthetic peptide substrates used to measure tryptase (*4*). Consequently, one needs to understand the subtle differences in the activities of these three enzymes and their interactions with inhibitors to measure their

From: *Methods in Molecular Biology, vol. 315: Mast Cells: Methods and Protocols*
Edited by: G. Krishnaswamy and D. S. Chi © Humana Press Inc., Totowa, NJ

activities. For example, tryptase requires heparin for its activity. Although tryptase is very stable in solutions containing 2 *M* NaCl, it is rapidly inactivated in buffers of physiological ionic strength in the absence of heparin. Additionally, CatG is inhibited by heparin.

Tryptase β is a well-established marker of human mast cell activation or degranulation *(5)*, and measurement of its enzymatic activity provides a simple method of detecting this process *(6–8)*. Measurement of tryptase activity works well with purified mast cells, but one must be aware that other trypsin-like proteases may cleave the synthetic peptide substrate used to measure tryptase activity and interfere.

Protocols for the assay of each enzyme will be given along with information to aid in distinguishing the activity of each enzyme with a particular substrate. Although a number of para-nitroanilide and fluorescent peptide substrates have been used to assay mast cell proteases, thiobenzyl ester substrates are more sensitive than para-nitroanilide substrates and easier to use than fluorescent substrates. Castillo et al. *(9)* were the first to demonstrate the sensitivity and utility of peptide thiobenzyl ester substrates and they developed several very useful substrates for measuring protease activities. Proteases cleave thiobenzyl esters at much higher rates than para-nitroanilides, yet the thiobenzyl esters are far less sensitive to autolysis at alkaline pH than ethyl or methyl esters *(10)*. Additionally, the benzene thiol product reacts with 5,5' dithiobis (2-nitro benzoic acid) (DTNB), also referred to as Ellman's reagent, to yield a yellow product (NBS [2-nitro-5-thiobenzoate anion]) that has a molar extinction coefficient of 13,600 cm^{-1} at 410 nm. The chemistry of these reactions is shown in **Fig. 1**. The sensitivities of thiobenzyl ester substrates relative to para-nitroanilide substrates can be seen by comparing k_{cat}/K_m values (substrate specificity constants) for the same peptide substrates (**Table 1**). For chymase the k_{cat}/K_m value with Succinyl-Ala-Ala-Pro-Phe-para-nitroanilide is 1×10^6 $M^{-1}s^{-1}$, whereas with Suc-AAPF-SBzl it is 16×10^6 $M^{-1}s^{-1}$, making the later substrate 16-fold more sensitive. Fluorescent substrates for tryptase have been developed with a 7-amino-4-carbamoylmethylcoumarin (ACC) fluorescent leaving group *(11)*. The most specific of these substrates was *N*-acetyl-Pro-Arg-Asn-Lys-AAC (Ac-PRNK–ACC) with a reported k_{cat}/K_m of 1.23×10^6 $M^{-1}s^{-1}$, which is only slightly higher than 0.836×10^6 $M^{-1}s^{-1}$ found for the simple Z-Lys-SBzl *(12)*. However, it must be pointed out that Ac-PRNK–ACC has the advantage that it is not readily cleaved by other trypsin-like enzymes, such as thrombin. By choosing the most specific peptide substrates and by using inhibitors to block interfering activities it is possible to assay different mast cell proteases. As knowledge increases regarding the specificities of these proteases more specific substrates will be developed.

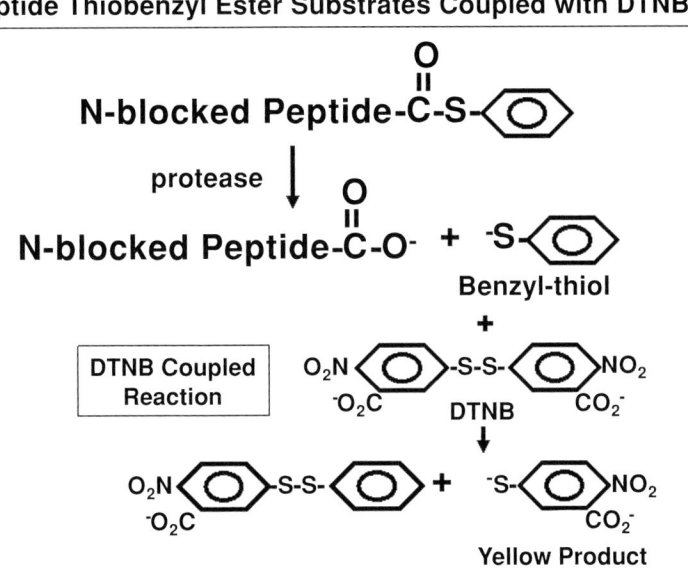

Fig. 1. The chemistry of thiolbenzyl ester substrate assays.

Table 1
Thiolbenzyl Ester Substrate Kinetic Constants

Protease	Substrate	k_m (μm)	k_{cat} (s^{-1})	k_{cat}/k_m $10^{-6} \times ^{-1}$s^{-1}	Ref
Tryptase	Z-K-SBzl	55	46	0.836	*(12)*
Chymase	Sus-AAPF-SBzl	22	363	16	*(27)*
Chymase	Suc-VPF-SBzl	48	400	8.3	*(28)*
CatG	Sus-AAPF-SBzl	48	14	0.3	*(27)*
CatG	Suc-VPF-SBzl	19	22	1.2	*(10)*

2. Materials

1. *N*-carbobenzoxy-Lysine thiobenzyl ester (Z-Lys-SBzl).
2. Succinyl-Ala-Ala-Pro-Phe-thiobenzyl ester (Suc-AAPF-SBzl).
3. DTNB.
4. Heparin.
5. Visible Plate Reader with kinetic capability at 405 or 410 nm.
6. Tryptase Assay Buffer: 0.1 *M* HEPES, 10% glycerol v/v, 0.1 mg/mL Heparin, 0.01% Triton X-100 v/v, 0.02% NaN$_3$ w/v, pH 7.5 (*see* **Note 1**).
7. 20 m*M* Z-Lys-SBzl; dissolve 17 mg in 2 mL of isopropyl alcohol (warming the tube in hot water aids dissolution; *see* **Note 2**).

8. 10 mM solution of DTNB; dissolve 40 mg in 10 mL of Tryptase Assay Buffer. The DTNB solution is stable for approx 1 wk when stored at 4°C, but if it becomes visibly yellow it should be discarded.

9. Tryptase Substrate Assay Solution; mix 0.87 mL of Tryptase Assay Buffer, 0.1 mL of DTNB solution, and 30 µL of the 20 mM Z-Lys-SBzl stock solution, along with 1 µL of octanol to prevent bubble formation (*see* **Note 3**).

10. Chymase Assay Buffer: 0.1 M HEPES, 1 M NaCl, 10% glycerol v/v, 0.1 mg/mL heparin, 0.01% Triton X-100 v/v, 0.02% NaN$_3$ w/v, pH 7.5. Because glycerol volumes are not easily measured, weigh 25 g of glycerol (density is 1.25 g/mL) into a 250-mL bottle on a top loading balance. Then add 150 mL of deionized water and mix before adding solids; 4.76 g of HEPES, 11.7 g of NaCl, 20 mg of heparin, 0.2 mL of 10% Triton X-100 in water, 40 mg of NaN$_3$, adjust pH to 7.5 with NaOH and dilute to 200 mL (*see* **Notes 1** and **4**).

11. 20 mM stock solution of the Suc-AAPF-SBzl chymase substrate; dissolve 12.2 mg in 1 mL of dimethylsulfoxide (DMSO; not soluble in isopropanol) and store at –20°C (*see* **Note 5**).

12. 10 mM solution of DTNB; dissolve 40 mg in 10 mL of Chymase Assay Buffer. The DTNB solution is stable for approx 1 wk when stored at 4°C, but if it becomes visibly yellow it should be discarded.

13. Chymase Substrate Assay Solution; mix 0.87 mL of Assay Buffer, 0.1 mL of DTNB solution, and 30 µL of the 20 mM Suc-AAPF-SBzl stock solution, along with 1 µL of octanol to prevent bubble formation (*see* **Note 3**).

3. Methods

3.1. Assay of Tryptase Activity

1. Pipet samples containing tryptase into microplate wells and dilute to 50 µL with Tryptase Assay Buffer.

2. Pipet 50 µL of buffer in Blank wells in place of sample.

3. Set up the plate reader software to read the desired plates at 405 or 410 nm in kinetic mode.

4. Set the plate reader to mix on high speed for 10 s prior to the first read. Readings at 410 nm are normally taken at 20-s intervals for 10 min.

5. Start assay reactions by quickly adding 50 µL of Substrate Assay Solution.

6. Readings at 405 or 410 nm are normally taken at 20-s intervals for 10 min, but these parameters can be adjusted based on the amount of enzyme present (*see* **Note 6**).

7. A plot of initial rates versus the amount of enzyme should be linear as shown in **Fig. 2**.

3.2. Assay of Chymase Activity

1. Follow the steps in **Subheading 3.1.** for assaying tryptase using the Chymase Substrate Assay Solution containing Suc-AAPF-SBzl and the Chymase Assay Buffer in place of the solution used to assay tryptase.

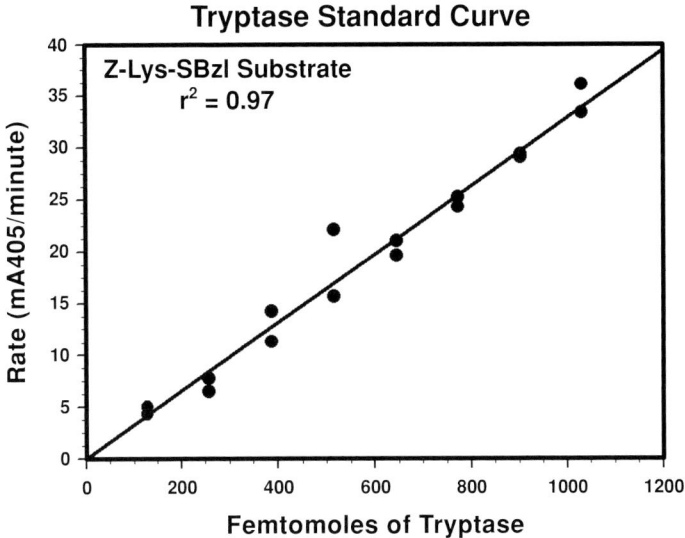

Fig. 2. Tryptase standard curve. Recombinant human tryptase beta was assayed using the Z-Lys-SBzl substrate as described. Rates were plotted against the amount of enzyme.

3.3. Application of the Assays to Human Mast Cells

1. The human leukemia mast cells lines HMC-1 *(13)* and a subclone of this cell line, designated 5C6 *(14)*, were analyzed for their content of tryptase and chymase activities. Cord blood-derived mast cells (CBDMCs) also were analyzed for these enzyme activities. The cells were generously provided by Drs. D. Chi and G. Krishnaswamy of East Tennessee State University *(15,16)*.

2. To measure the protease activities in cultured mast cells extracts of CBDMCs, HMC-1, and 5C6 cells were prepared. Preliminary work had shown that tryptase is very stable in high salt buffers at pH 6.1 and that Triton X-100, a nonionic detergent extracts additional tryptase and chymase activity from HMC-1 cells. Therefore, 10 mM MES; 2 M NaCl; 10% glycerol (v/v); 0.02% NaN$_3$, pH 6.1; with 0.1% Triton X-100 was chosen as the cell extraction buffer. One tube of each of HMC-1, 5C6 (10×10^6 cells each), and CBDMC (1×10^6 cells), which had been stored as frozen cell pellets, was suspended in 2 mL of cold extraction buffer. Cell suspensions were transferred to 10 mL of polypropylene tubes and homogenized using an Omni 2000 rotary tissue grinder at maximum speed for 10 s and placed on ice. The rotary tissue grinder breaks the cells and reduces the viscosity of the extracts by sheering the DNA. Homogenates were stored overnight at 4°C and soluble fractions were obtained by centrifuging the samples in the same 10-mL tubes in the Beckman R-20 rotor using rubber adaptors at 30,000g for 30 min. Each extract represented 5×10^6 cells/mL for HMC-1 and 5C6 cells and 0.5×10^6 cells/mL for CBDMCs. Assays for tryptase and chymase

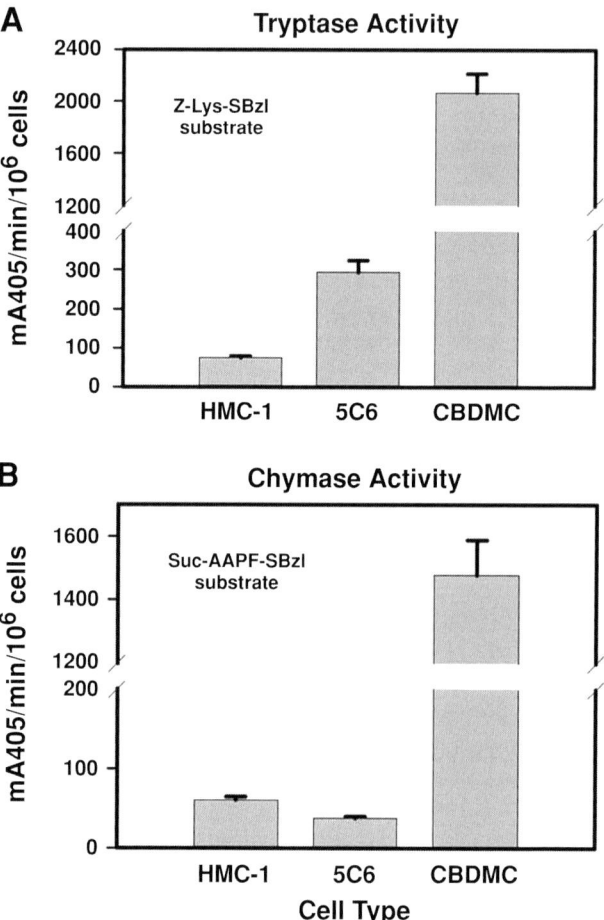

Fig. 3. Tryptase and chymase activities in mast cells. Extracts of two mast cell lines (HMC-1 and 5C6; 5×10^6 cells/mL) and CBDMC (0.5×10^6 cells/mL) were assayed for tryptase using Z-Lys-Bzl as described (**A**) and chymase using Suc-AAPF-SBzl (**B**) as described. Assays were performed in triplicate and the error bars are standard deviations from the mean.

activities were performed on 10–40 µL of extract, using the Z-Lys-SBzl substrate for tryptase and the Suc-AAPF-SBzl substrate for chymase. The results of these assays are shown in **Fig. 3A** and **3B**, respectively. Although CatG has been reported in human tissue-derived mast cells *(2,3)* and in the HMC-1 cell line *(17)*, the amount of CatG relative to chymase is unknown. Because, on the basis of their k_{cat}/K_m ratios, Suc-AAPF-SBzl is a 53-fold better substrate for chymase than for CatG, it can be concluded that most of the activity observed is attributable to chymase even if these chymotrypsin-like enzymes are present in equal concentrations. Additionally, HMC-1 cells seem to have much less CatG than chymase *(17)*, further indicating that the Suc-AAPF-SBzl substrate measures chymase, rather than CatG in this cell line. Although CatG activity might interfere with the measurement of tryptase and chymase activities, CatG does not cleave these synthetic substrates very rapidly and the amount of CatG in mast cells is probably low. Heparin is required for the stability of the active tryptase tetramer *(12,18)* and chymase is activated by heparin *(19)*. Whereas heparin has been shown to inhibit CatG *(20,21)*, the inclusion of heparin in the tryptase and chymase assay buffers would further reduce CatG activity.

3. Inhibitors can aid in distinguishing between different proteases, as demonstrated by Sheth et al. *(17)*, who used aprotinin (bovine pancreatic trypsin inhibitor; also known as Trasylol a product of Bayer, AG), which inhibits CatG, but not chymase. These workers also used a synthetic inhibitor of chymase called Y-40018 *(22)* that inhibits chymase by 100% and CatG by only approx 20%. As pharmaceutical companies develop new inhibitors of chymase and/or CatG as potential drugs, more specific inhibitors will become available. Tryptase is uniquely resistant to inhibition by the protease inhibitors present in human blood *(23)* and this property can be used to distinguish tryptase from other trypsin-like serine proteases.

4. As with any enzyme assay, running positive controls with known amounts of pure enzyme aids in standardizing the technique and for testing its application to the system of interest. Fortunately, recombinant human tryptase *(24)* is available from Promega (Madison, WI). Chymase and CatG purified from human tissues are commercially available, although recombinant forms not yet available. Active recombinant chymase has been expressed *(25)*, but there are no reports of recombinant CatG.

4. Notes

1. Because glycerol volumes are not easily measured, weigh 25 g of glycerol (density is 1.25 g/mL) into a 250-mL bottle on a top of a loading balance. Then, add 150 mL of deionized water and mix, before adding solids, 4.76 g of HEPES, 20 mg of heparin, 0.2 mL of 10% Triton X-100 in water, 40 mg of NaN_3, adjust pH to 7.5 with NaOH, and dilute to 200 mL. As mentioned earlier, heparin is required for tryptase stability, and we have found that glycerol also aids enzyme stability. Triton X-100 prevents the tendency of tryptase to bind to surfaces at lower ionic strengths.

2. Although Z-Lys-SBzl stock solutions can be prepared in DMSO, we have found that the substrate gives lower rates over time when stored in DMSO, whereas this does not happen when the isopropanol is used as the solvent. There was no indication that the substrate was hydrolyzing during storage in DMSO because the substrate buffer blanks did not increase during storage. Although we have not analyzed the chemistry associated with this loss of substrate function in DMSO, we do know that Z-Lys-SBzl is very stable in isopropaol.

3. The volume of Substrate Assay Solution prepared depends on the number of wells being used plus enough extra volume to allow pipetting. For example to assay 20

wells make up 1.2 mL of Substrate Assay Solution. A multichannel pipetor is useful for quickly adding the Substrate Solution when assaying a large number of wells, but there is more substrate wastage because extra volume must be in the buffer troughs used with multichannel pipetors.

4. The assay buffer for chymase is essentially the same as that used for tryptase with the addition of 1 M NaCl, which has been shown to increase activity *(26)*.

5. Suc-AAPF-SBzl has a 53-fold larger k_{cat}/K_m ratio for chymase than for CatG and the addition of heparin to the buffer activates chymase and inhibits CatG. Consequently, assays of mast cell extracts using the Suc-AAPF-SBzl substrate predominantly measure chymase with little interference from CatG.

6. Although we normally perform assays at room temperature (approx 22°C), higher temperatures, such as 37°C can be used. To obtain initial velocity measurements check the linearity of each reaction via linear regression. When the curves are not linear over the course of 10 min, initial velocities (or rates) usually can be obtained by using the data from the first 2 to 5 min. If the plots are not linear, repeat the assays using less enzyme (cell extract) so the initial velocities can be accurately determined.

Acknowledgments

The author is grateful for the assistance of Andrew Hull and Susannah Johnson, who performed portions of this work as part of their undergraduate research experiences. Appreciation is expressed to Dr. James Powers (Georgia Tech.) for introducing the author to thiolbenzyl ester substrates. This work was supported by NIH grant R15 AI45549.

References

1. Craig, S. S., Schechter, N. M., and Schwartz, L. B. (1989). Ultrastructural analysis of maturing human T and TC mast cells in situ. *Lab. Invest.* **60,** 147–157.

2. Schechter, N. M., Wang, Z. M., Blacher, R. W., Lessin, S. R., Lazarus, G. S., and Rubin, H. (1994). Determination of the primary structures of human skin chymase and cathepsin G from cutaneous mast cells of urticaria pigmentosa lesions. *J. Immunol.* **152,** 4062–4069.

3. Schechter, N. M., Irani, A. M., Sprows, J. L., Abernethy, J., Wintroub, B., and Schwartz, L. B. (1990). Identification of a cathepsin G-like proteinase in the MCTC type of human mast cell. *J. Immunol.* **145,** 2652–2661.

4. Polanowska, J., Krokoszynska, I., Czapinska, H., Watorek, W., Dadlez, M., and Otlewski, J. (1998). Specificity of human cathepsin G. *Biochim. Biophys. Acta* **1386,** 189–198.

5. Hogan, A. D. and Schwartz, L. B. (1997). Markers of mast cell degranulation. *Methods* **13,** 43–52.

6. Caughey, G. H., Lazarus, S. C., Viro, N. F., Gold, W. M., and Nadel, J. A. (1988). Tryptase and chymase: comparison of extraction and release in two dog mastocytoma lines. *Immunology* **63,** 339–344.

7. Kivinen, P. K., Kaminska, R., Naukkarinen, A., Harvima, R. J., Horsmanheimo, M., and Harvima, I. T. (2001). Release of soluble tryptase but only minor amounts of chymase activity from cutaneous mast cells. *Exp. Dermatol.* **10,** 246–255.

8. Lavens, S. E., Proud, D., and Warner, J. A. (1993). A sensitive colorimetric assay for the release of tryptase from human lung mast cells in vitro. *J. Immunol. Methods* **166,** 93–102.

9. Castillo, M. J., Nakajima, K., Zimmerman, M., and Powers, J. C. (1979). Sensitive substrates for human leukocyte and porcine pancreatic elastase: a study of the merits of various chromophoric and fluorogenic leaving groups in assays for serine proteases. *Anal. Biochem.* **99,** 53–64.

10. Powers, J. C. and Kam, C. M. (1995). Peptide thioester substrates for serine peptidases and metalloendopeptidases. *Methods Enzymol.* **248,** 3–18.

11. Harris, J. L., Niles, A., Burdick, K., et al. (2001). Definition of the extended substrate specificity determinants for beta-tryptases I and II. *J. Biol. Chem.* **276,** 34,941–34,947.

12. Addington, A. K. and Johnson, D. A. (1996). Inactivation of human lung tryptase: evidence for a re-activatable tetrameric intermediate and active monomers. *Biochemistry* **35,** 13,511–13,518.

13. Butterfield, J. H., Weiler, D., Dewald, G., and Gleich, G. J. (1988). Establishment of an immature mast cell line from a patient with mast cell leukemia. *Leuk. Res.* **12,** 345–355.

14. Weber, S., Babina, M., Kruger-Krasagakes, S., Grutzkau, A., and Henz, B. M. (1996). A subclone (5C6) of the human mast cell line HMC-1 represents a more differentiated phenotype than the original cell line. *Arch. Dermatol. Res.* **288,** 778–782.

15. Krishnaswamy, G., Hall, K., Youngberg, G., et al. (2002). Regulation of eosinophil-active cytokine production from human cord blood-derived mast cells. *J. Interferon Cytokine Res.* **22,** 379–388.

16. Krishnaswamy, G., Martin, R., Walker, E., et al. (2003). Moraxella catarrhalis induces mast cell activation and nuclear factor kappa B-dependent cytokine synthesis. *Front. Biosci.* **8,** a40–a47.

17. Sheth, P. D., Pedersen, J., Walls, A. F., and McEuen, A. R. (2003). Inhibition of dipeptidyl peptidase I in the human mast cell line HMC-1: blocked activation of tryptase, but not of the predominant chymotryptic activity. *Biochem. Pharmacol.* **66,** 2251–2262.

18. Schechter, N. M., Eng, G. Y., Selwood, T., and McCaslin, D. R. (1995). Structural changes associated with the spontaneous inactivation of the serine proteinase human tryptase. *Biochemistry* **34,** 10,628–10,638.

19. McEuen, A. R., Sharma, B., and Walls, A. F. (1995). Regulation of the activity of human chymase during storage and release from mast cells: the contributions of inorganic cations, pH, heparin and histamine. *Biochim. Biophys. Acta* **1267,** 115–121.

20. Ferrer-Lopez, P., Renesto, P., Prevost, M. C., Gounon, P., and Chignard, M. (1992). Heparin inhibits neutrophil-induced platelet activation via cathepsin G. *J. Lab. Clin. Med.* **119,** 231–239.

21. Ledoux, D., Merciris, D., Barritault, D., and Caruelle, J. P. (2003). Heparin-like dextran derivatives as well as glycosaminoglycans inhibit the enzymatic activity of human cathepsin G. *FEBS Lett.* **537,** 23–29.

22. Akahoshi, F., Ashimori, A., Sakashita, H., et al. (2001). Synthesis, structure-activity relationships, and pharmacokinetic profiles of nonpeptidic difluoromethylene ketones as novel inhibitors of human chymase. *J. Med. Chem.* **44,** 1297–1304.

23. Smith, T. J., Hougland, M. W., and Johnson, D. A. (1984). Human lung tryptase. Purification and characterization. *J. Biol. Chem.* **259,** 11,046–11,051.

24. Niles, A. L., Maffitt, M., Haak-Frendscho, M., Wheeless, C. J., and Johnson, D. A. (1998). Recombinant human mast cell tryptase beta: stable expression in Pichia pastoris and purification of fully active enzyme. *Biotechnol. Appl. Biochem.* **28,** 125–131.

25. Nakakubo, H., Fukuyama, H., Nakajima, M., et al. (2000). Secretory production of recombinant human chymase as an active form in Pichia pastoris. *Yeast* **16,** 315–323.

26. Schechter, N. M., Sprows, J. L., Schoenberger, O. L., Lazarus, G. S., Cooperman, B. S., and Rubin, H. (1989). Reaction of human skin chymotrypsin-like proteinase chymase with plasma proteinase inhibitors. *J. Biol. Chem.* **264,** 21,308–21,315.

27. Harper, J. W., Ramirez, G., and Powers, J. C. (1981). Reaction of peptide thiobenzyl esters with mammalian chymotrypsinlike enzymes: a sensitive assay method. *Anal. Biochem.* **118,** 382–387.

28. Powers, J. C., Tanaka, T., Harper, J. W., et al. (1985). Mammalian chymotrypsin-like enzymes. Comparative reactivities of rat mast cell proteases, human and dog skin chymases, and human cathepsin G with peptide 4-nitroanilide substrates and with peptide chloromethyl ketone and sulfonyl fluoride inhibitors. *Biochemistry* **24,** 2048–2058.

16

Mast Cell Histamine and Cytokine Assays

David S. Chi, S. Matthew Fitzgerald, and Guha Krishnaswamy

Summary

Mast cells are crucial to the development of chronic allergic inflammation and are likely to play a critical role in host defense. In this chapter methodology for histamine and cytokine assays is provided. Crosslinkage of IgE receptor I (FcεRI) on cord blood-derived mast cells by myeloma IgE and anti-human IgE is used to induce histamine release. Histamine levels were measured in the culture supernatants using an enzyme-linked immunosorbent assay. A human mast cell line (HMC-1), derived from a patient with mast cell leukemia, was activated with interleukin (IL)-1β to study cytokine production and gene expression. Cytokine gene expression was evaluated by reverse transcriptase polymerase chain reaction and cytokine production was assayed in culture supernatants using an enzyme-linked immunosorbent assay kit.

Key Words: Mast cells; cord blood-derived mast cells; IgE; IgE receptor; histamine; inflammation; enzyme-linked immunosorbent assay; reverse transcription polymerase chain reaction (RT-PCR); cytokines; RNA, IL-8.

1. Introduction

Mast cells are critical to the development of chronic allergic inflammation, as seen in allergic asthma *(1,2)*. Crosslinking of cell surface IgE bound to the high-affinity IgE-receptor I, FcεRI, leads to the rapid release of inflammatory mediators, including histamine, proteases, chemotaxins, and arachidonic acid metabolites, such as prostaglandins and leukotrienes *(3)*. Studies from several laboratories, including our own, have demonstrated the capacity of these cells to express certain cytokines regulating the inflammatory response *(4–7)*. Through their production of cytokines, chemokines, and inflammatory mediators, mast cells play an important role in various inflammatory and neoplastic states *(8)*.

In this chapter, crosslinkage of FcεRI by myeloma IgE and anti-human IgE are used to induce histamine release from human cord blood-derived mast cells

From: *Methods in Molecular Biology, vol. 315: Mast Cells: Methods and Protocols*
Edited by: G. Krishnaswamy and D. S. Chi © Humana Press Inc., Totowa, NJ

(CBDMCs *[7]*). Histamine levels will be measured in the culture supernatants using the enzyme-linked immunosorbent assay (ELISA). The procedure of growing human CBDMCs is detailed in Chapters 8 and 9. In this chapter, CBDMCs and human mast cell line (HMC-1) derived from a patient with mast cell leukemia *(9)* were activated with the cytokine interleukin (IL)-1β to induce IL-8 production and gene expression. IL-8 gene expression was evaluated by reverse transcriptase polymerase chain reaction (RT-PCR) whereas cytokine levels in culture supernatants were assayed by ELISA.

2. Materials

2.1. Histamine Release From Human CBDMCs by Crosslinkage of FcεRI With Myeloma IgE and Anti-Human IgE

2.1.1. Crosslinkage of FcεRI With Myeloma IgE and Anti-Human IgE

1. Human CBDMC media: DMEMF12 (Gibco Invitrogen, Carlsbad, CA) supplemented with 20% fetal bovine serum (Atlanta Biologicals, Atlanta, GA); $5 \times 10^{-5} M$ 2-mercaptoethanol (Fisher, Pittsburgh, PA); 0.5 mL of insulin–transferin–sodium selenite solution (Sigma-Aldrich, St. Louis, MO); 25 mM HEPES (Gibco, Carlsbad, CA); 300 nM PGE$_2$ (Cayman, Ann Arbor, MI); 100 ng/mL recombinant human IL-6 (kindly provide by Amgen, Thousand Oaks, CA); and 80 ng/mL stem cell factor (kindly provided by Amgen *[7]*).
2. 75-cm^2 flasks culture flasks, vented cap (Corning, Corning, NY).
3. Myeloma IgE (Calbiochem, San Diego, CA).
4. Anti-human IgE (Mouse IgM monoclonal antibody, Hybridoma Reagent Laboratory, Baltimore, MD).
5. Phosphate-buffered saline (PBS), pH 7.2.
6. Tyrode's solution: 124 mM NaCl, 4 mM KCl, 0.64 mM NaH$_2$PO$_4$, 1 mM CaCl$_2$, 0.6 mM MgCl$_2$, 10 mM HEPES buffer, and 0.03 % human serum albumin, pH 7.4.
7. Phorbol myristate acetate (PMA; 1 µg/mL stock solution, Sigma).
8. Centrifuge tubes (15 mL).
9. 12-well culture plate (Falcon).

2.1.2. Measurement of Histamine by ELISA

1. Immunotech Histamine Enzyme Immunoassay Kit (Beckman Coulter, Fullerton, CA), which includes a 96-well microtiter plate with lid (coated with monoclonal anti-histamine antibody), standards (six vials containing histamine ranging from 0 to 100 nM), control (one vial of histamine of known concentration), acylation reagent (one vial), dimethyl sulfoxide (one 3-mL vial to dissolve acylation reagent), acylation buffer (one 5-mL vial), histamine-release buffer (one vial to be reconstituted with 25 mL of distilled water), histamine–alkalin phosphatase conjugate (one vial to be reconstituted with conjugate diluent H), conjugate diluent H (one 25-mL vial), wash solution 20X (one 50-mL vial to be diluted to 1 L with distilled water), substrate buffer (one 30-mL vial), substrate (two 15-mg tablets of Para-nitrophenylphosphate, pNPP, to be dissolved in 30 mL of substrate buffer), and stop solution (one 6-mL vial of 1 N NaOH solution).

2. Plastic tube (15 mL and 50 mL).
3. Micropipets (20 µL, 200 µL, and 1000 µL).
4. Vortex-type mixer.
5. Microtiter plate shaker (350 rpm).
6. Microtiter plate washer (Bio-Tek, Winooski, VT).
7. Microtiter plate reader (405-414 nm, Dynatech MR5000, Chantilly, VA).
8. BioLinx 2.22 software (Dynex Technology, Chantilly, VA).

2.2. Growth of HMC-1 Cells

1. HMC-1 culture media: RPMI 1640 media supplemented with 2×10^{-5} *M* 2-mercaptoethanol (Sigma), 10 m*M* HEPES, gentamycin 50 µg/mL, 5 mg/mL insulin transferrin (Sigma), 2 m*M* L glutamine, and 5% heat-inactivated fetal bovine serum.
2. 75-cm^2 culture flasks, vented cap (Corning, Corning, NY).
3. Sterile serological pipet tips and pipets.
4. Incubator (37°C and 5% CO_2).
5. Cell culture hood.

2.3. Cytokine Production and Gene Expression in IL-1 β-Activated HMC-1 Cells

2.3.1. Activation of Mast Cells With IL-1 β

1. IL-1β (Sigma).
2. Micropipets and tips.
3. Cell culture media (*see* **Subheading 2.2.**).

2.3.2. RNA Extraction and Reverse Transcriptase Polymerase Chain Reaction

1. Micropipets (p200 and p1000) and tips.
2. Centrifuge tubes (1.5 mL).
3. Microcentrifuge and large centrifuge.
4. Ice and bucket.
5. RNA-Bee.
6. Chloroform (at 0°C).
7. Phenol-cholorform (*see* **Note 1**).
8. Tris-HCl (sterile, 0.1 and 0.5 *M*, pH 8.0).
9. *n*-propanol.
10. 75% ethanol + 0.1% DEPC.
11. 0.1% diethyl pyrocarbonate (DEPC) H_2O.
12. Spectrophotometer.
13. RT-PCR Kit (GeneAmp RNA PCR Core Kit, Applied Biosystems, Roche, Branchburg, NJ).

2.3.3. Cytokine Production in Culture Supernatants Using ELISA

1. Cytokine ELISA Kit (R&D Systems, Minneapolis, MN).
2. Same as **steps 2–8** in **Subheading 2.1.2.**

3. Methods

The methods described in **Subheadings 3.1.–3.3.** outline: (1) histamine release from human CBDMC by crosslinkage of FcεRI with myeloma IgE and anti-human IgE; (2) growth of HMC-1 cells; and (3) cytokine gene and protein expression in IL-1β-activated HMC-1 cells. For the method of growth of CBDMC, please *see* Chapters 8 and 9.

3.1. Histamine Release From Human CBDMCs by Crosslinkage of FcεRI With Myeloma IgE and Anti-Human IgE

3.1.1. Crosslinkage of FcεRI With Myeloma IgE and Anti-Human IgE

1. Human CBDMCs are developed from human cord blood and maintained in CBDMC media for approx 8–16 wk or until mature *(7)*.
2. Pipet 10 mL of CBDMC (5×10^5 cells/mL in CBDMC media) into each of the 75-cm^2 flasks. Treat CBDMC with 0 or 2 µg/mL final concentration of myeloma IgE by adding 0 (media control) or 20 µL of myeloma IgE (1 mg/mL) to the flask, and incubate at 37°C in a 5% CO_2 incubator overnight.
3. Pipet myeloma IgE-treated CBDMC into 15-mL centrifuge tubes (*see* **Note 2**) and centrifuge the tubes at 250*g* for 10 min at room temperature. Resuspend the cell pellet in 11 mL of PBS and do a cell count. Centrifuge the cell suspension and make up cell suspension at 1×10^6 cells/mL in Tyrode's solution.
4. Distribute 1.5 mL of CBDMCs into each well of 12-well culture plate in triplicate. Add anti human IgE antibody to the wells at a final concentration of 0 (media control) or 3 µg/mL (i.e., adding 0 or 2.25 µL of 2 mg/mL anti-IgE, respectively). For positive controls, CBDMCs are treated with PMA at 50 ng/mL final concentration (adding 75 µL of 1 µg/mL PMA). The culture is further incubated for 30 min.
5. The cell cultures are harvested, centrifuged at 250*g* for 10 min, and cell-free supernatants are collected and kept at –80°C for histamine assay. Cell pellet is suspended in 1 mL of distilled water, frozen and thawed twice, and centrifuged at 250*g* for 10 min. Cell lysates are collected and kept at –80°C for histamine assay (for determination of cell residual histamine content).
6. The experimental results are expressed as the percentage of histamine release relative to the total cellular histamine content. Histamine release (%) = $[(E - S) / (E + L)] \times 100$, where E (experimental release) is the histamine in the experimental sample, S (spontaneous release) is the histamine in the sample of cells in buffer, and L (cell lysate) is the histamine in cell lysate sample.

3.1.2. Measurement of Histamine by ELISA

1. Equilibrate reagents of the kit to room temperature before use.
2. Reconstitute: (1) acylation reagent in the required volume of dimethyl sulfoxide just before use; and (2) conjugate solution with diluent H. Also, dissolve one tablet of substrate in 15 mL of substrate buffer at least 30 min before use.

3. Perform acylation of standards, control, and samples: add 25 µL of acylation solution, 100 µL of standards, control and samples, and 25 µL of acylation buffer to clean plastic tubes, and vortex immediately.

4. Add 50 µL of acylated standard, control, or samples and 200 µL of enzymatic conjugate into antibody-coated wells (*see* **Note 3**), and incubate for 2 h at 2–8°C with constant shaking on a microtiter plate shaker.

5. Wash the microtiter plate wells three times with the wash solution using a microtiter plate washer. Alternatively, the washing can be carried out manually as following: 1) turn microtiter plate upside-down and shake vigorously over the sink, 2) fill the wells with the wash solution using a squeeze bottle, 3) repeat **steps 1** and **2** twice for a total of three washes, and 4) firmly tap the upside-down microtiter plate on clean absorbent paper.

6. Add 200 µL of substrate to all wells, cover plate with lid, and incubate for 30 min at 18–25°C with constant shaking.

7. Stop the reaction by adding 50 µL of stop solution to all wells.

8. Read the optical density (OD) of the wells at 405–414 nm using a microtiter plate reader, zero with the substrate blank (*see* **Note 4**).

9. Results are obtained by interpolation from standard curve, which is generating from BioLinx 2.22 software (*see* **Note 5**).

3.2. Growth of HMC-1 Cells

HMC-1 cells, established from a patient with mast cell leukemia, were graciously provided by Dr. J. H. Butterfield (Mayo Clinic, Rochester, MN *[9]*).

1. Cells (1 mL) taken out of the freezer are thawed, diluted in media (10 mL), and centrifuged to remove freezing media.

2. Reconstitute cell pellet to $1–2 \times 10^5$ cells/mL. Mast cells should be grown in vented cap culture flasks in a proliferating state at an optimal concentration of 2×10^5 cells/mL to 4×10^5 cells/mL *(6,10,11)*. Overcrowding of cells will decrease their viability.

3. Subculture cells every 3–4 d to a 1:15 dilution with fresh new media. Culture flasks should be laid on their bottom (not standing up) to maximize media surface area.

3.3. Cytokine Production and Gene Expression in IL-1 β-Activated HMC-1 Cells

3.3.1. Activation of Mast Cells With IL-1 β

1. Make a cell suspension at a concentration of 1×10^6 cells/mL.

2. One milliliter of HMC-1 is seeded in tissue culture dishes or 12- or 24-well tissue plates, depending on the experimental design. Cells in media alone serve as negative controls. A combination of PMA (50 ng/mL) and ionomycin (5 µM) is used as a positive control.

3. For IL-1β activation, add varying concentrations of IL-1β (1, 10, and 100 ng/mL) to wells containing mast cells, and swirl in a figure eight motion to evenly distribute the stimulant *(6,10,11)*.

4. For cytokine production, mast cell cultures are incubated at 37°C for 0, 24, and/or 48 h (as required), harvested in 1.5-mL centrifuge tubes, and centrifuged at 250*g* for 10 min to remove cell debris.

5. Cell-free supernatants are transferred to new tubes and stored at –70°C until ready for cytokine assay by ELISA (*see* **Note 6**).

6. For ribonucleic acid (RNA) extraction, activation is conducted for 3 h in tissue culture plates (*see* **Note 7**). The cells (a total of 2–4 million cells will give sufficient RNA) are then harvested and subjected to RNA preparation and analysis. RNA can be extracted at 0, 3, 6, 9, 12, or 24 h as needed (depending on experimental condition).

3.3.2. RNA Extraction

1. Centrifuge cells in 15-mL centrifuge tubes, discard supernatants (or save as the case may be), break pellet by flicking the bottom of the tube.

2. Add 1 mL of RNAzol to broken cell pellet and pipet up and down until a watery consistency is obtained. Transfer to 1.5-mL centrifuge tubes.

3. Add 100 μL of cold chloroform and shake for 1 min. Do not vortex.

4. Centrifuge for 15 min at 12,000*g* at 4° C.

5. Transfer top aqueous layer to a new 1.5-mL centrifuge tube (*see* **Note 8**).

6. Add approx 800 μL of phenol–chloroform and vortex.

7. Centrifuge for 5 min at 12,000*g* at 4°C.

8. Repeat **steps 5–7**.

9. Transfer top aqueous layer to a new 1.5-mL centrifuge tube and add approx 800 μL of cold chloroform to the sample. Vortex the tube.

10. Centrifuge for 5 min at 12,000*g* at 4°C.

11. Transfer top layer to a new 1.5-mL centrifuge tube and add 800 μL of cold n-propanol. RNA should start to precipitate. Vortex. Store at –20°C overnight.

12. The next day, centrifuge samples for 30 min at 12,000*g* at 4°C.

13. Discard supernatant and add 1 mL of 75% ethanol + 0.1% DEPC.

14. Vortex gently until RNA pellet rises and falls intact.

15. Centrifuge for 8 min at 10,000*g* at 4°C.

16. Discard supernatant and using a p200 micropipet remove any trace of liquid from RNA pellet.

17. Allow RNA pellet to air dry for 10 min at room temperature (*see* **Note 9**).

18. Add 20 μL of 0.1% DEPC H_2O to dissolve RNA. Read optical density on a spectrophotometer (*see* **Note 10**).

19. Apply 1000 ng of RNA (1000 ng RNA in 10 μL of DEPC H_2O and 2 μL of bromophenol blue; *see* **Note 11**) on a 2% agarose gel containing ethidium bromide and perform electrophoresis at 100 V for 30–45 min to ensure band equality and RNA integrity (**Fig. 1**).

3.3.3. RT-PCR

3.3.3.1. RT REACTION

1. Use **Table 1** to make an RT reagent cocktail, which is enough to run a sample for five different pairs of primers. Double the volume if a sample needs to be run for

IL-1β (ng/mL)

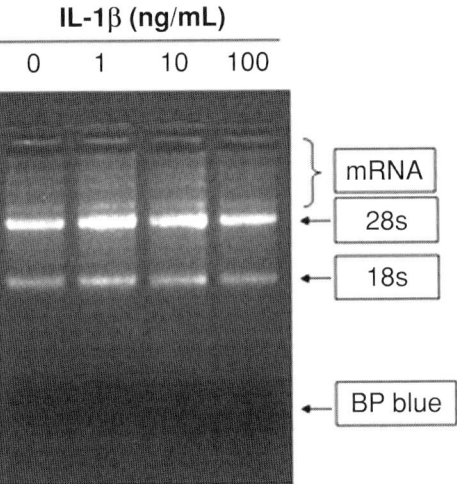

Fig. 1. RNA gel showing four RNA samples from HMC-1 stimulated with different concentrations of IL-1β. RNA (1000 ng) was diluted in 10 μL of DEPC water with 2 μL of bromophenol blue added and electrophoresis conducted on a 2% agarose gel containing ethidium bromide. The messenger RNA (mRNA) shows a ladder pattern because of the differing lengths. The 28S and 18S bands of rRNA are shown.

6–10 pairs of primers. Additionally, increase the volume by multiplying the sample number. For example, there are five RNA samples to be run with three primers. Because there are only three primers, one serving (18 μL of RT reagent cocktail) is required for each sample. For five RNA samples, we need 18 μL × 5 = 90 μL of RT reagent cocktail total. For better results, make one master mix of RT reagents, vortex, and distribute this to the five samples. To get enough RT reagent cocktail to distribute, add an extra serving (thus, 18 μL × 6 = 108 μL). Allow at least one extra sample for a housekeeping gene (*6,10,11*).

2. Label one RT-PCR tube for every RNA sample. Each tube will receive 18 μL of RT reagent cocktail and 1000 ng of RNA in 2 μL of dH$_2$O for every serving.

3. Centrifuge each tube for several seconds to collect the reagents and RNA to the bottom.

4. Add tubes to a thermal cycler at 42°C for 20 min, 99°C for 10 min and 5°C for 5 min to transcribe cDNA.

5. Remove tubes at this point or set thermal cycler for a 4°C soak until tubes can be removed.

3.3.3.2. PCR (*SEE* **NOTE 12**)

1. While samples are being run through the RT cycle, prepare the PCR reagent cocktail according to **Table 2** (*see* **Note 13**). Multiply the volume of reagents by [(number of samples + 1 extra) × number of primers] and combine all the reagents in a master mix. Vortex the PCR reagent cocktail.

Table 1
Reverse Transcriptase Reagent Cocktail

Reagent	Volume
10x buffer	2 μL
MgCl$_2$ (25 mM)	4 μL
dGTP (10 mM)	2 μL
dATP (10 mM)	2 μL
dCTP (10 mM)	2 μL
dTTP (10 mM)	2 μL
Oligonucleotide (50 μM)	1 μL
RNase inhibitor (20 U/μL)	1 μL
Reverse transcriptase (50 U/μL)	1 μL
dH$_2$O	1 μL
RNA (1000 ng total) in dH$_2$O	2 μL
Total	20 μL

2. Label the appropriate number of RT-PCR tubes and place them in a rack. Each tube will receive 2 μL of the up primer, 2 μL of the down primer (*see* **Note 14;** for equal RNA loading, at least one housekeeping gene primer should be added to your experiment, such as hypoxanthine phosphoribosyl transferase [HPRT]), 4 μL of RT product (after it has been transcribed to cDNA), and 42 μL of PCR reagent cocktail (*6,10,11*).
3. Briefly centrifuge each tube to collect all materials to the bottom of the RT-PCR tube. If the thermal cycler requires samples to be covered with ultra pure mineral oil, do so at this time.
4. Place tubes in thermal cycler and set temperature conditions and times according to primer specifications. Cycle number will depend on the amount of RNA present (usually 25–45 cycles is sufficient).
5. When cycles are complete transfer sample to new tube, label, and freeze at –20°C.
6. To visualize product, run 10 μL of product with 2 μL of bromophenol blue on a 2–3% agarose gel containing ethidium bromide at 100 V for 45–60 min (**Fig. 2**). Compare band lengths with a DNA ladder to ensure correct length of product. We use PhiX174 DNA/Hae III ladder (band sizes: 1353, 1078, 872, 603, 310, 281, 271, 234, 194, and 118 basepairs).
7. Cut bands and sequence if necessary.

3.3.4. Cytokine Measurement in Culture Supernatants Using ELISA

1. Cytokine measurements are done using a commercially available ELISA kit, which requires 50–200 μL of sample depending on the kit. Usually, 0.5-mL to 2-mL cultures in 6-, 12-, or 24-well tissue culture plates will provide enough supernatants for assays and generate enough product for detection (usually in the

Table 2
Polymerase Chain Reaction Reagent Cocktail

Reagent	Volume
10x buffer	4.8 µL
MgCl$_2$ (25 mM)	3.6 µL
dGTP (10 mM)	0.8 µL
dATP (10 mM)	0.8 µL
dCTP (10 mM)	0.8 µL
dTTP (10 mM)	0.8 µL
T. aq polymerase (5 U/µL)	0.2 µL
dH$_2$O	30.2 µL
Total	42 µL

pg/mL scale). Each ELISA kit comes with specific instructions and these should be followed very closely.

2. A standard dilution is prepared from reagents provided in the kit.
3. In a 96-well plate, add the standards and samples and incubate undisturbed for the indicated time.
4. Wash the wells with wash buffer (provided) and add the appropriate conjugate antibody (also provided). Incubate undisturbed for the indicated time and wash again.
5. A substrate solution should now be added which will change color if desired product is detected.
6. After a short incubation period, add stop solution and run on a spectrophotometer at 450 nm with a correction at 570 nm.
7. Generate a standard curve as shown in **Fig. 3**. Values from the ELISA will be interpolated or extrapolated from this curve.
8. Take numbers from duplicate or triplicate samples and calculate a mean and standard deviation or standard error. Repeat experiments for reproducibility.
9. **Figure 4** shows the results of IL-8 production in IL-1β activated HMC-1 cultures. Statistica for Windows (StatSoft, Tulsa, OK) is used for statistical analysis and Slidewrite Plus for Windows (Advanced Graphics Software, Encinitas, CA) for graph generation.

4. Notes

1. To prepare phenol–choroform: warm phenol to room temperature, place in 50°C waterbath to melt crystals. Pipet desired volume into appropriate sized flask. Add 8-hydroxyquinoline to a final concentration of 0.1%, and then add 1 mL of β-mercaptoethanol to every 100 mL of phenol. Then, add an equal volume of 0.5 M Tris-HCl (sterile, pH 8.0), cover with parafilm, and stir overnight. Aliquot phenol into sterile 50-mL tubes and add an equal volume of chloroform. Layer with 10 mL of 0.1 M Tris-HCl (pH 8.0) to prevent oxidation of the phenol. Wrap in foil to protect from light and store at 4°C.

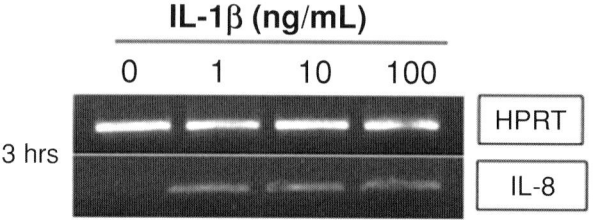

Fig. 2. RT-PCR gel showing expression of IL-8 in HMC-1. RNA from HMC-1 was subjected to RT-PCR with primers specific for human IL-8. Ten microliters of the PCR product with 2 µL of bromophenol blue was electrophoresed on a 3% agarose gel. Hypoxanthine phosphoribosyl transferase (HPRT) was used as a housekeeping gene.

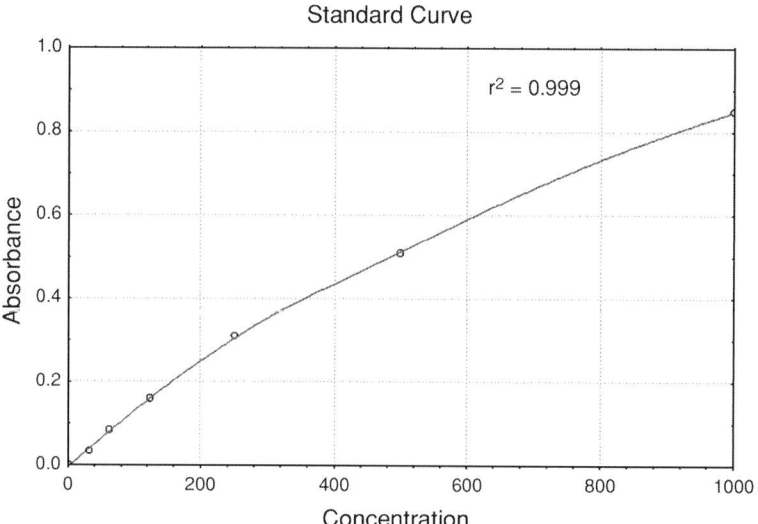

Fig. 3. Standard curve used for IL-8 ELISA analysis. A standard curve was constructed by plotting known concentrations of IL-8 on the x-axis against their respective absorbance at 450 nm corrected at 570 nm on the y-axis. The absorbance of the samples can be interpolated or extrapolated from this graph. Most computer software programs will calculate these values.

2. To increase yield of cells, rinse the flasks with 5 mL of PBS and add this residual cell suspension to the tube prior to centrifugation.

3. Leave one well empty to serve as a substrate blank. This substrate blank well should also be washed three times before addition of substrate.

4. Reading may be delayed for up to a maximum of 2 h at 18–25°C, if the plate is left in the dark and kept with its lid on in order to avoid evaporation.

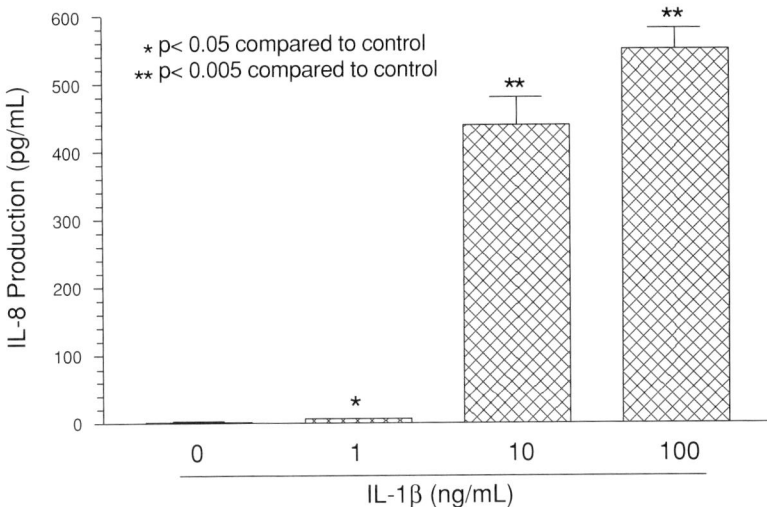

Fig. 4. A graph showing IL-8 production from HMC-1. Values taken from tripli-cate samples of HMC-1 treated with 1, 10, and 100 ng/mL of IL-1β were used to generate a mean and standard deviation. The data were analyzed by Student's two-tailed *t*-test.

5. If the OD of the sample is out of the range of the standard curve, the sample needs to be either diluted with assay buffer (in case the OD is lower than that of the highest standard) or concentrated with Amicon filter (in case the OD is higher than that of the lowest standard). In the current experiment, the supernatants are diluted to 1:500 before the histamine assay.

6. The time at which the cell supernatants will be harvested is a factor for consider-ing the cell concentration of cultures because mast cells proliferate quickly and begin to die when overcrowded. For cell supernatant harvests at 12 and 24 h, mast cell concentrations at 1×10^6 cells/mL work well and produce ample amounts of cytokine to be measured by ELISA. Experiments that require greater than 48 h incubation times work best with 0.5×10^6 cells/mL. Cell supernatant experiments should be performed in duplicate or triplicate and repeated for accuracy.

7. Sometime pretreatment of mast cells is required before activation with IL-1β. If pretreatment lasting longer than 12 h (such as treatment with glucocorticoids or dominant-negative plasmids), the culture should be done in the tissue culture flasks. If pretreatments lasting less than 12 h (such as treatment with actinomycin or nuclear factor-kB inhibitor), the culture can be done in 6 well plates or tissue culture dishes. In both cases, cell viability should be checked before subject to preparation for RNA extraction. HMC-1 is a more resilient cell than CBDMC and is more likely to tolerate vortexing. If cell viability becomes a concern, slowly invert tube to mix mast cells and stimulants instead of vortexing before culturing in culture flask, plate, or dish.

8. It is better to leave part of the aqueous layer than to transfer any of the interface or RNA-Bee.
9. Depending on humidity, RNA pellet may not dry at room temperature. In this case, use a vacuum pump to help evaporate pellet. Drying the pellet too long may reduce its ability to be redissolved.
10. A 260:280 nm ratio of 2 is best for the RNA preparation ($\geq$1.8 is acceptable; using 260 nm detects nucleic acids, whereas 280 nm detects proteins). A high 260:280 nm ratio (> 2.5) indicates phenol contamination, whereas a low 260:280 nm ratio indicates protein contamination. An absorbance at 230 nm indicates contamination with phenol or urea. An absorbance at 325 nm indicates particulate contamination or dirty cuvetes. If the RNA sample is contaminated with phenol, the phenol can be removed by the following procedure: (1) bring sample volume to 400 µL with 0.1% DEPC H_2O and mix; (2) add 500 µL of chloroform and vortex; (3) centrifuge at 12,000g for 5 min at 4°C; (4) remove aqueous layer with a pipet; (5) add 1/10 the volume with 3.0 M sodium acetate, pH 5.2, and mix; (6) double the sample volume with cold isopropanol and store overnight at –20°C; (7) centrifuge at 12,000g for 30 min at 4°C; (8) discard supernatant, add 1 mL of icecold 75% ethanol + 0.1% DEPC, and vortex (pellet should rise and fall intact); (9) centrifuge at 9,500g for 8 min at 4°C; (10) discard all liquid from RNA pellet and air dry at room temperature; (11) reconstitute RNA pellet with 20 µL of 0.1% DEPC H_2O; and (12) characterize RNA on a spectrophotometer.
11. To make bromophenol blue, mix 0.25 g of bromophenol blue in 30 mL of glycerol and 70 mL of dH_2O.
12. Real-time PCR may be considered. The recent introduction of fluorescence-based techniques to PCR has allowed the development of real-time PCR, also called QPCR or kinetic PCR. Unlike conventional PCR that uses an endpoint analysis of the amplicon, real-time PCR is based on the detection and quantitation of the PCR product as it is made, using either fluorogenic specific probes or double-stranded DNA binding fluorescent dyes such as SYBR Green. During the exponential phase of the amplification, the fluorescent signal increase is directly proportional to the amount of PCR product. The real-time PCR technology is increasingly used, because it offers significant advantages such as high sensitivity, wide quantification range, and good reproducibility.
13. Depending on the salt concentration required for your specific primers, the $MgCl_2$ volume may need to be changed.
14. Better results are obtained when equal volumes of the up and down primer are mixed in a microcentifuge tube, vortexed, and 4 µL of this mix is added to each tube. Primers were synthesized at the John Hopkins University School of Hygiene and Public Health DNA Synthesis Core Facility, Baltimore, MD.

Acknowledgments

This study was supported by USPHS grants AI-43310 and HL-63070, RDC grant (ETSU), State of Tennessee Grant 20233, AMGEN, Inc., and Ruth R. Harris Endowment (ETSU).

References

1. Costa, J. J., Weller, P. F., and Galli, S. J. (1997) The cells of the allergic response: mast cells, basophils, and eosinophils. *JAMA* **278,** 1815–1822.
2. Rossi, G. L. and Olivieri, D. (1997) Does the mast cell still have a key role in asthma? *Chest* **112,** 523–529.
3. Marone, G., Casolaro, V., Patella, V., Florio, G., and Triggiani, M. (1997) Molecular and cellular biology of mast cells and basophils. *Int. Arch. Allergy Immunol.* **114,** 207–217.
4. Church, M. K. and Levi-Schaffer, F. (1997) The human mast cell. *J. Allergy Clin. Immunol.* **99,** 155–160.
5. Bradding, P. (1996) Human mast cell cytokines. *Clin. Exp. Allergy* **26,** 13–19.
6. Krishnaswamy, G., Lakshman, T., Miller, A. R., Srikanth, S., Hall, K., and Huang, S. K. (1997) Multifunctional cytokine expression by human mast cells: regulation by T cell membrane contact and glucocorticoids. *J. Interferon Cytokine Res.* **17,** 167–176.
7. Krishnaswamy, G., Hall, K., Youngberg, G., et al. (2002) Regulation of eosinophil-active cytokine production from human cord blood-derived mast cells. *J. Interferon Cytokine Res.* **22,** 379–388.
8. Krishnaswamy, G., Kelley, J., Johnson, D., et al. (2001) The human mast cell: functions in physiology and disease. *Front. Biosci.* **6,** d1109–d1127.
9. Butterfield, J. H., Weiler, D., Dewald, G., and Gleich, G. J. (1988) Establishment of an immature mast cell line from a patient with mast cell leukemia. *Leukemia Res.* **12,** 345–355.
10. Fitzgerald, S. M., Lee, S. A., Hall, H. K., Chi, D. S., and Krishnaswamy, G. (2004) Human lung fibroblasts express Interleukin-6 in response to signaling after mast cell contact. *Am. J Respir. Cell Mol. Biol.* **30,** 585–593.
11. Huang, S. K., Krishnaswamy, G., Su, S. N., Xiao, H. Q., and Liu, M. C. (1994) Qualitative and quantitative analysis of cytokine transcripts in the bronchoalveolar lavage of patients with asthma. *Ann. N. Y. Acad. Sci.* **725,** 110–117.

17

Measurement of Mast Cell Cytokine Release by Multiplex Assay

Kevin F. Breuel and W. Keith De Ponti

Summary

Mast cells are highly responsive cells that are capable of secreting a variety of inflammatory mediators, including histamine, heparin, serine proteases, leukotrienes, prostaglandins, and thromboxanes. Studies from several laboratories have demonstrated that mast cells have the capacity to produce a variety of cytokines in response to various stimuli. Characterization of the cytokine profiles in mast cells has routinely been determined by the performance of individual enzyme-linked immunosorbent assays. This process is expensive, time-consuming, and requires a great deal of material to characterize multiple cytokines. In this chapter, we describe a multiplex cytokine assay to detect 17 cytokines simultaneously in 50 µL of culture supernatant derived from stimulated human cord blood-derived mast cells.

Key Words: Mast cells; cord blood-derived mast cells; Luminex®; xMAP™; Bio-Plex 17-plex cytokine assay; cytokines; microsphere; multiplex.

1. Introduction

Human mast cells are dynamic, tissue-dwelling cells that are capable of producing a plethora of biological mediators, including histamine, heparin, serine proteases, leukotrienes, prostaglandins, thromboxanes *(1–9)*, and a number of proinflammatory cytokines *(1,10–14)*. The identification and quantification of mast cell cytokine production traditionally has been determined by the performance of enzyme-linked immunosorbent assays (ELISAs *[13–15]*). However, assessment of mast cell cytokine production using ELISA methodology has one or more limitations, including: (1) the ability to measure only one cytokine at time; (2) the need for a large sample volume to measure multiple cytokines; (3) the time commitment to perform sequential cytokine assays; and (4) the cost to perform multiple ELISAs to quantify multiple cytokines.

From: *Methods in Molecular Biology, vol. 315: Mast Cells: Methods and Protocols*
Edited by: G. Krishnaswamy and D. S. Chi © Humana Press Inc., Totowa, NJ

Advances in microsphere technology have led to the development of flow cytometric assays, which allow the simultaneous detection of as many as 100 analytes in a single microtiter well *(16–20)*. Recently, several companies have developed commercially available cytokine assays that use the Luminex® (Austin, TX) Multi-Analyte Profiling (xMAP™) technology to simultaneously measure as many as 22 individual cytokines in a single microtiter well (*see* **Note 1**). In this chapter, we describe the Bio-Plex assay procedure for the simultaneous determination of 17 human cytokines (interleukin [IL]-1β, IL-2, IL-4, IL-5, IL-6, IL-7, IL-8, IL-10, IL-12, IL-13, IL-17, tumor necrosis factor [TNF]-α, interferon-gamma [IFN-γ], granulocyte colony-stimulating factor [G-CSF], granulocyte macrophage colony-stimulating factor [GM-CSF], monocyte chemoattractant protein-1 [MCP-1], and macrophage inflammatory protein-1 β [MIP-1β]) in media collected from human cord blood-derived mast cells (CBDMCs) cultured in vitro.

2. Materials

2.1. Isolation and Generation, Confirmation, and Activation of Human CBDMCs

1. Human BDMCs, provided kindly by Drs. Guha Krishnaswamy and David S. Chi.
2. IBL medium: Modified Dulbecco's modified Eagle's medium containing 10 μg/mL insulin, 10 μg/mL transferrin, 5 10^{-5} M 2-mercaptoethanol, 25 mM HEPES, and 2.6 ng/ml NaSeO$_3$ (Atlanta Biologicals, Atlanta, GA).
3. IBL+ medium: IBL medium supplemented with 5% fetal bovine serum (Atlanta Biologicals), 80 ng/mL human recombinant stem cell factor (rSCF; Amgen, Thousand Oaks, CA), 50 ng/mL human rIL-6 (Amgen), and prostaglandin E$_2$ (PGE$_2$; Sigma, St. Louis, MO).
4. Thyrode's Solution: 124 mM NaCl, 4 mM KCl, 0.64 mM NaH$_2$PO$_4$, 1 mM CaCl$_2$, 0.6 mM MgCl$_2$, 10 mM HEPES, and 0.03% human serum albumin.
5. 75-cm^2 flasks.
6. Incubator for culturing cells at 37°C and 5% CO$_2$.

2.2. Performance of the Bio-Plex Human 17-Plex Cytokine Assay

1. Luminex 100™ system with XYZ platform (Luminex, Austin TX).
2. Bio-Plex™ Human Cytokine 17-Plex Panel (Bio-Rad, Hercules, CA).
3. Bio-Plex™ Buffer kit for assay (Bio-Rad Laboratories).
4. Titer Plate Orbital Shaker (Lab-line, Melrose Park, IL.).
5. Millipore MultiScreen Resist Vacuum Manifold, MAVM0960R (Millipore, Billerica, MA).
6. Thermodine Maxi Mix II Vortexer, M37615 Mixer, (Barnstead International, Dubuque, IA).
7. Mini Ultrasonik™ sonicator (Dentsply Ceramco, Burlington, NJ).
8. 55 mL of Sterile Solution Basin (Cole-Parmer, Vernon Hills, IL).
9. Eppendorf Research Pro Multichannel Pipetter (Eppendorf, AG, Hamburg, Germany).

10. Eppendorf Repeater® pro pipetter (Eppendorf, AG).
11. Eppendorf centrifuge 5417R (Eppendorf, AG).
12. Gilson Pipetman® p20, and p200 pipettors (Gilson, Middleton, WI).

2.3. Analysis of Cytokine Data

1. Luminex Data Collector software, version 1.7, build 69 (Luminex).
2. Bio-Plex Manager data reduction software (Bio-Rad).
3. Slidewrite Plus data analysis software for Windows, version 5.0 (Advanced Graphics Software, Encinitas, CA).

3. Methods

The methods described in **Subheadings 3.1.–3.5.** outline: (1) the isolation and generation, confirmation, and activation of CBDMC; (2) the setting up and calibrating of the Luminex instrument; (3) the performance of the Bio-Plex Human 17-plex cytokine assay; (4) the analysis of cytokine data; and (5) results.

3.1. Isolation and Generation, Confirmation, and Activation of CBDMCs

CBDMCs were isolated and generated, confirmed, and activated as previously described by Krishnaswamy et al. *(10)*. The methods for the isolation and generation, confirmation, and activation are briefly described in **Subheadings 3.1.1.–3.1.3.**

3.1.1. Isolation and Generation of CBDMCs

Heparinized umbilical cord blood was obtained and processed as previously described by Saito et al. *(21)* and Krishnaswamy et al. *(10)*. Mononuclear cell fractions were isolated by centrifugation and re-suspended in 75-cm^2 flasks containing IBL+ medium and cultured in an atmosphere of 5% CO_2 in air at 37°C.

3.1.2. Confirmation of CBDMCs

The cells were used when there was 100% uniformity in morphology of the cells. They were further confirmed to be 90% pure by immunohistochemical staining for tryptase.

3.1.3. Activation of the Human Mast Cells

Cells were treated with either Phorbol 12-myristate 13-acetate + Ionomycin (PMA/Iono) or IgE followed by anti-IgE to stimulate cytokine production. The combination of PMA and Iono have been previously shown to increase mast cell cytokine production *(10,12)*. Crosslinking of cell surface IgE bound to high-affinity IgE receptor, FCŒμRI, leads to expression of various cytokines *(10,11)*. Mast cells (100,000/mL) were cultured in Tyrode's solution in 75-cm^2 flasks. Cells were treated with media alone, PMA/Iono, or anti-IgE for 24 h before the supernatant was collected into a microcentrifuge tube and frozen at –80°C. Cells treated with anti-IgE were sensitized overnight with myeloma IgE.

3.2. Setting Up and Calibrating the Luminex 100 System

Before running the Bio-Plex 17-plex cytokine assay on the Luminex 100 instrument, it is necessary to perform the start-up maintenance and instrument calibration procedure. These procedures are briefly described in **Subheadings 3.2.1.** and **3.2.2.**

3.2.1. Setting Up the the Luminex 100 System

1. Turn on the Luminex 100 instrument, XY platform and the Luminex SD (Sheath Delivery System) and start the Luminex data acquisition software and initiate the "warmup" feature to allow the optics to properly warm-up.
2. During the warm-up period, approx 30 min, the lines must be checked for vacuum leaks; waste and sheath fluid connections must form a tight seal; the sheath fluid container must be adequately full; and waste fluid container should be empty.
3. Prime and flush the system with alcohol, which provides the opportunity to both get the fluidics ready and clean for the assay, and make sure that there are no bubbles in the fluid lines within the machine.
4. Wash the system twice with sheath fluid to rinse the alcohol out of the system and prepare the fluidics properly for the calibration.
5. Using a 96-well plate and three spacers, set the probe height for the Luminex 100 system.

3.2.2. Calibrating the Luminex 100 System

1. Place five drops of fresh classification and reporter calibrators, respectively, into two separate wells of a 96-well plate.
2. Verify or enter the correct classification and reporter calibrator target values and initiate the calibration program.
3. Upon completion, verify that both the classification and reporter calibrations were successful and then wash the fluidics lines four times with sheath fluid.

3.3. Performance of the Human Bio-Plex 17-Plex Cytokine Assay

Samples were prepared and assayed according to the Bio-Plex cytokine assay instruction manual *(22)* with modifications. Permission was granted by Bio-Rad Laboratories to reproduce the assay protocol as a part of the sample preparation section. The protocol listed below reflects material preparation necessary to perform an entire 96-well microtiter plate on cell culture supernatants.

3.3.1. Sample Preparation

1. Twelve hours before the assay, remove the samples and aliquoted sample medium from the –80°C freezer and place into the refrigerator (4°C) to thaw.
2. Centrifuge the samples at 2151g for 5 min and aliquot the supernatant to a separate microcentrifuge tube (*see* **Note 2**).
3. Immediately place the samples on ice and maintain on ice throughout the assay procedure.

4. If samples are expected to have cytokine concentrations greater than the highest standard point on the standard curve, dilute them appropriately with culture medium (*see* **Note 3**).

3.3.2. Standard Preparation

1. Perform a quick-spin of the lyophilized multiplex cytokine standard.
   Prepare a 50,000 pg/mL standard stock solution by adding 500 µL of the cell culture medium.
2. Gently vortex the reconstituted standard solution for 5 s, place on ice, and incubate for 30 min.
4. Prepare a broad range eight-point standard curve covering the concentrations between 1.95 and 32,000 pg/mL (*see* **Note 4**) by performing the following dilutions in 1.5-mL microcentrifuge tubes:

   a. Prepare the 32,000 pg/mL standard solution by adding 128 µL of the stock solution into 72 µL of culture medium and vortex gently to mix.
   b. Prepare the 8000 pg/mL standard solution by adding 50 µL of the 32,000 pg/mL standard solution (a) to 150 µL of culture medium and vortex gently to mix.
   c. Prepare the 2000 pg/mL standard solution by adding 50 µL of the 8000 pg/mL standard solution (b) to 150 µL of culture medium and vortex gently to mix.
   d. Prepare the 500 pg/mL standard solution by adding 50 µL of the 2000 pg/mL standard solution (c) to 150 µL of culture medium and vortex gently to mix.
   e. Prepare the 125 pg/mL standard solution by adding 50 µL of the 500 pg/mL standard solution (d) to 150 µL of culture medium and vortex gently to mix.
   f. Prepare the 31.3 pg/mL standard solution by adding 50 µL of the 125 pg/mL standard solution (e) to 150 µL of culture medium and vortex gently to mix.
   g. Prepare the 7.8 pg/mL standard solution by adding 50 µL of the 31.3 pg/mL standard solution (f) to 150 µL of culture medium vortex gently to mix.
   h. Prepare the 1.95 pg/mL standard solution by adding 50 µL of the 7.8 pg/mL standard solution (g) to 150 µL of culture medium and vortex gently to mix.

5. Use culture medium only for the zero point of the standard.
6. Place standard solutions on ice until use.

3.3.3. Conjugated Bead Preparation

1. Vortex the stock anti-cytokine conjugated beads for 15–20 s at medium speed.
2. Sonicate the stock anti-cytokine conjugated beads for 30 s (*see* **Note 5**).
3. Prepare 6 mL of anti-cytokine conjugated bead working solution (enough to perform an entire 96-well plate) by adding 240 µL of 25X stock anti-cytokine conjugated beads to 5.76 mL of Bio-Plex assay buffer in a 10-mL tube.
4. Wrap the tube in aluminum foil to protect the beads from light and place on ice (*see* **Note 6**).

3.3.4. Preparation of 96-Well Filter Plate and Samples for Multiplex Bead, Detection Antibody, and Streptavidin–PE Incubations

1. Pre-wet the 96-well filter plate by adding 100 µL of wash solution to each well.

    a. Allow the plate to soak for 15–30 s.

    b. Place the plate on the Millipore filtration unit and apply 3 mm Hg pressure to empty the wells (*see* **Note 7**).

    c. Remove the filter plate and gently blot the bottom of the plate onto paper towels twice to remove any excess fluid before continuing with the assay.

2. Vortex the working anti-cytokine bead solution 15–20 s and add 50 μL of the working bead solution to all 96 wells.

3. Filter the wells utilizing the Millipore filtration vacuum unit.

4. Add 100 μL working wash solution (Bio-Plex buffer A) to each well to wash, filter and repeat. Remove the filter plate and blot the bottom of the filter plate twice on clean paper towels to remove excess liquid (*see* **Note 8**).

5. Place the filter plate onto a plastic plate holder (*see* **Note 9**), gently mix and vortex the standards and pipet 50 μL of each standard (in duplicate) into their assigned well of the plate.

6. Gently mix and vortex each sample and pipet 50 μL, in duplicate, into the appropriate wells. Pipet tips should be changed after each sample.

7. Cover the plate with the cover and aluminum foil, place it on the orbital shaker, and incubate for 30 min at room temperature (*see* **Note 10**).

8. Twenty minutes after initiating the incubation in **step 12**, prepare the biotinylated detection antibody by gently vortexing the multiplex detection antibody (50X) stock solution.

    a. Perform a quick-spin of the detection antibody.

    b. Dilute the 120-μl, tube of 25X biotinylated detection antibody concentrate 50-fold with 2.88 mL of Bio-Plex detection antibody diluent A to make a total of 3 mL 1X working detection antibody.

9. At the end of the 30-min incubation, place the plate on the plate filter and apply a vacuum to remove the solution from the wells.

10. Wash three times with 100 μL of working wash solution/well (Bio-Plex wash buffer A) and blot as previously described in **step 8**.

11. Briefly vortex the biotinylated detection antibody (prepared in **step 13**) and pipet 25 μL into each well of the plate.

12. Cover the plate with the cover and aluminum foil, place it on the orbital shaker and incubate for 30 min at room temperature.

13. During the last 10 min of the incubation, prepare the streptavidin-PE working solution.

    a. Perform a quick-spin of the streptavidin–PE stock solution (100X).

    b. Dilute the 60 μL of 100x streptavidin–PE concentrate 100-fold with 5.94 mL of Bio-Plex assay buffer A.

14. At the end of the 30-min incubation, remove the cover from the plate and filter the solution from the wells using the filter apparatus.

15. Wash the beads in the filter plate three times with 100 μL of working wash solution and blot after each wash (Bio-Plex wash buffer A), as in **step 8**.

16. Vortex the streptavidin–PE working solution and then pipet 50 μL to each well.

17. Cover the plate, wrap in aluminum foil, and incubate on the orbital shaker for 10 min at room temperature.
18. After 10 min, place the plate on the filter apparatus to remove the streptavidin–PE solution.
19. Wash the plate three times with the working wash solution, being careful to blot the plate after each wash.
20. Pipet 125 μL of Bio-Plex assay buffer in each well, cover the plate and shake on the orbital shaker for 30 s, slowly increasing the speed to a maximum of 1100 rpm.
21. Load the plate into the Luminex XYP platform (*see* **Note 11**).
22. Set up the Luminex instrument using the Luminex Data Collector software
    a. Set the instrument to remove 50 μL of sample.
    b. Set total events to equal the number of analytes in the multiplex (X) 100.
    c. Assign the bead regions for each cytokine according to the package insert.
    d. Set the inclusion gates at 8000 and 15,000.
23. Run the Luminex 100™ instrument and collect the median fluorescent intensity data utilizing the Luminex Data Collector Software.

3.4. Data Reduction and Presentation

Median fluorescent intensity data was imported into the Bio-PlexManager software to perform data reduction. Standard curves were generated and cytokine concentrations were interpolated for each sample utilizing a 5-parameter curve fit equation. Utilizing Slidewrite Plus Data Analysis Software, the data are presented as the mean ± standard error for each treatment group (**Figs. 1–4**).

3.5. Results

Data validating the use of a multiplex cytokine assay procedure to simultaneously measure cytokine production in stimulated CBDMC are presented in **Figs. 1–4**. Data for IL-6 were collected; however, because the medium was supplemented with IL-6, the measured concentrations for all samples were greater than the linearity of the curve and therefore they are not included in the results. Co-incubation of CBDMCs with PMA/Iono significantly ($p < 0.05$) increased the concentrations of IL-1β, IFN-γ, TNF-α, GM-CSF, G-CSF, IL-2, IL-4, IL-5, IL-7, IL-10, IL-12, IL-13, and IL-17 as compared with those cultured with media alone (**Figs. 1–4A**). Similarly, treatment of CBDMCs with IgE/anti-IgE significantly ($p < 0.05$) increased the concentrations of IL-8, MIP-1, and MCP-1β as compared to those cultured with media alone (**Fig. 4B,D**).

4. Notes

1. The Luminex Multi-Analyte Profiling (xMAP) technology is based on the development of 100 distinct sets of color-coded beads that serve as the solid support to build a conventional immunoassay. The Bio-Rad 17-plex cytokine assay is designed

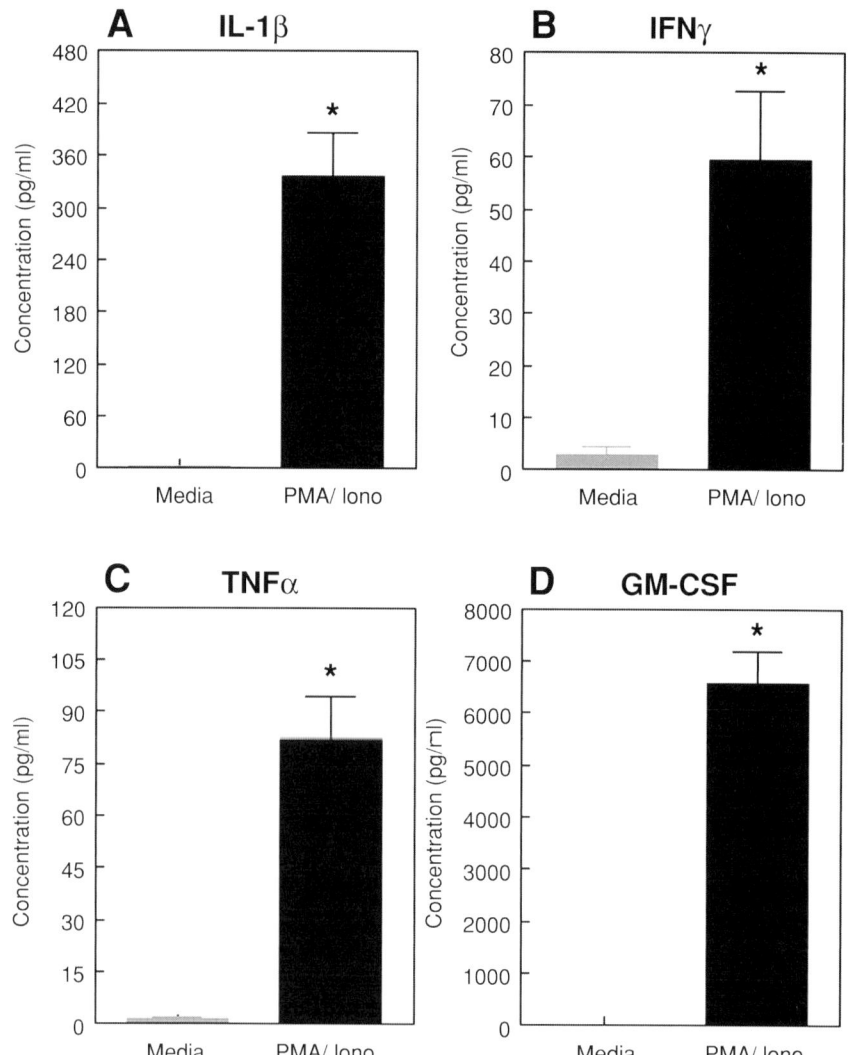

Fig. 1. Treatment of cord blood-derived mast cells (CBDMCs) with PMA/Iono
increased media levels of IL-1β, IFN-γ, TNF-α, and GM-CSF. CBDMCs incubated
in media alone served as the negative control. Each bar represents the mean ± SEM for
each treatment group (*$p < 0.05$ vs media).

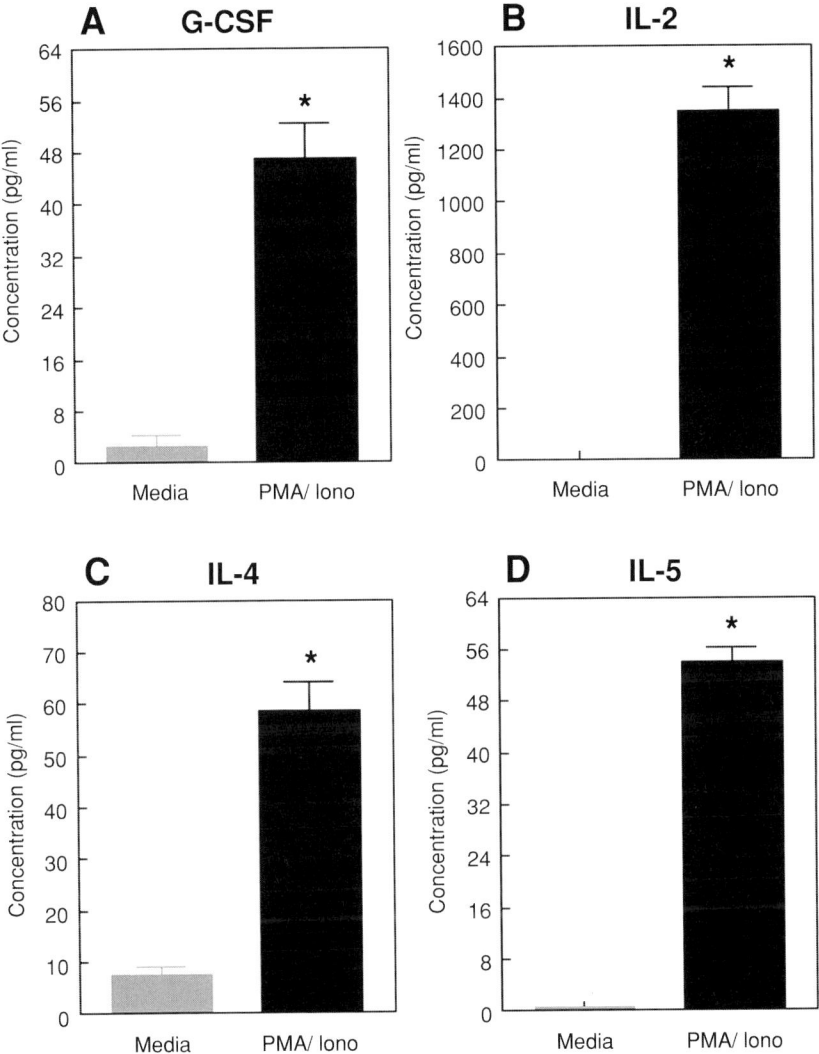

Fig. 2. Treatment of cord blood-derived mast cells (CBDMCs) with PMA/Iono increased media levels of G-CSF, IL-2, IL-4, and IL-5. CBDMCs incubated in media alone served as the negative control. Each bar represents the mean ± SEM for each treatment group (*$p < 0.05$ vs media).

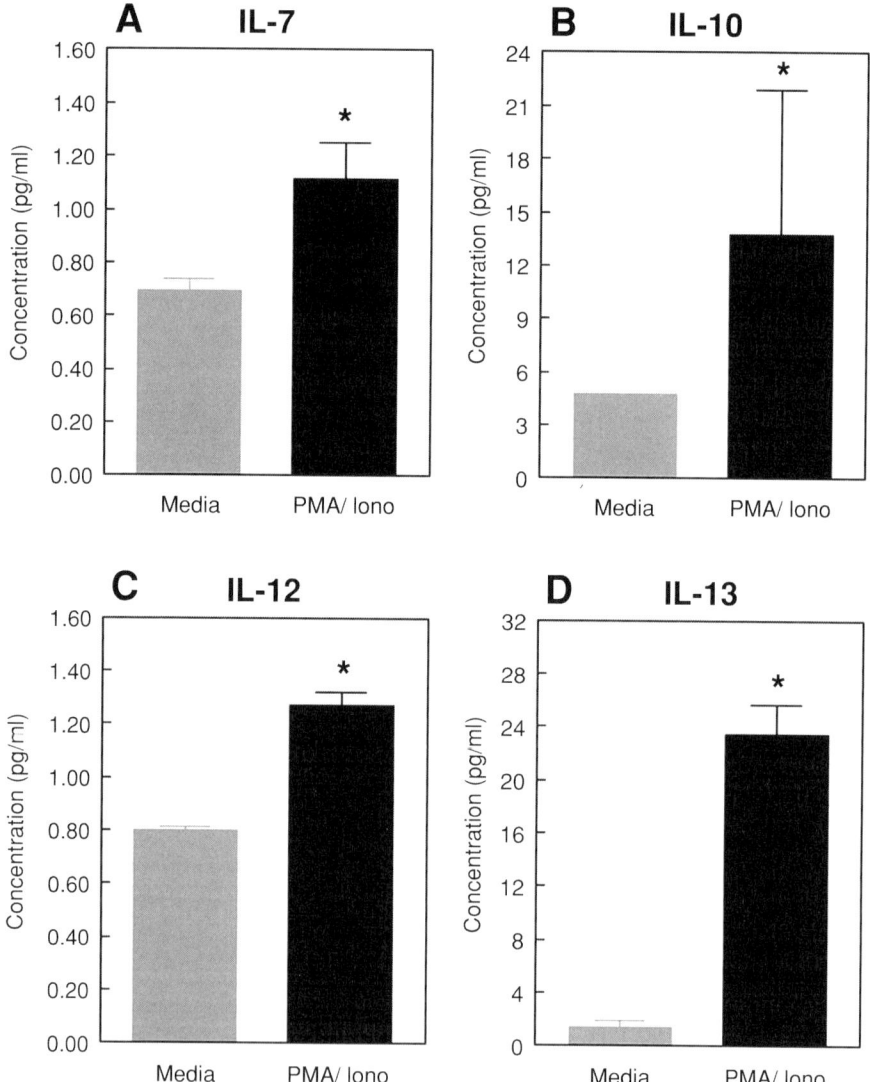

Fig. 3. Treatment of cord blood-derived mast cells (CBDMCs) with PMA/Iono increased media levels of IL-7, IL-10, IL-12, and IL-13. CBDMCs incubated in media alone served as the negative control. Each bar represents the mean ± SEM for each treatment group (*$p < 0.05$ vs media).

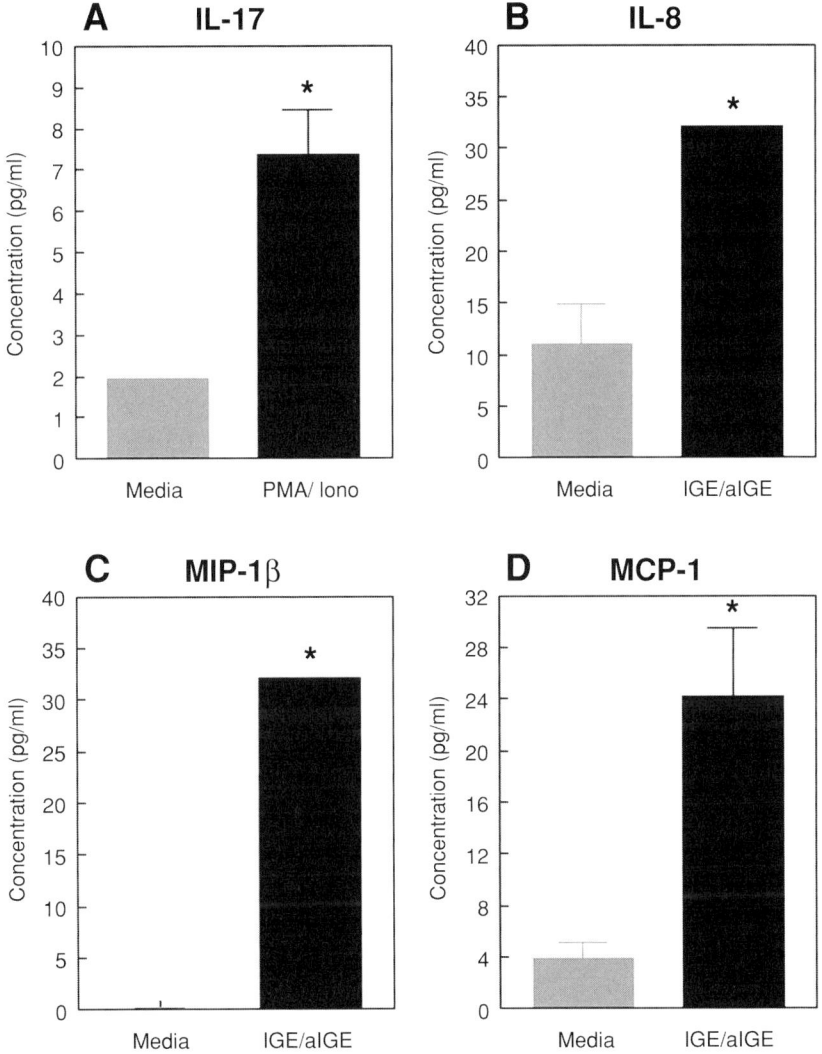

Fig. 4. Treatment of cord blood-derived mast cells (CBDMCs) with PMA/Iono increased media levels of IL-17, whereas IgE/anti-IgE increased media levels of IL-8, MIP-1β, and MCP-1. CBDMCs incubated in media alone served as the negative control. Each bar represents the mean ± SEM for each treatment group (*$p < 0.05$ vs media).

in a conventional capture sandwich immunoassay format. Cytokine-specific antibodies are covalently coupled to color coded 5.6-μm beads. The antibody-coupled beads are incubated with known (standards) and unknown (sample) amounts of cytokine. After a series of brief washes to remove unbound protein a biotinylated detection antibody specific for a different epitope on the cytokine is added to the beads. The reaction mixture is detected by the addition of streptavidin-phycoerythrin, which binds to the biotinylated detection antibodies. The solution in each well is drawn up into the flow-based Luminex system, which identifies and quantifies each cytokine.

2. Cell culture samples routinely contain varying amounts of debris. It is imperative that the sample is centrifuged prior to performance of the multiplex assay. If needed, samples may be centrifuged at 12,000g for 15 min. This step assures that the sample is free of debris which might alter the assay or clog the Luminex 100 instrument. Additionally, centrifugation also will assure that any sample trapped in the lid or on the side of the tube is spun to the bottom.

3. It is important to maintain the same matrix for the standards and samples. If it is anticipated that the cytokine levels are higher than the highest standard, dilute the sample with the same culture media used in the experiment. It is best to collect and freeze an additional 50-mL aliquot of the culture medium used for the experiment in order to assure identical sample matrixes at the time of assay performance.

4. If possible, fine tune the range of standards to cover the anticipated concentrations of cytokines. Ideally, it is best if most samples have values that are read from the middle of the standard curve. If the sample values cannot be estimated reliably, then a broad range for the standard curve should be established.

5. Sonication separates out individual beads from the agglomeration of beads that occurs when the beads are left in one position for a period of time. Failure to separate the beads will hinder the assay performance and will clog the Luminex 100 instrument.

6. The xMAP technology uses fluorescent dye in the assay procedure. Repeated exposure of the beads to light will alter the performance of the assay by decreasing the mean fluorescent intensity measured by the Luminex 100 instrument.

7. To avoid tearing the filters on the bottom of the 96-well filter plate, keep the vacuum for the filter plate set to less than 5 mm Hg of pressure. Keeping the vacuum at a constant 3 mm Hg of pressure insures safe operation of the apparatus on the filter plate.

8. It is important to thoroughly blot the bottom of the filter plate on paper towels after each filtration. This helps prevent cross-contamination and the loss of fluids from inside the microtiter wells.

9. Great care should be taken to keep the bottom of the 96-well plate from touching another surface during performance of the assay. Failure to do so will result in cross-contamination between wells and the wicking of fluids from inside the well during incubation steps. A plastic plate holder can be used so that the undersides of the wells do not touch any surfaces beneath them. If a plastic plate holder is not available, the plastic cover from a 96-well plate can be turned upside-down and placed under the filter plate.

10. During incubation steps, the plate should be covered with the either the plastic lid provided with the plate, or an adhesive plate sealer/tape specially designed for 96-well plates. The covered plate should then be wrapped in aluminum foil to protect it from light. After placing the plate on the orbital shaker, the speed should be increased gradually from 0 to 1000 rpm, maintained for 30 s, and reduced to 300 rpm for the remaining incubation time. Gradually increasing the speed will assure thorough mixing of the reagents and will reduce splashing of them onto the sides of the microtiter wells.

11. If the filter plate cannot be read immediately, it can be covered, wrapped in aluminum foil, and stored at 4°C for up to 24 h. Before reading the plate should be shaken at 1100 rpm for 30 s.

References

1. Abraham, S. N. and Malaviya, R. (1997) Mast cells in infection and immunity. *Infect. Immun.* **65,** 3501–3508.
2. Barrett, K. E. (1992) Effect of histamine and other mast cell mediators on T84 epithelial cells. *Ann. N. Y. Acad. Sci.* **664,** 222–231.
3. Cairns, J. A. and Walls, A. F. (1996) Mast cell tryptase is a mitogen for epithelial cells. Stimulation of IL-8 production and intercellular adhesion molecule-1 expression. *J. Immunol.* **156,** 275–283.
4. Galli, S. J. (1993) New concepts about the mast cell. *N. Engl. J. Med.* **328,** 257–265.
5. Hebda, P. A., Collins, M. A., and Tharp, M. D. (1993) Mast cell and myofibroblast in wound healing. *Dermatol. Clin.* **11,** 685–696.
6. Malaviya, R., Malaviya, R., and Jakschik, B. A. (1993) Reversible translocation of 5-lipoxygenase in mast cells upon IgE/antigen stimulation. *J. Biol. Chem.* **268,** 4939–4944.
7. Sugimoto, K., Kasuga, F., and Kumagai, S. (1994) Effects of B subunit of cholera toxin on histamine release from rat peritoneal mast cells. *Int. Arch. Allergy Immunol.* **105,** 195–197.
8. Kelley, J. L., Chi, D. S., Abou-Auda, W., Smith, J. K., and Krishnaswamy, G. (2000) The molecular role of mast cells in atherosclerotic cardiovascular disease. *Mol. Med. Today* **6,** 304–308.
9. Krishnaswamy, G., Kelley, J., Johnson, D., et al. (2001) The human mast cell: functions in physiology and disease. *Front Biosci.* **6,** D1109–D1127.
10. Krishnaswamy, G., Hall, K., Youngberg, G., et al. (2002) Regulation of eosinophil-active cytokine production from human cord blood-derived mast cells. *J. Interferon Cytokine Res.* **22,** 379–388.
11. Shakoory, B., Fitzgerald, S. M., Lee, S. A., Chi, D. S., and Krishnaswamy, G. (2004) The role of human mast cell-derived cytokines in eosinophil biology. *J. Interferon Cytokine Res.* **24,** 271–281.
12. Hahn, S. and Moroni, C. (1994) Modulation of cytokine expression in PB-3c mastocytes by IBMX and PMA. *Lymphokine Cytokine Res.* **13,** 247–252.
13. Bradding, P., Roberts, J. A., Britten, K. M., et al. (1994) Interleukin-4, -5, and -6 and tumor necrosis factor-alpha in normal and asthmatic airways: evidence for the human mast cell as a source of these cytokines. *Am. J. Respir. Cell Mol. Biol.* **10,** 471–480.

14. Krishnaswamy, G., Lakshman, T., Miller, A. R., et al. (1997) Multifunctional cytokine expression by human mast cells: regulation by T cell membrane contact and glucocorticoids. *J. Interferon Cytokine Res.* **17,** 167–176.

15. Church, M. K. and Levi-Schaffer, F. (1997) The human mast cell. *J. Allergy Clin. Immunol.* **99,** 155–160.

16. Kellar, K. L. and Douglass, J. P. (2003) Multiplexed microsphere-based flow cytometric immunoassays for human cytokines. *J. Immunol. Methods* **279,** 277–285.

17. Prabhakar, U., Eirikis, E., and Davis, H. M. (2002) Simultaneous quantification of proinflammatory cytokines in human plasma using the LabMAP assay. *J. Immunol. Methods* **260,** 207–218.

18. Carson, R. T. and Vignali, D. A. (1999) Simultaneous quantitation of 15 cytokines using a multiplexed flow cytometric assay. *J. Immunol. Methods* **227,** 41–52.

19. de Jager, W., te Velthuis H., Prakken, B. J., Kuis, W., and Rijkers, G. T. (2003) Simultaneous detection of 15 human cytokines in a single sample of stimulated peripheral blood mononuclear cells. *Clin. Diagn. Lab Immunol.* **10,** 133–139.

20. Martins, T. B., Pasi, B. M., Pickering, J. W., Jaskowski, T. D., Litwin, C. M., and Hill, H. R. (2002) Determination of cytokine responses using a multiplexed fluorescent microsphere immunoassay. *Am. J. Clin. Pathol.* **118,** 346–353.

21. Saito, H., Ebisawa, M., Tachimoto, H., et al. (1996) Selective growth of human mast cells induced by Steel factor, IL-6, and prostaglandin E2 from cord blood mononuclear cells. *J. Immunol.* **157,** 343–350.

22. Bio-Rad Laboratories. *Bio-Plex Cytokine Assay Instruction Manua*l. Rev D. 7–1-2003. Bio-Rad Laboratories, Inc., Richmond, CA

18

Assays for Histamine-Releasing Factors
From Identification and Cloning to Discovery of Binding Partners

Jacqueline M. Langdon and Susan M. MacDonald

Summary

When using a model to study disease, it may be advantageous to identify molecules responsible for biologic functions observed in the model to better understand the disease process being studied. The late phase reaction is used as a model for chronic inflammation, and the histamine releasing activity observed from late phase fluids was thought to be an important factor in the propagation of symptoms that remain in both the late-phase reaction and in chronic inflammation, when the offending antigen is no longer present. Purification from biologic fluids and identification may be helpful in understanding the role of the histamine-releasing factors in inflammation. Once the specific molecule is identified and cloned, techniques such as yeast two-hybrid screens and co-immunoprecipitation experiments can be used to identify binding partners and further elucidate the role of the cloned molecule. The purification and cloning of *human recombinant histamine-releasing factor* and the subsequent yeast two-hybrid screen and co-immunoprecipitation will be described to illustrate how any functionally defined molecule can be investigated.

Key Words: Late-phase reaction (LPR); human recombinant histamine releasing factor (HrHRF); basophils; cloning; yeast two-hybrid system; co-immunoprecipitation.

1. Introduction

The late-phase reaction (LPR) is a model for chronic allergic inflammation for many reasons, including the pattern of cellular influx. Specifically, an influx of eosinophils, monocytes, and basophils occurs, and these cells are known to be activated and hyper-responsive to stimuli *(1,2)*. Although many characteristics of the LPR are well documented, the stimulus for the activation of basophils, as well as the reason why only some allergic individuals have a LPR are still unclear. Since Theueson et al. in 1979 *(3)*, histamine-releasing factors (HRFs),

From: *Methods in Molecular Biology, vol. 315: Mast Cells: Methods and Protocols*
Edited by: G. Krishnaswamy and D. S. Chi © Humana Press Inc., Totowa, NJ

or molecules that cause basophils to release histamine, have been under study by many groups including our own. Our HRF initially was defined by the direct release of histamine from the basophils of a subset of allergic donors *(4)*. Clinical data demonstrating the presence of HRF in skin blister fluids after antigen challenge *(5)*, as well as in nasal lavages during the LPR *(6)*, indicated that identifying the molecule in these biological fluids responsible for causing the histamine release was a crucial step to understanding the mechanisms of the LPR. Fortunately, HRF also was found in cellular supernatants of several cell lines, including the macrophage-like cell line U937 *(7)*, which we used to identify the actual molecule responsible for the histamine release observed *(8)*. Herein, we will describe the approaches and methods used to identify a molecule of defined function from biological fluids, clone this molecule and then use this recombinant protein to search for binding partners that would further elucidate the functions of the molecule.

2. Materials

1. U937 cell line (American Type Culture Collection).
2. Chromatography equipment.
3. Column Buffers (CB): for Sepahadex G75 CB: 0.01 M Tris-HCl, 0.15 M NaCl, pH 7.4; Mono Q CB: 0.02 M Tris-HCl, pH 8.0, with HCl; and for Superdex CB (1X PIPES): 25 mM PIPES, 110 mM NaCl, 0.5 mM KCl, pH 7.3 with NaOH.
4. Dialysis tubing.
5. Sodium dodecyl sulfate-polyacrylamide gel electrophoresis (SDS-PAGE) gels, buffers, and equipment.
6. Transfer buffer: 12 mM Tris, 96 mM glycine, 20% methanol.
7. Polyvinylidene difluoride membrane.
8. Coomassie blue.
9. Access to a sequencing facility.
10. Custom oligonucleotide primers.
11. Reverse transcriptase polymerase chain reaction (RT-PCR) kit.
12. Agarose and ethidium bromide.
13. Deoxyribonucleic acid (DNA) purification kits.
14. Restriction enzymes, T7 DNA polymerase, and T4 DNA ligase.
15. Bacterial expression vectors (e.g., pGEX-2T, pRSET)
16. *Escherichia coli* strains (e.g., JM109, DH5α, BL21 [DE3]).
17. LB medium: 10 g of tryptone, 5 g of yeast extract, 10 g of NaCl, and 1 L of water.
18. Phosphate-buffered saline (PBS).
19. Triton X-100.
20. Glutathione agarose.
21. Antibiotics for selection (e.g., Ampicillin, Zeocin™; Invitrogen).
22. Isopropyl-β-ᴅ-thio-galactopyranoside (IPTG).
23. Elution buffer: 5 mM reduced glutathione, 50 mM Tris-HCl, pH 7.5.
24. Yeast two-hybrid kit and cDNA expression library.

25. Yeast medium: a) YC: 0.12% yeast nitrogen base, 0.5% ammonium sulfate, 1% succinic acid, 0.6% NaOH, 2% glucose, 0.01% of adenine, arginine, cysteine, leucine, lysine, threonine, tryptophan, and uracil, 0.005% aspartic acid, histidine, isoleucine, methionine, phenylalanine, proline, and serine, with 2% agar for plates; and b) YPAD: 1% yeast extract, 2% peptone, 2% D-glucose, 0.1 g of adenine, with 2% agar for plates.
26. Y-DER™ Yeast DNA Extraction Kit (Pierce).
27. Protease Inhibitor Cocktail (BD-Pharmingen).
28. Nitrocellulose.
29. Antibodies to fusion protein tags and/or molecules of interest (e.g., anti-GST [z-5, Santa Cruz Biotechnology], anti-Express [Invitrogen], anti-HRF, control rabbit IgG, and HRP-tagged secondary antibodies.)
30. Chemiluminescent substrate.
31. RIPA 50: 50 mM Tris-HCl, 50 mM NaCl, 1% Nonidet P-40, 1% sodium deoxycholate, 0.1% SDS, 2 mM ethylene diamine tetraacetic acid.
32. Protein A Sepharose 4 Fast Flow (Amersham Biosciences).
33. Stripping buffer: 70 mM SDS, 60mM Tris-HCl, pH 6.7.

3. Methods

The methods in **Subheadings 3.1.–3.4.** describe: (1) the purification and identification of a functionally defined molecule from biological fluids; (2) the cloning and expression of the molecule in *E. coli*; (3) the use of the yeast two-hybrid system to identify a binding partner; and (4) the confirmation of this protein–protein interaction using co-immunoprecipitation experiments.

3.1. Purification and Identification of a Functionally Defined Molecule

In the search for a causative agent responsible for a specific bioactivity, in our case histamine release, the general approach is to remove the maximum amount of overall protein, while maintaining the function of interest by sequential purification steps. Our strategy involved monitoring total protein by absorbance readings (A_{280}) and function by histamine-release assays using basophils from our subpopulation of allergic donors. The purification steps were: (1) repetitive column chromatography; followed by (2) gel electrophoresis.

3.1.1. Repetitive Column Chromatography

1. Culture the U937 cell line to obtain 50 L of supernatant containing histamine release activity.
2. Concentrate the supernatant to 14 mL and apply to a Sephadex G75 gel filtration column (5 × 90 cm) with a bed volume of 1.8 L in 0.01 M Tris-HCl, 0.15 M NaCl, pH 7.4.
3. Collect 140–13-mL column fractions and monitor the protein concentration by A_{280} and the bioactivity by histamine release.

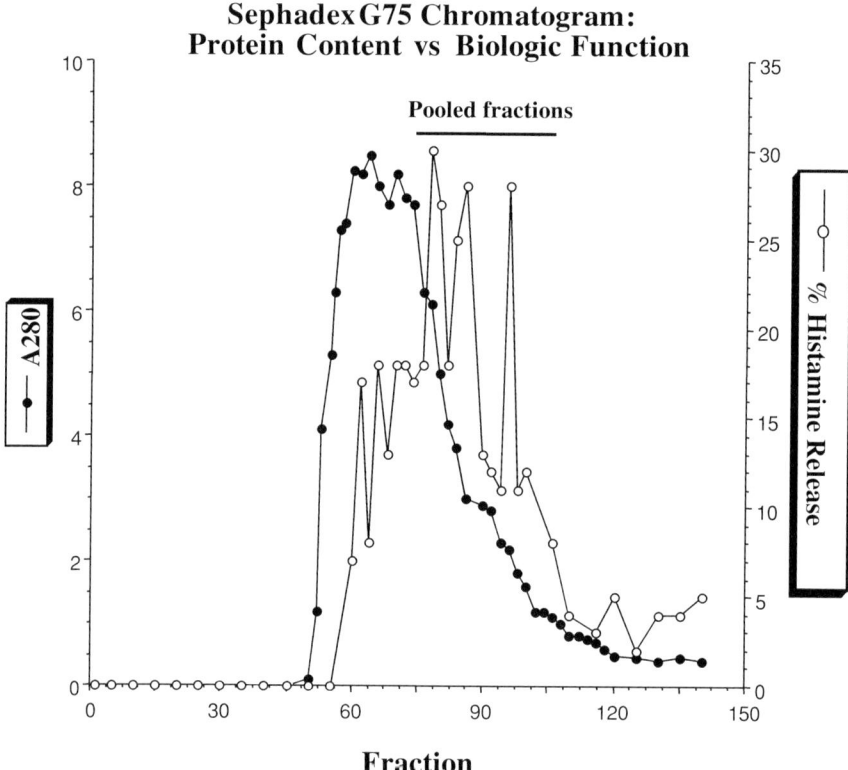

**Sephadex G75 Chromatogram:
Protein Content vs Biologic Function**

Fig.1. Example of column chromatography using size-exclusion Sephadex 675 is shown. The protein tracing (●) is demonstrated to be predominately separated from the biologic activity (○, histamine release). Fractions were pooled (tubes 72–100) to maximize biologic activity and minimize protein contamination.

4. The histamine release assay is routinely used in our laboratory *(4)*, but any functional measure that is of interest can be used to track the purification, for example, with a commercially available ELISA.
5. **Figure 1** shows the graph of these chromatography parameters and the fractions chosen to be further purified. This is a typical graph used to determine the column fractions of interest based on retaining maximal function and minimal protein.
6. Pool, concentrate, and dialyze the bioactive fractions into the MONO Q CB.
7. Perform several chromatographic runs on a MONO Q anion exchange column in 0.2 *M* Tris-HCl, pH 8.0 with an increasing salt gradient from 0 to 1 *M* NaCl.
8. Collect 30–2-mL column fractions and monitor the fractions as described above.
9. Pool the bioactive fractions from all of the MONO Q runs, concentrate, and dialyze against the Superdex CB.
10. Run numerous Superdex columns in 1X PIPES and collect 65–2-mL column fractions.

11. Monitor as previously described and pool and concentrate the active fractions for gel electrophoresis (*see* **Note 1**).

3.1.2. Gel Electrophoresis

1. Electrophoris the concentrated column fractions on SDS-PAGE using standard methods.
2. Blot onto a polyvinylidene difluoride membrane and stain with Coomassie blue.
3. Excise the visible bands from the membrane and send to an institutional core or a commercial laboratory for amino-terminal sequencing.
4. Once the sequence is obtained, online resources such as the NCBI Entrez page (http://www.ncbi.nlm.nih.gov) are useful for determining if the sequence matches a known sequence in a data base. In our case, a search matched one sequence to a protein in the data base with no known function called translationally controlled tumor protein (accession no. X16064, Swiss-Prot no. P13693).

3.2. Cloning and Expression in E. coli

To confirm that the sequence obtained from the database is responsible for the bioactivity of interest, the following can be performed: (1) subclone the sequence from the data base into an *E. coli* expression vector; (2) express the recombinant protein in *E. coli* as a tagged fusion protein; and (3) purify the recombinant protein by affinity chromatography and test the biologic function (*see* **Note 2**).

3.2.1. Subclone the Sequence into an E. coli Expression Vector

1. Amplify the protein of interest using RT-PCR from the cDNA of a primary cell or cell line that makes the protein. For our protein, we used the monocytic cell line U937.
2. Design custom oligonucleotide primers using the sequence from the data bank with the addition of restriction sites to the 5' and 3' ends (*see* **Note 3**). For example, the primers we used were: 5' primer, 5'-AAAAGGATCCATGATCAT CTACCGGGACC-3; 3' primer, 5'-AAAGAATTCTTAACATTTCTCCAT–3'. These primers include a *Bam*H1 site on the 5' end and *Eco*R1 site on the 3' end.
3. Amplify the PCR product using the manufacturer's standard protocol and PCR conditions based on the custom oligonucleotides (*see* **Note 4**).
4. Run a 1% agarose gel with 0.5 µg/mL ethidium bromide to visualize the band, and then excise the PCR product from the gel.
5. Purify the PCR product using a commercially available kit and then restrict both the PCR product and the vector, pGEX-2T in our case, with the specific restriction enzymes for 1 h at 37°C.
6. Ligate the restricted PCR product in frame with GST in the pGEX-2T vector (*see* **Note 5**).
7. Perform standard bacterial transformations according to the manufacturer's specifications (*see* **Note 6**).

3.2.2. Express the Recombinant Protein

1. Express the protein in *E. coli* cells by inoculating a 100-mL culture of LB with 50 µg/mL ampicillin with a single colony from the transformation and shake overnight at 37°C.
2. Add the 100-mL overnight culture to 1 L of LB with 50 µg/mL ampicillin and grow for an additional 3 h, shaking at 37°C.
3. Induce the protein production with 0.1 m*M* IPTG for 4 h shaking at 37°C (*see* **Note 7**).
4. Spin the cultures at 3500*g* for 15 min. Discard the supernatant and store the pellets at –20°C until purification.

3.2.3. Purify the Recombinant Protein and Test the Function

1. Resuspend the cell pellets in 25 mL of PBS and lyse by sonication on ice.
2. Spin the lysates at 10,000*g* for 10 min.
3. Add Triton X-100 to the lysates at a 1% final concentration and combine with a 50% slurry of glutathione agarose to a 1% final concentration.
4. Wash three times with 50 mL of PBS in a batch method by spinning at 500*g* for 5 min.
5. Elute the GST fusion protein from the agarose with 3–2-mL washes of 5 m*M* reduced glutathione elution buffer in a batch method with 3–5 min 500*g* spins.
6. Dialyze the free glutathione out of the sample with a buffer compatible with your functional assay before determining function or protein levels.
7. The biologic function of the cloned HrHRF was tested using our histamine release assay *(4)*, but again, any functional marker could be used depending on the protein of interest.

3.3. The Yeast Two-Hybrid System

The yeast two-hybrid system is a method for detecting interaction between proteins, and can be used to discover novel protein interactions (*see* **Note 8**). Generally, the protein of interest is subcloned into a plasmid to form a fusion protein with a DNA-binding domain (DBD) and then cotransformed into yeast with a relevant cDNA library in a plasmid containing the activation domain (AD). If there is a protein interaction between the protein of interest, also known as the bait, and one of the library proteins, the DBD and AD are brought together in the nucleus of the yeast and transcriptional activation is restored. This activation can be monitored by expression of reporter genes downstream, such as lacZ and/or a marker for nutritional auxotrophy. The activation of lacZ is measured by a screen for β-galactosidase activity, and the auxotrophic activation is determined by colony growth on YC media deficient for the specific auxotrophic marker. The transcriptional activation markers will depend upon the strain of yeast used, and the media specifications will vary accordingly. Numerous manufacturers have kits and prepared cDNA libraries to facilitate this type of investigation. The kits are complete with detailed instructions on methods specific for the yeast two-hybrid system, therefore this section will describe the steps and troubleshoot this method. This section will outline: (1) the construction of a bait plasmid; (2) the co-transformation of the bait with a cDNA library; (3) the screen for transcription activation; and (4) the identification of positive clones.

3.3.1. Construction of a Bait Plasmid

1. Subclone the protein of interest, HrHRF, in frame with the DBD to create a fusion protein (DBD/HrHRF). The protein expression and yeast DBD vectors may have multiple cloning sites that will allow a direct restriction and ligation from the protein expression vector directly into the yeast DBD vector. If this strategy is not viable, design a cloning strategy as described in **Subheading 3.2.1.** using a PCR-amplified product with additional restriction sites to make the DBD/HrHRF fusion protein in frame.
2. Maintain and propagate the DBD/HrHRF yeast vector in *E. coli*.
3. Sequence the fusion protein to insure the cloning strategy was successful before proceeding.
4. Transform the bait DBD/HrHRF plasmid into yeast alone and with an empty library vector, as described in **Subheading 3.2.2.**, and screen the DBD/HrHRF fusion protein for non-specific activation of the reporter genes, as described in **Subheading 3.3.3.**, before proceeding with library screening (*see* **Note 9**).

3.3.2. Co-Transformation of the Bait With a cDNA Library

1. Co-transform the yeast with the DBD/HrHRF vector and the library vector using standard small scale yeast transformation.
2. Briefly, repeat the small-scale transformations in order to screen the desired number of clones, approx 10 million in our case were screened to give a good representation of the library (*see* **Note 10**).
3. To determine the number of clones you have screened, plate a portion of your transformation on YC media containing selection markers for both the Bait vector and Library vector. We used the antibiotic Zeocin to select for the DBD vector and the auxotrophic marker TRP-1 to select for the Library vector. The media we used was YC, minus tryptophan, plus Zeocin.

3.3.3. Screen for Transcription Activation

Screen for protein interactions by plating the transformations on YC media deficient for the auxotrophic marker for transcriptional activation. This will vary depending on the yeast strain used, but in our case it was histadine deficient media (YC–histadine). Further screen colonies detected by the selective plates for β-galactosidase expression. Specifically, restreak each colony from the auxotrophic selective media plate onto duplicate plates. Keep one plate to propagate the clones of interest and the other to screen for β-galactosidase activity (*see* **Note 11**). A filter lift assay is quick and allows screening of numerous clones at one time (*9*).

3.3.4. Identification of Positive Clones

1. To identify the proteins responsible for the interaction with the bait protein, HrHRF, isolate the plasmid DNA from double-positive yeast clones. Using a commercially available kit, such as Y-DER™ Yeast DNA Extraction Kit, will facilitate this step. Yeast cells are difficult to lyse, and the standard methods involve harsh and time-consuming treatments. Regardless, the quality and quantity of plasmid DNA isolated from the yeast clone is not sufficient for sequencing.

2. To obtain sequence quality DNA, transform the extracted yeast DNA into *E. coli* using a standard bacterial transformation according to the manufacturer's specifications.

3. Grow *E. coli* mini preps from single colonies from the transformation and isolate the plasmid DNA using a commercially available kit. Numerous DNA purification kits are available, so check with the sequencing facility that you will use for the preferred method.

4. After sequencing, search data bases for a match to the sequence, as suggested in **Subheading 3.1.2.** (*see* **Note 12**). Check the open reading frame of the sequences of interest to determine if the predicted protein is translated. Our library screen and data base search yielded one sequence match which was elongation factor-1δ *(10)*.

3.4. Confirmation of the Interaction of Molecules by Co-Immunoprecipitation

Protein interactions identified in yeast two-hybrid screens require validation in another system. The protein–protein interaction can be confirmed by co-immunoprecipitating the original bait protein with the newly identified interactor from cellular lysates. The yeast vector used for the cDNA library in the yeast two-hybrid screen is not suitable for protein expression, so the interactors of interest are subcloned into an *E. coli* expression vector. The recombinant protein is then used for co-immunoprecipitation experiments. This section will outline: (1) the subcloning of the interactor for protein expression; and (2) the co-immunoprecipitation of the bait and the yeast two-hybrid identified proteins.

3.4.1. Subcloning of the Interactor for Protein Expression

1. Subclone the interactor from the yeast library vector into a bacterial expression vector. Choose a vector that will allow the protein of interest to be produced as a recombinant fusion protein with a convenient tag. Choose a tag based on available antibodies, ability of the antibodies to immunoprecipitate, and the ease of purification depending on the co-immunoprecipitation strategy (*see* **Note 13**). The protein expression and yeast vectors may have multiple cloning sites that will allow a direct restriction and ligation from the yeast vector directly into the chosen protein expression vector. If this strategy is not viable, design a cloning strategy as described in **Subheading 3.2.1.** using a PCR-amplified product with additional restriction sites to produce the fusion protein in frame.

2. Perform standard bacterial transformations according to the manufacturer's specifications.
3. Grow *E. coli* mini preps from the transformations, lyse the cell pellet in SDS/PAGE sample buffer, and run a Western blot.
4. Use antibodies to the tag or the protein of interest in a Western blot analysis to check for expression of the recombinant protein at the predicted size (*see* **Note 14**). Alternatively or in addition, isolate the plasmid DNA from a mini prep and sequence the fusion protein to insure that the cloning strategy was successful.
5. Produce the protein as described in **Subheading 3.2.2.**

3.4.2. Co-Immunoprecipitation of Proteins

1. Lyse the *E. coli* cell pellet from the protein production in RIPA 50 buffer with protease inhibitor cocktail and freeze thaw the cell suspension three times, switching from an ethanol bath with dry ice to a 37°C water bath.
2. Spin the lysates at 14,000g for 5 min and save the supernatant in two equal aliquots.
3. Preclear both lysates with 80 µL of a 50% slurry of protein A Sepharose 4 Fast Flow beads and 1 µg of control IgG antibody for 2 h rotating at 4°C to reduce nonspecific binding.
4. Spin the lysates at 1000g for 3 min and save the supernatant.
5. Add 1.5 µg of affinity purified GST-HrHRF fusion protein, prepared as described in **Subheading 3.2.3.** and rotate at 4°C for 16 h.
6. Add 1 µg of either control rabbit IgG or rabbit anti-GST antibody and rotate for 5 h at 4°C.
7. Add 40 µL of protein A Sepharose 4 Fast Flow Bead to each and rotate for 2 h at 4°C.
8. Wash the beads three times in 1 mL of RIPA 50 and spin for 5 min at 14,000g at 4°C.
9. Resuspend the beads in 40 µL of 2X SDS/PAGE sample buffer with 5% β-mercaptoethanol, boil for 5 min, and spin at 14,000g for 5 min.
10. Electrophoris the immunoprecipitation supernatants from each of the beads on SDS-polyacrylamine gels using standard methods.
11. Blot onto nitrocellulose and Western blot with mouse anti-fusion protein. We used anti-Express antibody. Strip the same blot with stripping buffer for 1 h at 65°C and Western blot with monoclonal anti-HrHRF. If the specific antibody immunoprecipitation lane is positive for both Western blots, while the control lane is clear, the protein–protein interaction is confirmed. We confirmed the interaction between HRF and elongation factor-1δ (*10*).

4. Notes

1. The repetitive chromatography strategy was designed to maximize recovery using size separation such as Sephadex and Superdex. The Mono Q column was run to separate the molecules using charge. We had previously determined using DE-52 batch elution that our protein bound an anion exchange column, and therefore the MONO Q column was used. Note that some proteins may require a cation exchange column for separation using charge. Loading volumes are depen-

dent on the bed volume of the column, and increasing length of chromatography columns can increase separation. The number of column runs depends on the total protein of the sample and the capacity of the column *(11)*. For all concentrations and dialysis a low molecular weight cut off was used because the size of the protein of interest was unknown.

2. When choosing an *E. coli* expression vector, consider making a tagged recombinant fusion protein that will facilitate protein purification. We used a glutathione-*S*-transferase (GST) tag in the pGEX-2T expression vector to make a GST fusion protein. Purification by GST affinity chromatography is simple and provides good yields and purity. In addition, the pGEX-2T has a thrombin cleavage site that allows for removal of the GST tag from the protein of interest. This cleavage can be helpful when proving the biologic function is to the result of the protein of interest and not the tag.

3. Primer design can be done on-line with programs provided by the commercial laboratories which make custom oligonucleotides, but these programs do not always allow for the addition of restriction sites. Consequently, we usually design them manually (*see* **Note 4**). When choosing restriction sites, check internal restriction sites of your protein to insure that your restriction enzymes do not cleave the protein of interest. Again, this can be done manually, or with the aid of computer software. Also, make sure that the restriction enzymes chosen have compatible restriction buffers. Manufacturers of the restriction enzymes provide the information regarding buffer compatibility.

4. Custom oligonucleotide, or primer design can be performed manually using the criteria described below which was developed by H. Halcem Smith and B. Vonakis (personal communication). The primers should be 19–26 bases and contain 8-12 Gs or Cs, so that 40–60% of the nucleotides are either G or C. The primers should contain either a G or a C anchor at both the 3' and the 5' ends. The melting temperature (T_m) should be between 60 and 75°C. The T_m is calculated using the formula T_m (°C) = 4(G +C) + 2(A+T). Do not have four of the same nucleotides consecutively or four consecutive Gs and Cs in the primer. Visually check the secondary structure to avoid hairpins, which occur when the primer has complementary sequences within the primer that would fold onto itself. In addition, check that there are no complementary sequences between the primer pairs that would allow them to hybridize to each other, creating primer dimers. When using these criteria for custom oligonucleotide design, the following PCR conditions can be used: 30 cycles of denature/anneal/amplify, specifically, 95°C for 1 min, 60°C for 1 min, and 72°C for 1 min, followed by a 3-min extension at 72°C and a 4°C soak.

5. PCR expression cloning can be very effective strategy for cloning; sometimes however, the enzymes do not efficiently restrict small PCR generated products. Therefore, it may be helpful to TA clone, using the sticky ends of the PCR product. Place the protein of interest into an intermediate vector specifically designed for TA cloning, and then subclone the protein of interest into the desired expression vector using the multiple cloning sites.

6. Several *E. coli* strains can be used for protein expression, including but not limited to JM109, DH5-α, and BL21(DE3). Some strains are optimized for protein expression, such as the BL21(DE3), but are not stable and require a fresh transformation for each protein expression. Choosing a strain such as DH5-α, which can be saved as a glycerol stock after the initial transformation, may save time.

7. Kinetics of optimal protein expression should be determined individually for each recombinant protein. A time coarse to determine optimal protein expression can be done by inoculating the culture as described and then removing small aliquots of the culture before induction with IPTG and then subsequently every hour. These samples can be lysed and then run on SDS-PAGE to identify the protein band of interest.

8. The yeast two-hybrid system has several pit falls. There are often many false positives that have sequences that do not correspond to any protein. These include, but are not limited to, known proteins that are inserted backwards into the vector. In addition, false negatives occur when previously observed interactions are not detected in the library screen. Also, the nature of the system requires that the interaction occur in a yeast nucleus, and this may be unfavorable for plasma membrane protein interactions. Other potential approaches, especially for extracellular interactions would include chemical crosslinking and co-immunoprecipitations using cells that are known to interact with the protein of interest.

9. If the bait nonspecifically activates the reporter genes or is lethal to the yeast strain, alternative strategies are possible. For example, there are many strains of yeast that can be used in the yeast two-hybrid system, and another strain may be more suitable. In addition, you can try using only a portion of your protein as bait, and then recheck the activation markers.

10. Large-scale co-transformations can also be performed; however, they are not as efficient as repetitive small scale yeast co-transformations.

11. The complete library screening generates numerous positive clones; therefore, the accuracy of labeling and maintaining the generated clones is important. The master plates of positive clones can be kept wrapped in Parafilm at 4°C but should be processed as soon as possible to determine whether any clones are of interest. Practically, small-scale co-transformations may be repeated after completion of the final analysis of positive clones.

12. The retrieval of yeast DNA, followed by the transformation in *E. coli* and sequencing, is time consuming and expensive. Consequently, positive interactors may be selectively screened based on the strength of the reporter. For example, only sequence clones with strong β-galactosidase interactions that appear before 30 min. This strategy is based on the observation that the strength of reporter may indicate strength of the protein interaction *(12)*.

13. When designing a strategy for co-immunoprecipitations be careful to chose an antibody which has been proven to immunoprecipitate. Commercial antibodies have this property designated in some cases, and technical support can provide specific protocols. In our case, an antibody to the GST tag was used to immuno-

precipitate. Consequently, the yeast two-hybrid identified protein was subcloned into an expression vector containing a tag other than GST. To simplify the Western blot analysis of the co-immunoprecipitation, it is best to use a primary antibody from a species different from that used to immunoprecipitate. In the case where the same species antibody is used in both the immunoprecipitation and Western blot, the secondary antibody used in the Western blot will crossreact with the IgG in the IP lanes, and may interfere with band detection, depending on the size of the molecule. The amount of antibody used in this protocol is determined to be effective with a minimum of nonspecific binding compared to control antibodies. The conditions for each immunoprecipitation may vary, and should be determined by trying different amounts of antibodies and proteins to optimize the reaction.

14. Western blot analysis generally involves a blocking step, an incubation with primary antibody to the tag or protein of interest, an incubation with a secondary labeled antibody and development with a chemiluminescent substrate, with washes in between each step. The exact conditions of the general steps vary for each antibody, and include, but are not limited to, different blocking agents, washing buffers, incubation times and antibody dilutions. Commercially available antibodies are provided with Western blotting protocols, but conditions should be optimized for the application.

Acknowledgments

These studies were supported by NIH grant R01 A132651 to Susan MacDonald. We thank Dr. Becky Vonakis and Ms. Halecm-Smith for their primer design protocol.

References

1. Viksman, M. Y., Liu, M. C., Schleimer, R. P., and Bochner, B. S. (1994) Application of flow cytometric method using autofluorescence and a tandem fluorescent dye to analyze human alveolar macrophage surface markers. *J. Immunol. Methods* **172**, 17–24.
2. Naclerio, R. M., Meier, H. C., Kagey-Sobtka, A., et al. (1983) Mediator release after nasal airway challenge with allergen. *Am. Rev. Respir. Dis.* **128**, 597–602.
3. Thueson, D. O., Speck, L. S., Lett-Brown, M. A., and Grant, J. A. (1979) Histamine releasing activity (HRA) I. Production by mitogen- or antigen-stimulated human mononuclear cells. *J. Immunol.* **123**, 626–632.
4. MacDonald, S. M., Lichtenstein, L. M., Proud, D., Plaut, M., Naclerio, R. M., and Kagey-Sobotka, A. (1987) Studies of IgE-dependent histamine releasing factors: heterogeneity of IgE. *J. Immunol.* **139**, 506–512.
5. Warner, J. A., Pienkowski, M. M., Plaut, M., Norman, P. S., and Lichtenstein, L. M. (1986) Identification of histamine releasing factor(s) in the late phase of cutaneous IgE-mediated reactions. *J. Immunol.* **136**, 2583–2587.
6. Plaut, M., MacDonald, S. M., Naclerio, R. M., et al. (1986) Characterization of human IgE-dependent histamine releasing factors. *Fed. Proc.* **45**, 243A.

7. Plaut, M., Liu, M. C., Conrad, D. H., Proud, D., and MacGlashan, D. W. (1986) Histamine release from human basophils is induced by IgE-dependent factor(s) derived from human lung macrophages and an Fcε receptor-positive human B cell line. *Trans. Assoc. Am. Phys.* **98,** 305–312.

8. MacDonald, S. M., Rafnar, T., Langdon, J., and Lichtenstein, L. M. (1995) molecular identification of an IgE-dependent histamine-releasing factor. *Science* **269,** 688–690.

9. Breeden, L. and Nasmyth, K. (1985) Regulation of the yeast HO gene. *Cold Spring Harbor Symp. Quant. Biol.* **50,** 643–650.

10. Langdon, J. M., Vonakis, B. M., and MacDonald, S. M. (2004) Identification of the interaction between the human recombinant histamine releasing factor/ translationally controlled tumor protein and elongation factor-1 delta (also know as eElongation factor-1B beta). *Biochim. Biophys. Acta* **1688,** 232–236.

11. Campbell, D. H., Garvey, J. S., Cremer, N. E., and Sussdorf, D. H., eds. (1970) Column Chromatography, in *Methods in Immunology.* W. A. Benjamin, Inc., New York, NY, pp. 104–110.

12. Estojak, J., Brent, R., and Golemis, E. A. (1995) Correlation of two-hybrid affinity data with in vitro measurements. *Mol. Cell. Biol.* **15,** 5820–5829.

19

Assays for Nitric Oxide Expression

William L. Stone, Hongsong Yang, and Min Qui

Summary

The purpose of this chapter is to review the analytical methodology specifically associated with studying the role of nitric oxide (NO) in mast cell physiology and biochemistry. The methodology for measuring cellular secretion of nitric oxide with Griess Reagent will be described in detail, as well as the use of 4,5-diaminofluorescein diacetate for continuous monitoring of nitric oxide production in live cells. We will point out the limitations of the analytical techniques and also indicate areas in which promising analytical techniques have not yet been applied to the study of mast cell physiology, that is, new research opportunities. In addition to reviewing the methodology associated with measuring NO itself, we will briefly touch upon some analytical methods important in characterizing the biochemical products formed from nitric oxide (e.g., 3-nitrotyrosine).

Key Words: Mast cells; nitric oxide; peroxynitrite; Griess reagent; nitrite; nitrate; nitric oxide synthase; 4,5-diaminofluorescein diacetate (DAF-2A); 2-(4-carboxyphenyl)-4,4,5,5-tetramethylimidazoline-1-oxyl-3-oxide (carboxy-PTIO).

1. Introduction

A number of excellent reviews have been published on the general techniques for measuring nitric oxide (NO) in biological systems (*1,2*). NO is a simple gaseous, diatomic free radical molecule that has a wide array of physiological functions, for example, a neuromessenger in the central nervous system, a modulator of blood pressure, a regulator of gastric motility, and a killer of airborne pathogens in the lung. NO can easily diffuse through biological membranes and between subcellular organelles because of its small size and lack of charge. It is synthesized by many cells types, including mast cells and macrophages, which play critical roles in immunity and inflammation (*3*).

Mast cells are widely distributed in many tissue types and have very specialized secretory functions. They play a key role in allergic responses and inflammation (*4*). Knowledge of how NO modulates mast cell functions has been

From: *Methods in Molecular Biology, vol. 315: Mast Cells: Methods and Protocols*
Edited by: G. Krishnaswamy and D. S. Chi © Humana Press Inc., Totowa, NJ

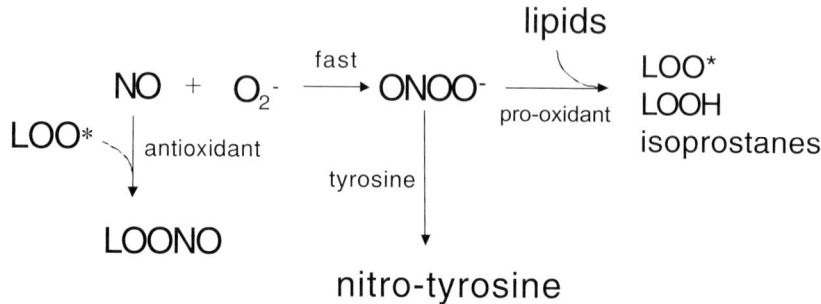

Fig. 1. Nitric oxide (NO) acts as an antioxidant by quenching lipid peroxyl radicals (LOO*). Peroxynitrite (ONOO−) is, however, a pro-oxidant that reacts with lipids to form lipid hydroperoxides (LOOH), lipid peroxyl radicals, and isoprostanes. Peroxynitrite also can react with tyrosine residues on proteins to form nitro-tyrosine.

rapidly expanding in recent years, and excellent reviews are available *(5,6)*. It is now clear that mast cells are both a target and a source of NO *(6)*.

NO is a free radical because it has an unpaired electron in its 2p-π orbital. Despite being a free radical, nitric oxide is a very effective antioxidant *(7,8)*. As shown in **Fig. 1**, NO can rapidly react with superoxide radical (O_2^{-*}) to form peroxynitrite (ONOO−), which is potent pro-oxidant capable of promoting lipid peroxidation *(9)*. Peroxynitrite may have extremely important effects on mast cell functions *(5)*. Peroxynitrite arising from mast cells in the lung could cause pulmonary capillary leakage and thereby play a critical role in the pathophysiology of pulmonary disease *(10)*.

The presence of peroxynitrite in biological systems can be detected by measuring 3-nitrotyrosine, which is formed by the reaction of peroxynitrite and tyrosine residues on protein *(11,12)*. A new sensitive and specific assay has been developed *(11)* for measuring the 3-nitrotyrosine levels in proteins by quantitative conversion into a pentafluorobenzyl derivative which is then detected using negative ion chemical ionization gas chromatography/mass spectrometry. This important analytical methodology has not yet been employed to study mast cell physiology. It is interesting, however, that increased levels of 3-nitrotyrosine have been found in the exhaled breath condensate of patients with asthma *(13)*.

NO in biological systems are generated either by an inducible form of nitric oxide synthase (iNOS) or a constitutive form (cNOS). cNOS enzymes synthesize low levels of NO but do so in a rapid fashion whereas iNOS synthesizes much higher levels of NO and does so over a prolonged time interval. All NOS enzymes catalyze the five electron oxidation of L-arginine to yield equimolar quantities of NO and L-citrulline (*see* **Fig. 2**). NOS activity also requires the

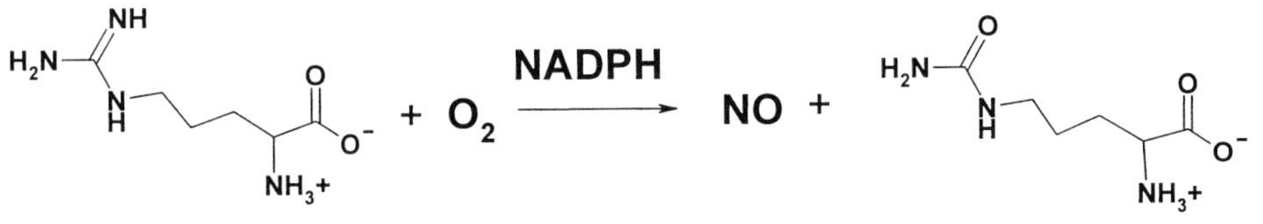

Fig. 2. Nitric oxide synthase uses L-arginine, oxygen, and NADPH to form nitric oxide and L-citrulline.

presence of (6R)-5,6,7,8-tetrahydrobiopterin (BH_4) as a cofactor. BH_4 has been identified as a critical factor in the production of NO by mast cells *(14)*. The high levels of NO produced by iNOS are subsequently oxidized to reactive nitrogen oxide species (RNOS) at a very rapid rate (reactions 1 and 2).

$$NO + O_2 \rightarrow NO2/N2O3 \text{ (aq)} \rightarrow NO_2^-/NO_3^- \tag{1}$$

$$NO + O_2^{-*} \rightarrow ONOO^- \text{ (aq)} \rightarrow NO_2^-/NO_3^- \tag{2}$$

For most immunological cells, iNOS is the primary enzyme involved in NO synthesis. Moreover, many of the immunological and inflammatory effects of NO produced by iNOS are the indirect result of RNOS which rapidly react with cellular thiols to form nitrosothiols (RS-NOs) which could modulate numerous cell signaling pathways *(15)*. Akaike et al. *(15)* have described a specific and highly sensitive high-performance liquid chromatography method for detecting RS-NOs.

Mast cells are reported to have both an iNOS and a cNOS form *(6)*. Gilchrist *(16)* found that unstimulated rat peritoneal mast cells (PMC) express low levels of cNOS mRNA but neither mRNA for iNOS nor neuronal nitric oxide synthase (nNOS). However, stimulation with antigen, interferon (IFN)-γ, or anti-CD8 antibody was found to up-regulate iNOS mRNA expression in these cells as was confirmed by *in situ* reverse transcription polymerase chain reaction *(16)*.

NO plays a key role in modulating many important mast cell functions *(5,6,17–19)*. For example, NO suppresses antigen-induced mast cell degranulation, mediator release, and cytokine expression *(17)*. To study the role of NO in modulating mast cell functions, it is important to look at conditions in which either exogenous or endogenous sources of NO are used *(17)*.

A wide variety of chemical NO donors are available to study the role of exogenous NO. For example, NO generating ions of the general structure R_2N-[N(O)NO]⁻, called diazeniumdiolates, have been developed by the National Cancer Institute (http://home.ncifcrf.gov/lcc/nitricoxide/aboutNOresearch. asp). These NO ions generate NO at physiological pH, with half-lives ranging from 2 s to 20 h. 3-Morpholino-sydnonimine is also a well-known NO donor and it also simultaneously releases superoxide radicals and is therefore useful for probing the biological effects of peroxynitrite generation (*see* reaction 2).

Before detailing a number of specific methodologies, it is important to discuss some general analytical considerations. NO is very unstable in biological systems and has a physiological half life of only 1–40 s. It is, therefore, very difficult to measure NO itself and most assays are therefore based on the determination of the stable end products of NO, that is, NO_2- and NO_3-. The activity of NOS enzymes can, however, be determined by the formation of L-citrulline (*see* **Fig. 2**). Most assays for measuring the stoechiometric production of NO and L-citrulline from L-arginine by NOS enzymes are based on radiolabeled arginine, that is, L-[3H]-arginine or L-[14C]-arginine *(20)*. For example, Combet et al. *(21)* have carefully described a discontinuous assay based on the formation of L-[3H]-citrulline from L-[3H]-arginine. These investigators were careful to demonstrate the specificity of the NOS activity by using a specific NOS inhibitor, that is, NG-monomethyl-L-arginine monoacetate (L-NMMA). NOS assays based on radiolabeled L-arginine are quite sensitive. Carlberg et al. *(22)* have developed an assay for nNOS (found on mast cells) based on the HPLC determination of L-citrulline. This nonradioactive method has a detection limit of 0.1 pmol L-citrulline.

The production of L-citrulline is particularly useful for measuring NOS activity in isolated enzyme preparations or cultured cells. It is, however, more subject to difficulties when used with whole tissues where both unlabeled substrate could be present and alternative enzymatic means of forming L-citrulline from radiolabeled L-arginine (e.g., arginase- and ornithine transcarbamylase-mediated reactions *[23]*). Giraldez and Zweier has attempted to address these issues *(23)* but these problems must be kept in mind as an intrinsic limitation of all L-arginine conversion assays.

Holstein et al. *(24)* have used a monoclonal antibody directed against L-citrulline for immunocytochemical staining in tissues section. Combined with specific antibodies to the various NOS enzymes, this is a powerful method for looking at the tissue distribution of both NOS proteins and their enzymatic activity *(24)*.

Chemiluminescence is an extremely sensitive technique and has been used to measure very low levels of NO on a real time basis. Chemiluminescence is the result of the transformation of chemical energy into light energy. NO is readily oxidized to NO_2 in the presence of O_3 (ozone) and this reaction (reaction 3) produces a quantity of light for each molecule of oxidized NO, which can be measured using a photomultiplier tube or solid state device. Under carefully controlled circumstances, the light level in the reaction chamber is proportional the concentration of NO in the sample.

$$NO + O_3 \rightarrow NO_2 + O_2 + h\nu \qquad (3)$$

The chemiluminescence technique is so sensitive that is has been used to monitor nitric oxide in breath and therefore has been clinically useful in monitoring inflammation in asthma *(25)*. There is a considerable body of evidence suggesting that mast cells play a key role in asthma *(26–29)*. Moreover, it is likely that lung mast cells contribute to the NO measured in breath but this remained as active area of research *(10,13)*.

As mentioned previously, nitrite and nitrate are the primary stable end products of NO in aqueous systems. Nitrite can be measured by the absorbance of the magenta-colored azo dye formed from NO_2^- and Griess reagent. Gilchrist et al. *(16)* have used the Griess assay to measure the release of NO from rat PMCs. In unstimulated PMCs, the production of NO is very low and only after stimulation with IFN-γ (800 U/mL) or anti-CD8 antibody (5 µg/mL) was the production of NO very significant. The NOS inhibitor L-NMMA (at a concentration of 100 µM) was able to block the production of NO, indicating that mast cell NOS was the specific source. Griess reagent can be purchased but is exceedingly easy and cost efficient to make oneself.

2. Materials

2.1. NO Based on Cellular Nitrite (NO_2^-) and Nitrate (NO_3^-) Secretion Into Culture Medium

1. Griess reagent is prepared by mixing equal volumes of reagent (a) and (b). Reagent (a) is 1% sulfanilamide (S 9251 Sigma) in 5% phosphoric acid (P5811, sigma-aldrich.com), prepared by adding 3.5 mL of 85% H_3PO_4 (Sigma) to 100 mL with distilled water and then dissolving 1.0 g of sulfanilamide. Reagent (b) is 0.1% *N*-1-naphthylethylenediamine dihydrochloride (NEDD; cat. no. 22,248,-8 from sigma-aldrich.com), prepared by dissolving 100 mg of NEDD in 100 mL of distilled water. These two reagents should be stored at 4°C in light protected plastic bottles and are stable for approx 4 mo.
2. β-NADPH (N 7785, sigma-aldrich.com).
3. Nitrate reductase EC 1.7.1.2) (N 7265, from *Aspergillus niger*, sigma-aldrich.com).
4. L-glutamate dehydrogenase (49392, sigma-aldrich.com).
5. α-ketoglutaric acid disodium salt dihydrate (75892, sigma-aldrich.com).
6. Ammonium chloride (A 9434, sigma-aldrich.com).
7. 2-(4-Carboxyphenyl)-4,4,5,5-tetramethylimidazoline-1-oxyl-3-oxide potassium salt (carboxy-PTIO potassium salt, C221, sigma-aldrich.com) stock solution (10 mg/mL) is prepared in pH 9.0, 0.1 M sodium phosphate buffer.
8. Carboxy–PTIO stock solution (10 mg/mL).
9. RMPI-1640 without phenol red (11835-030, Invitrogen, Carlsbad, CA)
10. Fetal bovine serum (FBS; Atlanta Biologicals, Atlanta, GA; *see* **Note 1**).
11. Phosphate-buffered saline: 150 mM, pH 7.4 (cat. no. 10010-23, Invitrogen).
12. Penicillin–streptomycin (cat. no. 15140-122, Invitrogen).
13. Sterile 96-well microplates.
14. Microplate VIS absorbance reader.
15. CO_2 (5%) cell incubator set at 37°C.

2.2. Continuous Monitoring of NO Production Using DAF-2A Diacetate

1. A 5 mM stock solution of 4,5-diaminofluorescein diacetate (DAF-2 diacetate) (cat. no. 85165, www.caymanchem.com) is made in tissue molecular biology grade dimethyl sulfoxide (DMSO), i.e., 1 mg of DAF-2 diacetate in 450 µL of DMSO. This stock solution is further diluted with culture medium (phenol red free) to give a final concentration of 10 µM DAF-2A diacetate.
2. Dimethyl sulfoxide (DMSO; cat. no. D 8418, sigma-aldrich.com).
3. RMPI-1640 without phenol red (cat. no. 11835-030, Invitrogen).
4. The cell culture medium is made be mixing 45.0 mL of RPMI-1640 (with bicarbonate), 5.0 mL of FBS, 0.5 mL of 1.0 M pH 7.4 HEPES and 0.25 mL of penicillin–streptomycin.
5. FBS (Atlanta Biologicals).
6. Penicillin–streptomycin (cat. no. 15140-122, Invitrogen).
7. 1 M HEPES buffer solution (15630-080, GibcoBRL, NY).
8. Sterile 96-well microplates (*see* **Note 2**).
9. CO_2 (5%) incubator set at 37°C.
10. Microplate fluorescent reader with temperature regulation capabilities such as the FLUOstar Galaxy (now sold as the FLUOstar OPTIMA) (BMG Labtechnologies, Durham, NC).

3. Methods

3.1. Griess Reagent Assay for Nitrite (Only) in Culture Medium

1. Cells are grown in 96-well microplates with tissue culture medium containing RPMI-1640 (without phenol red) and 10% FBS. The culture medium is made by mixing 45.0 mL of RPMI-1640, 5.0 mL FBS, and 0.25 mL of penicillin–streptomycin.
2. After 4 to 18 h of incubation (5% CO_2, 95% air at 37°C), a 50-µL aliquot of the cell culture medium (containing the nitrite to be assayed) is transferred to a new 96-well plate containing 50 µL of Griess reagent (a) and 50 µL of Griess reagent (b) per well (*see* **Notes 3** and **4**).
3. After mixing and incubating for 10 min, the absorbance of the wells is measured at 543 nm against a blank containing fresh growth medium (not in contact with cells) and Griess reagent. The absorbance spectrum of the colored azo compound is fairly broad and a plate reader with a filter from 520 to 550 nm can be used.
4. A standard curve should be obtained with known concentrations of NO_2^-. It is important to make up the standards in the same matrix used for the experimental samples, for example, cell culture medium.

3.2. Griess Reagent Assay for Nitrite Plus Nitrate in Culture Medium

The Griess assay measures only nitrite, yet it is important to measure total nitrite plus and nitrate since both are produced by NO in aqueous conditions. This can be accomplished by adding bacterial nitrate reductase and NADPH to reduce nitrate to nitrite, that is, $NO_3^- + NADPH \rightarrow NO_2^- + NADP^+ + H_2O$.

This, however, creates a new analytical problem since any excess NADPH interferes with the Griess reaction. Fortunately, the excess NADPH can be removed by using an enzymatic reaction consuming NADPH such as L-glutamate dehydrogenase (NH3 + 2-oxoglutarate + NADPH → L-glutamate + H2O + NADP [20]).

1. A 50 µL sample of the cell culture medium is placed in well (96-well microplate) and incubated with a 5 µL sample of the stock nitrite reductase (2 U added to 150 µL of pH 7.4 PBS buffer) and a 5 µL of the stock 300 µM NADPH solution (2.5 mg of beta-NADPH Na$_4$ in 10 mL of distilled water) for 30 min at room temperature. This reduces NO$_3$– to NO$_2$– (*see* **Note 5**).
2. 5 µL aliquots of L-glutamate dehydrogenase (40 U/mL), ammonium chloride (1.5 M) and α-ketoglutaric acid disodium salt dihydrate (60 mM freshly prepared) are added to each well to be assayed and incubated for 15 min at room temperature to remove any excess NADPH.
3. The NO$_2$– plus NO$_3$– is now assayed using 50 µL Griess of reagent (a) and 50 µL of reagent (b).
4. After incubating for 10 min, the absorbance of the wells is measured at 543 nm against a blank containing 50 µL of fresh-growth medium (not in contact with cells) but treated in manner identical to the sample cell growth medium (that was in contract with cells). A standard curve should be obtained with known concentrations of NO$_2$– and NO$_3$–.

3.3. An Improved Technique Using Carboxy PTIO

An improved method for the detection of NO has been developed by Amano and Noda *(30)* based on the use of a nitric oxide radical scavenger, 2-(4-carboxyphenyl)-4,4,5,5-tetramethylimidazoline-3-oxide-1-oxyl (carboxy PTIO) and the Griess reagent. The addition of carboxy PTIO to stimulated cells increases the amount of NO$_2$– because carboxy PTIO rapidly reacts with NO to form NO$_2$– (and not NO$_3$–), which is then assayed using the Griess reaction *(31)*. Carboxy-PTIO has also been used as a scavenger of NO and, thereby, to test the roles of NO in various physiological functions. Nevertheless, the metabolic alterations induced by carboxy-PTIO have not been fully elucidated. It is known that carboxy-PTIO completely inhibits peroxynitrite-induced formation of 3-nitrotyrosine from free tyrosine as well as nitration of bovine serum albumin *(32)*.

Figure 3 shows the effect of carboxy-PTIO (160 µM) on the secretion of NO$_2$– (measured by the Griess assay) by unstimulated, LPS stimulated, IFN-γ-stimulated, and lipopolysaccharide plus IFN-γ-stimulated RAW264.7 murine macrophages as a function of time. Clearly, carboxy-PTIO almost doubles the sensitivity of the Griess assay. A 5 µL aliquot of stock carboxy-PTIO is added per 3 mL of the cell growth medium (final concentration of 53 µM) and, after incubation at 37°C aliquots of the medium are assayed as detailed in **Subheading 3.1.**

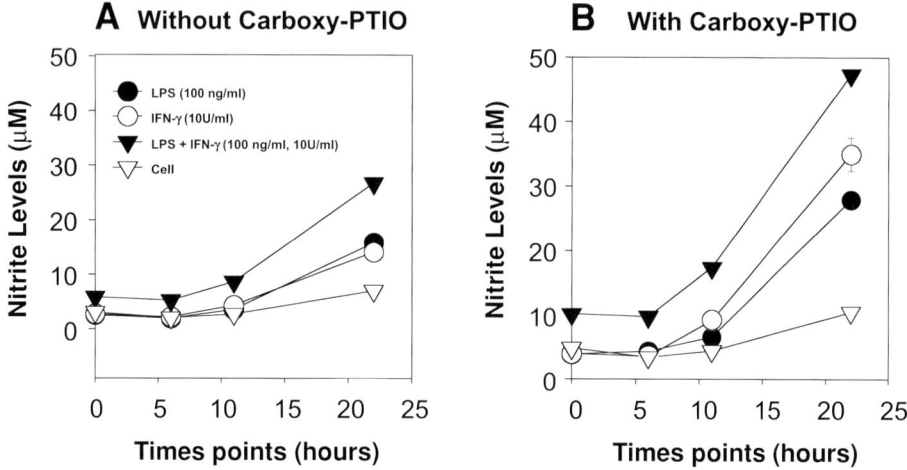

Fig. 3. The effect of carboxy-PTIO on nitrite secretion in cells stimulated with lipopolysaccharide (LPS), interferon (IFN)-γ, and the combination of both LPS and IFN-γ. (**A**) without carboy-PTIO; (**B**) with carboxy-PTIO.

3.4. Continuous Monitoring of NO Production in Live Cells Using DAF-2A Diacetate Fluorescent Indicator

Most assays based on measuring NO in cell culture medium are not sufficiently sensitive to detect the low NO output from cNOS. Kojima et al. *(33,34)* have developed membrane-permeable DAF-2 diacetate (DAF-2 DA) as a means of studying NO production in live cells. When DAF-2 DA is loaded into cells, its ester bonds are hydrolyzed by intracellular esterase, generating DAF-2, which remains essentially nonfluorescent until it reacts with the nitrosonium cation (produced by spontaneous oxidation of nitric oxide) to form a fluorescent heterocycle, which becomes trapped in the cytoplasm of the cell. Fluorescence in the cells increases in a NO concentration-dependent manner. We have routinely used DAF-2 diacetate to continuously measure NO production in stimulated macrophages cultured in 96-well microplates. For continuous monitoring, cells must be maintained at 37°C and pH 7.4 while in the plate reader. Therefore, it is important to use a microplate fluorescent reader with temperature regulation (at 37°C) capabilities such as the FLUOstar Galaxy (now sold as the FLUOstar OPTIMA from BMG Labtechnologies, Durham, NC). To maintain a pH 7.4 outside of the CO_2 incubator (where pH is usually maintained by bicarbonate-CO_2 equilibrium), it is important to have 10 mM HEPES present in the culture. Cells typically are incubated with the culture medium containing 10 μM DAF-2 diacetate (in the culture medium) for 30 min and fluorescence then continuously monitored using an excitation wavelength of 485 nm and an emission wavelength of 520 nm (*see* **Note 6**).

Gilchrist et al. *(14)* have used confocal laser scanning microscopy in live PMCs to study the production of NO using DAF-2. Confocal microscopy is efficient at rejecting out of focus fluorescent light and provides an image coming from a thin section of the cells. By scanning many thin sections, it is possible to construct a three-dimensional distribution of the fluorescent dye. Using this technique, Gilchrist *(14)* found distinct intracellular distributions of NO production in mast cells depending upon the type of stimulant being used (IgE or IFN-γ). The combination of confocal analysis with the use of NO sensitive dyes is a very powerful technique, particularly where a primary cell population of mast cells could be contaminated by small amounts other NO producing cells, such as macrophages.

4. Notes

1. FBS and all other reagents should be free of endotoxin because endotoxin is likely to be a stimulant for mast cells. It is important, therefore, to order FBS certified to have very low levels of endotoxin. Endotoxin values are reported in endotoxin U/mL (EU/mL) and 1 EU of endotoxin is approx 0.1 ng of endotoxin standard.

2. The optimal microplates for fluorescent assays should black with clear bottoms. This enhances the signal-to-noise ratio. Corning (Corning, NY) has sterile, tissue culture-treated, black 96-well assay plates with a clear bottom (cat. no. 3603).

3. This methods assumes that the cells to be assayed are adherent to the wells. If this is not the case, a centrifugation step should be performed to isolate cell-free medium.

4. Marzinzig *(35)* modified the Griess reaction by replacing sulfanilamide with dapsone (4,4'-diamino-diphenylsulfone). This modification, along with ultrafiltration of the samples, resulted in an enhanced sensitivity to measure NO_2- down to 0.2 μ*M*. The detection limit was further improved to 10 n*M* when NO_2- was identified by the fluorochrome 2,3-diaminonaphthalene *(35,36)*. Moreover, with the 2,3-diaminonaphthalene method, one also can use bacterial reductase to reduce nitrate to nitrite and thereby provide an excellent accounting of NO secretion into cell culture medium.

5. An alternative method to reduce nitrate is with vanadium(III) *(37)*.

6. Rathel et al. *(38)* have optimized the use of the fluorescent probe DAF-2 to reliably measure nanomolar levels of NO is the culture medium from cells expressing cNOS. In particular, these investigators used low concentrations of DAF-2 (0.1 μ*M*) to reduce DAF-2 auto-fluorescence, and they also subtracted the DAF-2 auto-fluorescence from the total fluorescence measured. In these experiments, an excitation wavelength of 495 nm and an emission wavelength of 515 nm were used. The amount of DAF-2 used in these experiments (0.1 μ*M*) is sufficient to measure up to 200 n*M* NO.

Acknowledgments

This work was supported by the U.S. Army Medical Research and Material Command under Contract/Grant/Intergovernmental Project Order DAMD17-98164001 (to W.L. Stone).

References

1. Yamamura, T. (1996) [Techniques for measurement of nitric oxide in biological systems: principles and practice]. Nippon Yakurigaku Zasshi. *Japanese J. Pharmacol.* **107**, 173–182.
2. Leone, A. M., Rhodes, P., Furst, V., and Moncada, S. (1995) Techniques for the measurement of nitric oxide. *Methods Mol. Biol.* **41**, 285–299.
3. Coleman, J. W. (2001) Nitric oxide in immunity and inflammation. *Int. Immunopharmacol.* **1**, 1397–1406.
4. Krishnaswamy, G., Kelley, J., Johnson, D., et al. (2001) The human mast cell: functions in physiology and disease. *Front Biosci.* **6**, D1109–D1127.
5. Forsythe, P., Gilchrist, M., Kulka, M., and Befus, A. D. (2001) Mast cells and nitric oxide: control of production, mechanisms of response. *Int. Immunopharmacol.* **1**, 1525–1541.
6. Bidri, M., Feger, F., Varadaradjalou, S., Ben Hamouda, N., Guillosson, J. J., and Arock, M. (2001) Mast cells as a source and target for nitric oxide. *Int. Immunopharmacol.* **1**, 1543–1558.
7. Rubbo, H., Radi, R., Anselmi, D., et al. (2000) Nitric oxide reaction with lipid peroxyl radicals spares alpha-tocopherol during lipid peroxidation. Greater oxidant protection from the pair nitric oxide/alpha-tocopherol than alpha-tocopherol/ascorbate. *J. Biol. Chem.* **275**, 10,812–10,818.
8. Kanner, J., Harel, S., and Granit, R. (1991) Nitric oxide as an antioxidant. *Arch. Biochem. Biophys.* **289**, 130–136.
9. Rubbo, H., Radi, R., Trujillo, M., et al. (1994) Nitric oxide regulation of superoxide and peroxynitrite-dependent lipid peroxidation. Formation of novel nitrogen-containing oxidized lipid derivatives. *J. Biol. Chem.* **269**, 26,066–26,075.
10. Gaston, B., Drazen, J. M., Loscalzo, J., and Stamler, J. S. (1994) The biology of nitrogen oxides in the airways. *Am. J. Respir. Crit. Care Med.* **149**, 538–551.
11. Jiang, H. and Balazy, M. (1998) Detection of 3-nitrotyrosine in human platelets exposed to peroxynitrite by a new gas chromatography/mass spectrometry assay. *Nitric Oxide (Print)* **2**, 350–359.
12. Kooy, N. W., Lewis, S. J., Royall, J. A., Ye, Y. Z., Kelly, D. R., and Beckman, J. S. (1997) Extensive tyrosine nitration in human myocardial inflammation: evidence for the presence of peroxynitrite. *Crit. Care Med.* **25**, 812–819.
13. Hanazawa, T., Kharitonov, S. A., and Barnes, P. J. (2000) Increased nitrotyrosine in exhaled breath condensate of patients with asthma. *Am. J. Respir. Crit. Care Med.* **162**, 1273–1276.
14. Gilchrist, M., Hesslinger, C., and Befus, A. D. (2003) Tetrahydrobiopterin, a critical factor in the production and role of nitric oxide in mast cells. *J. Biol. Chem.* **278**, 50,607–50,614.
15. Akaike, T., Inoue, K., Okamoto, T., et al. (1997) Nanomolar quantification and identification of various nitrosothiols by high performance liquid chromatography coupled with flow reactors of metals and Griess reagent. *J. Biochem.* **122**, 459–466.

16. Gilchrist, M., Savoie, M., Nohara, O., Wills, F. L., Wallace, J. L., and Befus, A. D. (2002) Nitric oxide synthase and nitric oxide production in in vivo-derived mast cells. *J. Leukocyte Biol.* **71,** 618–624.

17. Coleman, J. W. (2002) Nitric oxide: a regulator of mast cell activation and mast cell-mediated inflammation. *Clin. Exp. Immunol.* **129,** 4–10.

18. Gaboury, J. P., Niu, X. F., and Kubes, P. (1996) Nitric oxide inhibits numerous features of mast cell-induced inflammation. *Circulation* **93,** 318–326.

19. Iikura, M., Takaishi, T., Hirai, K., et al. (1998) Exogenous nitric oxide regulates the degranulation of human basophils and rat peritoneal mast cells. *Int. Arch. Allergy Immunol.* **115,** 129–136.

20. Hevel, J. M. and Marletta, M. A. (1994) Nitric-oxide synthase assays. *Methods Enzymol.* **233,** 250–258.

21. Combet, S., Balligand, J. L., Lameire, N., Goffin, E., and Devuyst, O. (2000) A specific method for measurement of nitric oxide synthase enzymatic activity in peritoneal biopsies. *Kidney Int.* **57,** 332–338.

22. Carlberg, M. (1994) Assay of neuronal nitric oxide synthase by HPLC determination of citrulline. *J. Neurosci. Methods* **52,** 165–167.

23. Giraldez, R. R. and Zweier, J. L. (1998) An improved assay for measurement of nitric oxide synthase activity in biological tissues. *Anal. Biochem.* **261,** 29–35.

24. Holstein, G. R., Friedrich, V. L., and Martinelli, G. P. (2001) Monoclonal L-citrulline immunostaining reveals nitric oxide-producing vestibular neurons. *Ann. N. Y. Acad. Sci.* **942,** 65–78.

25. DeNicola, L. R., Kissoon, N., Duckworth, L. J., Blake, K. V., Murphy, S. P., and Silkoff, P. E. (2000) Exhaled nitric oxide as an indicator of severity of asthmatic inflammation. *Pediatr. Emerg. Care* **16,** 290–295.

26. Broide, D. H., Gleich, G. J., Cuomo, A. J., et al. (1991) Evidence of ongoing mast cell and eosinophil degranulation in symptomatic asthma airway. *J. Allergy Clin. Immunol.* **88,** 637–648.

27. Carroll, N. G., Mutavdzic, S., and James, A. L. (2002) Distribution and degranulation of airway mast cells in normal and asthmatic subjects. *Eur. Respir. J.* **19,** 879–885.

28. Shichijo, M., Inagaki, N., Nakai, N., et al. (1998) The effects of anti-asthma drugs on mediator release from cultured human mast cells. *Clin. Exp. Allergy* **28,** 1228–1236.

29. Kraneveld, A. D., van der Kleij, H. P., Kool, M., et al. (2002) Key role for mast cells in nonatopic asthma. *J. Immunol.* **169,** 2044–2053.

30. Amano, F. and Noda, T. (1995) Improved detection of nitric oxide radical (NO.) production in an activated macrophage culture with a radical scavenger, carboxy PTIO and Griess reagent. *FEBS Lett.* **368,** 425–428.

31. Goldstein, S., Russo, A., and Samuni, A. (2003) Reactions of PTIO and carboxy-PTIO with *NO, *NO2, and O2⁻*. *J. Biol. Chem.* **278,** 50,949–50,955.

32. Pfeiffer, S., Leopold, E., Hemmens, B., Schmidt, K., Werner, E. R., and Mayer, B. (1997) Interference of carboxy-PTIO with nitric oxide- and peroxynitrite-mediated reactions. *Free Radical Biol. Med.* **22,** 787–794.

33. Kojima, H., Sakurai, K., Kikuchi, K., et al. (1998) Development of a fluorescent indicator for nitric oxide based on the fluorescein chromophore. *Chem. Pharm. Bull. (Tokyo)* **46,** 373–375.

34. Kojima, H., Nakatsubo, N., Kikuchi, K., et al. (1998) Detection and imaging of nitric oxide with novel fluorescent indicators: diaminofluoresceins. *Anal. Chem.* **70,** 2446–2453.

35. Marzinzig, M., Nussler, A. K., Stadler, J., et al. (1997) Improved methods to measure end products of nitric oxide in biological fluids: nitrite, nitrate, and S-nitrosothiols. *Nitric Oxide (Print)* **1,** 177–189.

36. Misko, T. P., Schilling, R. J., Salvemini, D., Moore, W. M., and Currie, M. G. (1993) A fluorometric assay for the measurement of nitrite in biological samples. *Anal. Biochem.* **214,** 11–16.

37. Miranda, K. M., Espey, M. G., and Wink, D. A. (2001) A rapid, simple spectrophotometric method for simultaneous detection of nitrate and nitrite. *Nitric Oxide (Print)* **5,** 62–71.

38. Rathel, T. R., Leikert, J. J., Vollmar, A. M., and Dirsch, V. M. (2003) Application of 4,5-diaminofluorescein to reliably measure nitric oxide released from endothelial cells in vitro. *Biol. Proc. Online* **5,** 136–142.

20

Immunohistological Detection of Growth Factors and Cytokines in Tissue Mast Cells

Zhenhong Qu

Summary

The relative rarity of mast cells (MCs) and the rich content of heparin in the cytoplasmic granules of MCs pose technical challenges in reliably detecting growth factors (GFs) or cytokines in MCs by conventional immunohistological stain (IHS) methods. A variety of polypeptide growth factors are characterized by high-affinity to heparin. Binding of GFs to MC granules during detection can lead to highly specific yet falsely positive results that cannot be easily discovered by conventional procedure controls. Many reagents used in IHS detection or related experiments contain GFs and are potential nonphysiological sources of the detected GFs in MCs. In addition, heparin also exhibits high binding affinity to avidin and streptavidin, key components of the most widely used IHS detection and amplification system. Although biotin–avidin-free detection systems are readily available and are highly recommended for the future studies in this field, the vast majority of the studies of GFs in MCs in the literature have used biotin–avidin-based methods. In this chapter, the inherent technical pitfalls related to the aforementioned features of MCs, and suggested solutions are presented. They are intended to provide technical assistance to investigators in this field and to help interpret the results of the past studies in the literature.

Key Words: Growth factors; basic fibroblast growth factor (bFGF); transforming growth factor (TGF)-β; tumor necrosis factor (TNF)-α; stem cell growth factor (SCF); immunohistochemistry; avidin–biotin complex (ABC); interleukin (IL)-4; interleukin (IL)-6; interleukin (IL)-10; vascular endothelial growth factor (VEGF).

1. Introduction

The challenge in developing a reliable and reproducible detection method for growth factors (GFs) in tissue mast cells (MCs) arises from two aspects of MC biology. The first is the relative rarity of MCs in most types of tissue and their morphological ambiguity on routine hematoxylin–eosin (H&E) stain, which makes it very difficult to appreciate the magnitude of MC infiltration and to reliably attribute a positive stain for a growth factor to MCs. The second

From: *Methods in Molecular Biology, vol. 315: Mast Cells: Methods and Protocols*
Edited by: G. Krishnaswamy and D. S. Chi © Humana Press Inc., Totowa, NJ

is the rich heparin content of MCs. Heparin is a sulfated polysaccharide synthesized by MCs and stored in the secretory granules *(1)*. Heparin within the MC granules permits the binding of avidin (streptavidin), immunoglobulin *(2)*, and GFs *(3,4)*. The abundant proteoglycans (e.g., heparin) in MCs potentially may result in a false-positive stain for GFs through two major mechanisms. First, proteoglycans are known to have high affinity to avidin *(5–8)*. Thus, when a biotin–avidin-base immunohistological staining (IHS) is used for detection, falsely positive results are likely to occur. In fact, peroxidase-conjugated avidin has been used to detect MCs *(5–7)*. Experienced investigators have learned to ignore such stains of MCs. However, when MCs are the focus of study, this can be a major hurdle. Fortunately, this type of false-positive stain is easy to identify by using appropriate procedural controls and is not very difficult to eliminate. Second, the heparin also has high affinity to a variety of GFs, especially those so called "heparin-binding growth factors" *(4)*, such as the fibroblast growth factor (FGF) family *(4,9)* and vascular endothelial growth factor (VGF *[10,11]*). Binding of exogenous GFs to MC heparin during the staining process may lead to a highly specific but falsely positive stain that cannot be uncovered by any conventional procedure controls, including preadsorption control. This is probably the most evasive and poorly documented pitfall in IHS of GFs in MCs. The source of the exogenous GFs may come from nonproteolytic enzymes used for antigen retrieval. For example, hyaluronidase extracted from bovine testis is rich in basic fibroblast growth factor (bFGF *[12,13]*). Testicular tissues also express SCF *(14,15)* and vascular endothelial growth factor *(16)*. Another common source of exogenous GFs is sera routinely used to block nonspecific tissue binding sites in IHS *(17,18)*. Many investigators have used 10–50% serum for the blocking step *(19–21)* or prolonged incubation with antibodies diluted in the serum-containing solution *(22)*. Given the GFs-enriching capacity of heparin in MCs, it is not hard to appreciate the potential problem, that is, exogenous GFs from the enzymes and/or serum bind to MC heparin and subsequently are detected by IHS as "MC-produced" GFs.

In this chapter, I will introduce general protocols modified to address the problems arising from these two aspects. It is my experience and my point of view, shared by many other investigators, that for a given GF or cytokine, the success of an IHS largely depends on tissue fixation, antigen-retrieval if applicable, and the type of primary antibodies used, that is to say, an IHS method or protocol successfully detecting a GF in other type of cells or tissue is also applicable to MCs in detecting the same GF given that the above mentioned pitfalls are avoided. For this reason, only a list of key steps of IHS protocols for GF and cytokine detection in the literature with references are included **Table 1**. Investigators are referred to these protocols for details. Although the proposed protocols and related comments focus on GF detection in MCs, the gen-

Table1
Growth Factor Antibodies and Key Components of IHS

Antibody to	Antibody type	Antibody source	Fixation	Antigen retrieval [b]	Detection method [c]	Ref.
bFGF [a]	Polyclonal	Santa Cruz	10% NBF	1	ABC	*(23–25)*
IL-3 [a]	Polyclonal	Chemicon	10% NBF	4	SAB	*(26)*
IL-4	Monoclonal, polyclonal	R&D System	10% NBF	2 or 3	ABC	*(27)*
IL-6	Monoclonal, polyclonal	R&D System	10% NBF	2	ABC	*(27)*
IL10	Monoclonal, polyclonal	R&D System	10% NBF	2	ABC	*(27)*
PDGF-A	Monoclonal	Zymogenetics	10% NBF	4	ABC	*(28)*
SCF [a]	Polyclonal	Genzyme and Amgen	Methanol	N/A	ABC	*(29,30)*
TGF-β1	Monoclonal	Santa Cruz,	10% NBF	2 and 5	ABC	*(24,31)*
TGF-β2	Polyclonal	Genzyme				
TNF-a [a]	Polyclonal	R&D System	10% NBF	3	SAB, ABC	*(32,33)*
VEGF [a]	Polyclonal, monoclonal	Santa Cruz	10% NBF	1 or 6	ABC	*(23,34)*
VEGF [a]	Polyclonal	Oncogene	10% NBF	7 or 8	ABC	*(35,36)*

[a] IHS results confirmed simultaneously by *in situ* hybridization.
[b] Antigen-Retrieval Methods (recommended):
  1. Heat in microwave at 98°C for 20 min in 10 m*M* sodium citrate buffer (pH 6.0).
  2. Heat in microwave for 15 min (three 5-min treatments) at 650 W in 1 m*M* di-sodium ethylene diamine tetraacetic acid solution (pH 8.0).
  3. Heat in a pressure cooker (Lakeland Plastics, Cumbria, UK) at full power for 5 min in 10 m*M* sodium citrate buffer (pH 6.0).
  4. Incubate with 0.1% pepsin (Sigma, cat. no. P-6887) in 0.01 *N* HCl for 20 min at 37°C
  5. Heat in microwave on high power for 8 min in 10 m*M* citrate buffer (pH 6.0).
  6. Incubated with 0.125% trypsin (10 min at 25°C)
  7. Heat in pressure cooker for 10 min in citrate buffer 0.1 *M*, pH 6.0.
  8. Heat in microwave at 50% power three times for 5 min in 10 m*M* sodium citrate buffer (pH 6.0).
[c] Detection/Amplification System: ABC, Avidin–biotin complex method; SAB = Streptavidin–biotin method.
  PDGF, platelet-derived growth factor; TGF, transforming growth factor; VEGF, vascular endothelial growth factor.

eral principles and the specific recommendations or technical tips are applicable to immunohistological detection of other macromolecules in different cell types. They are therefore intended not only to assist investigators in the future but also to help researchers critically interpret the results of the past studies in the literature of this field.

2. Materials

2.1. Reagents

1. 10% Neutral buffered formalin (NBF; cat. no. 23-245684, Fisher Scientific, Pittsburgh, PA).
2. Antibodies, primary (*see* **Table 1**).
3. Antibodies, biotinylated, specific for rabbit IgG (PK-6101), mouse IgG (PK-6102), goat IgG (PK-6105) (Vectastain® ABC kit, Vector Laboratories, Burlingame, CA).
4. Affi-Gel® Heparin Gel (153-6173, Bio-Rad Laboratories, Hercules, CA).
5. Anti-human tryptase (IgG1, 105 µg/mL; cat. no. M-7052, DakoCytomation, Carpinteria, CA).
6. Biømeda Crystal/Mount (cat. no. BM-M03, Fisher Scientific).
7. Crystal Bovine serum albumin (BSA; cat. no. B-6917, Sigma, St. Louis, MO).
8. DAB tablets (3,3'-diaminobenzidine tetrahydrochloride; cat. no. D-5905, Sigma).
9. Fast Red Kit (cat. no. CK-0802-20 or HK182-5K, BioGenex, San Ramon, CA).
10. Glass slide, Probe-On plus (Fisher Scientific).
11. Hyaluronidase type V (cat. no. H-6254, Sigma).
12. Imidazole (1,3-diaza-2,4-cyclopentadiene), C3H4N2, FW = 68.08 (I-0125, Sigma).
13. Mayer's hematoxylin (non-alcohol-based; cat. no. HK100-9K, BioGenex).
14. Nickel chloride (hexahydrate NiCl-6H2O, FW = 237.7; cat. no. N-5756, Sigma).
15. Normal horse, goat and rabbit sera (Sigma or Vector Laboratories).
16. Pepsin (cat. no. P-6887, Sigma).
17. Protein block (serum-free; cat. no. X0909, DakoCytomation).
18. Proteinase K (cat. no. S3020, DakoCytomation).
19. *p*-phenylenediamine (cat. no. P-6001, Sigma).
20. Streptavidin–biotin blocking kit (cat. no. SP-2002, Vector Laboratories).
21. Steptavidin–fluorescein isothiocyanate (FITC; cat. no. SA-5001, Vector Laboratories).

2.2. Stock (10X) and Working (1X) Buffers

1. Phosphate-buffered saline (PBS) stock (10X): Mix the following:

Sodium phosphate (monobasic), FW=137.99:	2.2 g	(16 mM)
Sodium phosphate (dibasic) FW = 141.96:	12.0 g	(84 mM)
Sodium chloride FW = 58.44:	85.0 g	(1.45 M)
Distilled water (dH$_2$O)	1000 mL	

   pH should be 6.8–7.1 (unadjusted), solution is stable in RT for at least 6 mo. PBS working solution (1X):
   Dilute the stock PBS with dH$_2$O near a ratio of 1:10 (e.g., add 100 PBS stock to 700 dH$_2$O). Adjust the pH to 7.3 using 25% sodium phosphate dibasic and then add dH$_2$O to total final volume of 1000 mL.

2. Tris-buffered saline (TBS) stock (X10):

   a. Tris stock solution (10X): 0.5 M Tris-HCl, pH 7.6

Tris-base (FW = 212.14)	60.55 g	(0.5 M)

Distilled water (dH$_2$O) 1000 mL
Adjust the pH to 7.5 with concentrated HCl.

b. NaCl stock solution (10X):

Sodium chloride (FW = 58.44)   87.66 g   (1.5 *M*)
Add dH$_2$O to a volume of 1000 mL

c. Working TBS (1X) solution: 0.05 *M* Tris-HCl, 0.15 NaCl, pH 7.6

Tris stock	NaCl stock	dH$_2$O	Final Volume
100 mL	100 mL	800 mL	1000 mL

Check pH again, adjust to pH 7.5 if necessary using HCl.

3. Acetate buffer (for hyaluronidase):

Na acetate (trihydrate) (FW.136.08)   1.3 g   (0.1 *M*)
NaCl (FW.58.44)   0.88 g   (0.15 *M*)
Add dH$_2$O to 100 mL
Adjust pH with acetic acid to pH 5.2–5.5

2.3. Blocking Solution, Antibody Diluent, and Washing Buffer

1. Antibody diluents (= blocking solution): PBS–0.05% Tween-20 with 3% BSA, 2% serum and 0.05% NaN$_3$.

PBS (1X) or TBS	100 mL
BSA (crystal) 3 g Normal serum (or sera)	2 mL (Heparin-adsorbed)
NaN$_3$	50 mg (or 10 mg thimerosal)
Tween-20	50 µL

Adjust pH to 7.2–7.3, with 0.1 N HCl (*see* **Note 1**). Filter through 0.2 µm and store at 4°C. The solution is stable for at least 2 mo.

2. Blocking solution: same as antibody diluent (i.e., PBS–0.05% Tween-20 with 3% BSA, 2% serum, and 0.05% NaN3). Commercially available Serum-free blocking solution (e.g., Protein Block, DakoCytomation, X0909) is a preferred alternative.
3. Washing solution: PBS (or TBS) containing 0.05% Tween-20.
4. For ABC complex: PBS (or TBS) with 0.1% Tween-20.

2.4. Antigen Retrieval Solutions

1. Hyaluronidase solution: Hyaluronidase type V (Sigma, H-6254): 2 mg/mL in 0.1 *M* acetate buffer (0.15 *M* NaCl and 0.1 *M* sodium acetate, adj. with HCl to pH 5.2). This solution is aliquoted into 3–5 mL/vial and stored at –20°C.
2. Pepsin solution: 0.1% in 0.01 *N* of HCl, also stored at –20°C.

Pepsin (Sigma P-6887)	0.1 g
dH$_2$O	99 mL
1 *N* HCl	1 mL

Dissolve pepsin in dH$_2$O completely before adding HCl. Store at –20°C.

3. Solutions for heat-retrieval: *see* **Table 1**.

2.5. Chromogen Substrates

1. Diaminobenzidine tetrahydrochloride (DAB):

Imidazole (Sigma, I-0125)	136 mg	(0.1 M)
PBS (pH 7.5)	20 mL	(155 mM)
DAB (1 tablet, Sigma D-5905)	10 mg	(0.5 mg/mL)
30% H_2O_2	20 µL	(0.03%)

   Incubate for 10 min in darkness.

   Alternatively, dissolve diaminobenzidine tetrahydrochloride in TBS at 0.6 mg/mL. This solution may be stored at 4°C for several weeks. Immediately before use add concentrated H_2O_2 to a final concentration of 0.01%.

2. Fast Red (chromogen for alkaline phosphatase): Fast Red Kit (CK-0802-20; BioGenex San Ramon, CA). Follow the vendor's instruction. Alternatively, dissolve 2 mg of naphthol-AS-MX phosphate (Sigma, cat. no. N-4875) in 0.2 mL of dimethylformamide in a glass tube. Add 9.8 mL of 0.1 M Tris (pH 8.2). This buffer is stable at 4°C for several weeks. Immediately before staining, dissolve Fast Red TR salt (Sigma, F-1500) at a concentration of 1 mg/mL and filter directly onto the slide. Levamisole may be added to the substrate solution at a final concentration of 1 mM.

3. Steptavidin-FITC (Vector Laboratories, cat. no. SA-5001).

2.6. Mounting Medium

1. Biømeda Crystal/Mount from Fisher Scientific (cat. no. BM-M03, Fisher Scientific).
2. Fisher Permount Mounting Medium (cat. no. SP15-100, Fisher Scientific).

3. Methods
3.1. Single Immunostain on Sequential Tissue Sections

1. Tissue fixed with 10% NBF for 1–2 d at 4°C, routinely processed and embedded in paraffin.
2. Cut the paraffin sections at 2–3 µm and lay the sections on Probe-on Plus or poly-L-lysine coated slides. Group alternating sections into two sets for different antibodies (i.e., sections 1, 3, and 5 for tryptase; and sections 2, 4, and 6 for GF/cytokine).
3. Melt the paraffin sections at 58°C for 45 min in a humidity chamber.
4. De-paraffinization and re-hydration at room temperature (RT):

   Xylene, 4 min × 4
   100% ethanol, 3 min × 3
   90% ethanol, 5 min × 1
   75% ethanol, 5 min × 1
   50% ethanol, 5 × 1
   dH$_2$O, 2 min twice (do not put in a buffer, *see* **Note 2**)

5. Antigen retrieval: for individual growth factor detection (*see* **Table 1**). For MC Tryptase: digestion in 0.2% type V hyaluronidase in 0.1 M acetate buffer for 30 min at RT (*see* **Note 3**).

6. Briefly rinse with tap water, then in PBS–0.05% Tween-20 for 10 min.
7. Incubated in the blocking solution at RT for 20 min (*see* **Note 4**).
8. Tap off the blocking solution (do not wash) then incubate with anti-tryptase at 1:400 dilution overnight at 4°C. For other GF antibodies (*see* **Table 1**).
9. Rinse with PBS–0.05% Tween-20; then wash with PBS–0.05% Tween-20 for 5 min three times at RT.
10. Incubate for 60 min at RT with biotinylated secondary antibody in antibody diluent at the dilution recommended by the vendor. The secondary antibody solution is stable for at least 5 d.
11. Quench endogenous horseradish peroxidase (HRP): soak in PBS containing 2% H_2O_2 or 0.65% (0.1 M) NaN_3 for 15 min (*see* **Note 5**).
12. Rinse and wash with PBS-0.05% Tween-20 for 5 min for three times at RT (*see* **Note 6**).
13. Prepare the streptavidin–HRP with PBS–0.1% Tween-20 following the vendor's instruction (*see* **Note 7**).
14. Incubate in streptavidin–HRP solution for 40 min at RT.
15. Rinse with PBS–0.05% Tween-20; then wash with PBS–0.05% Tween-20 for 5 min three times at RT.
16. Color-development in the following substrate solution for 10 min at RT in the darkness (*see* **Note 8**): 5 mg of DAB in 10 mL of PBS containing 0.068 g of imidazole (=ca. 0.1 M), (50 µL of 8% $NiCl·6H_2O$, optional), and 10 µL of 30% H_2O_2 (prepared freshly).
17. Rinse in tap water to stop the color reaction.
18. Counter stain with Mayer's hematoxylin.
19. Soak in 0.05% NH_4OH_3 in dH_2O for 1 min and rinse in water.
20. Dehydrate through graded alcohol and clear in xylene.

> 75% ethanol, 5 min × 1
> 90% ethanol, 5 min × 2
> 100% ethanol, 3 min × 3
> Xylene, 4 min × 4

21. Mount and cover with cover slip in Fisher Permount Mounting Medium (Fisher Scientific, cat. no. SP15-100).
22. Localization of the GF stain in MCs can be assessed by identifying the MCs (on anti-tryptase-labeled slide) and GF-positive cells on the adjacent sequential sections labeled by anti-GF antibody.

3.2. Double Immunostain for Growth Factor/Tryptase

1. Tissue fixed with 10% NBF for 1–2 d at 4°C, processed and embedded in paraffin.
2. Paraffin sections cut at 4–5 µm and placed on Probe-on Plus or poly-L-lysine-coated slides. Prepare three slides per set for each antibody.
3. Melt the paraffin sections at 58°C for 45 min in a humidity chamber.
4. De-paraffinization and re-hydration:

> Xylene 4 min × 4
> 100% ethanol, 3 min × 3

90% ethanol, 5 min × 1
75% ethanol, 5 min × 1
50% ethanol, 5 min × 1
dH2O 2 min × 2 (do not put in any buffer)

5. Antigen retrieval if required (*see* **Table 1** for individual antibodies).
6. Rinse with tap water, then in PBS–0.05% Tween-20 for 10 min.
7. Incubate in the blocking solution at RT for 20 min.
8. Tap off the blocking solution (do not wash) then incubate with appropriate primary antibody overnight at 4°C.
9. Rinse with and wash in PBS–0.05% Tween-20: 5 min once and 10 min twice
10. Incubate in appropriate biotinylated secondary antibody for 60 min at RT.
11. Rinse with and wash in PBS–0.05% Tween-20: 5 min once and 10 min twice.
12. Incubate with ABC-AP for 40 min at RT.
13. Rinse with and wash in PBS–0.05% Tween-20: 5 min once and 10 min twice.
14. Soak in TBS–0.05% Tween-20 for 5 min.
15. Color-development with Fast Red for 30 min at RT.
16. Rinse and wash with dH$_2$O for 2 min at RT.
17. Counter-stain with Meyer's hematoxylin at RT (*see* **Note 9**).
18. Rinse with running tap water to eliminate all residual hematoxylin.
19. Soak slides in NH$_4$OH$_3$ for 1 min at RT; then rinse with dH$_2$O.

Second Labeling for Tryptase

20. Antigen retrieval by incubation in 0.2% type V hyaluronidase in 0.1 *M* acetate buffer for 30 min at RT (*see* **Note 3**).
21. Rinse and wash with dH$_2$O for 2 min twice.
22. Incubated in the blocking solution at RT for 20 min (*see* **Note 10**).
23. Incubate with anti-tryptase at 1:50 for 60 min at RT. Use one previously labeled slide for anti-tryptase, one for non-immune mouse IgG and one with omission of IgG. The later two are controls.
24. Rinse with and wash in PBS–0.05% Tween-20 for 5 min once and 10 min twice.
25. Incubate with biotinylated horse anti-mouse (Vectastain Æ) at 1:200 for 60 min at RT.
26. Rinse with and wash in PBS with 0.05% Tween-20 for 5 min a total of five times.
27. Incubate with streptavidin-FITC at 1: 50 dilution in PBS with 0.05% Tween-20 for 40 min at RT
28. Rinse with and wash in TBS–0.05% Tween-20 at pH 8.5 for 5 min twice (*see* **Note 11**). Briefly review slide under fluorescent microscope to evaluate the intensity of FITC relative to Fast Red.
29. Co-localization of a GF/cytokine can be identified under light/fluorescent microscope. Data collection by photography or cell count.
30. Cover with Crystal Mount, then bake for 15 min at 80°C in an oven.

3.3. General Considerations

1. Selection of buffer:

Table 2
Comparison of PBS and Tris Buffer Saline for IHS

Features/buffer	PBS	TBS
Nature	Inorganic, nonreactive	Organic buffer, often reactive
Shelf life	Longer (>2 mo)	Short
pKa	7.2	8.3
pH tolerance to	Undesired acid	Undesired base
Preparation	Simple	More cumbersome
Inhibition to AP	Theoretic inhibition to AP	No
Delay FITC fading	No	Preferred (at pH > 8.5)
DAB colors	Brown and black	Yellow, brown, and black

A buffer plays a key role in providing an environment for interactions of macromolecules during IHS. Unfortunately, it is a frequently overlooked component, especially after the commercially available buffers have gained popularity. In the author's personal experience, errors in buffer preparation are among the most difficult to detect but easiest to correct. Three major aspects should be considered when selecting and preparing a buffer: salt concentration (ionic strength), buffering capacity (pH stability), and the surface tension imparted by detergents. For example, salt concentration affects both specific antibody-antigen and the nonspecific binding. As a general rule, an increase in salt concentration can reduce nonspecific staining. The pH of a buffer also plays a critical role. Most biological macromolecules are zwitter molecules that carry anionic or cation (negative or positive electrical) charge depending on the pH of environment. Avidin, for example, is strongly charged at pH 7.3, and may bind to tissue macromolecules including proteoglycans nonspecifically by charge. An increase of buffer pH to 9.2, for example, has been shown to effectively eliminate nonspecific binding of avidin to MC granules (*8*). It often surprises many that correction of buffer errors could make such a significant improvement of stain quality. Two representative buffers, PBS and TBS, are the most commonly used for IHS. They are, therefore, used as examples in **Table 2** to illustrate aspects to be taken into consideration when choosing a buffer for IHS.

2. Selection of the detection/amplification system:

The success of immunostain resides on stable specific binding of antibody to the antigen (i.e., GFs and cytokines), which is largely determined by tissue fixation, antigen retrieval, and the primary antibody. The main differences among various detection/amplification systems are the sensitivity and signal-noise ratio. Therefore, the selection of a particular detection system is largely personal preference rather than technical necessity. The presence of avidin or streptavidin in a detection system, however, often results in nonspecific staining of MCs. Avidin has two distinct disadvantages when used for IHS. It has a high isoelectric point of 10.0–10.5 and is therefore positively charged at neutral pH (*38*). Consequently, it may bind nonspecifically to negatively charged structures tissue components. The second disadvantage is that avidin is a glycoprotein and reacts with molecules such as heparin *(38)*. For this reason, avidin–biotin-based detection systems should be avoided altogether, especially when frozen tissue sections are used. The biotin–avidin-based system (ABC method) is used as an example in this chapter because the system is used in the vast majority of studies in the literature. A variety of avidin–biotin-free alternative detection systems are available and give excellent results. The readers are strongly encouraged to choose and adapt to these avidin-free detection/amplification systems for the immunohistological detection of GFs/cytokines in MCs.

3. Selection of the protocol:

After a detection/amplification system is selected, consideration of a specific protocol should be the next step which involves three aspects: (1) whether single IHS on sequential sections or double IHS on the same section for GF and tryptase should be used; (2) whether the GF or tryptase should be stained first; and (3) whether Fast Red or fluorescein isothiocyanate (FITC) should be used for the first labeling. Although single IHS of sequential tissue sections has the advantage of procedural simplicity, easy troubleshooting, and a permanent record, it takes an enormous amount of time to determine the co-localization of the GF and tryptase immunostainings on sequential sections. On the basis of personal experiences in studying inflammatory condition in the joint, lung, nasal mucosa, and eye, data collection from double IHS using Fast Red and FITC for visualization is much less time-consuming and the results are much more accurate than that from single IHS. The disadvantage of the double IHS, however, is the second staining with FITC cannot be kept permanently. To circumvent this problem, one may consider double IHS on two sets of sequential sections, one set stained first by anti-GF visualized with Fast Red, then stained by anti-trypase visualized by FITC, and the other set stained first by anti-tryptase visualized with Fast Red then stained by anti-GF visualized with FITC. Data can be collated immediately after the ISH. Co-localization of GF and tryptase is mutually confirmatory from these two sets, and the permanently retained Fast Red color (representing the GF in one set and tryptase in the other) still allows future re-assessment of the co-localization results because they are sequential sections. The determination of which target molecule to be stained first depends on their relative abundance and sensitivity to antigen retrieval. As a general rule, the macromolecule in low abundance and with antigenicity labile to heat and enzymatic treatment should be immunostained first. Tryptase appears to be quite abundant in MCs relative to most GFs and cytokines and its antigenicity (for DakoCytomation's clone AA1 antibody) has been shown to be resistant to heat and some enzymatic treatments.In the proposed double immunostaining protocol, it is therefore stained after the GF (*see* **Subheading 3.2.**). Finally, for similar reasons, FITC has to be used for the second IHS because it cannot tolerate heat or enzymatic treatment, and multiple blocking, quenching and washing steps.

4. Selection of conjugating enzyme (HRP vs alkaline phosphatase):

Table 3
Comparing Alkaline Phosphatase to HRP for IHS

Features/ enzymes	Alkaline phosphatase	HRP
Endogenous	Gastrointestinal, placenta, prostate	Bone marrow, inflamed tissues
Size/molecular weight	Much larger	Small
Charge at pH 7.3	Minimally charged	Strongly charged
Inhibition of endogenous	Difficult and reversible	Easy and irreversible
Substrate color options	Fewer options	More options
Fluorescent substrate	No	Yes (Fast Red)

HRP has several intrinsic features that impart drawbacks to the IHS. First, endogenous peroxidase is much more prevalent in tissues than (alkaline phosphatase) AP. Second, HRP is much smaller than AP and tend to diffuse locally. Third, several subtypes of HRP are used for IHS with wide range of isoelectric point. Type IV HRP, for example, has an isoelectric point of 9.1 and carries strong positive charge at the neutral pH. This often leads to nonspecific binding to tissue components. As the results, nonspecific staining is more likely when HRP is used. Fourth, HRP has less substrate color options in IHS than AP. However, endogenous HRP can be easily inhibited irreversibly and is less frequently encountered in gastrointestinal system, placenta and prostate. It is therefore particularly applicable to the IHS of these tissues and for double staining. Because of its smaller size, HRP also is preferred for IHS en block and immunocytochemistry where cell permeability becomes a major determinant of the successful stain. AP should be used for IHS in cells or tissues that are rich in endogenous peroxidase and can not be blocked with H_2O_2/methanol (often not suitable for cryostat section because of antigenic denaturation by methanol) such as human bone marrow, spleen, peripheral blood, and tissues that are heavily infiltrated with neutrophils and/or eosinophils. The features of these two commonly used enzymes are summarized in **Table 3**.

5. Selection of substrate chromogens:
   Selection of a substrate chromogen should be based on the visibility (density) of the color, solubility, enhancibility, stability and, for double or triple immunostaining, compatibility with other chromogens or fluorescent dyes. Extensive review of this topic is beyond the scope of this chapter. Two most commonly used chromogens, DAB and Fast Red, are used as examples to highlight the point (*see* **Table 4**). DAB, for example, offers a distinct color spectrum from golden yellow to black depending on the buffer pH and additional additives. It alone can be used in double immunostaining to visualize two different antigen-antibody complexes conjugated with one enzyme (HRP) provided that they are not colocalized subcellularly. The color intensity of DBA can be enhanced markedly if so desired. Measured by antibody concentration used, the detection sensi-

Table 4
Comparison of DAB and Fast Red as Substrate Chromogens for IHS

Features/chromogens	DAB	Fast Red
Enzyme	HRP	AP
Color variation	Golden, brown to black	Red, no other variation
Potential carcinogenic	Yes	No
Intensity enhancement	Yes, up to 10-fold *(37)*	No or only minimally
Double stains with FITC	Not compatible	Yes, excellent compatibility
Organic solvents	Resistant (insoluble)	Organic-soluble

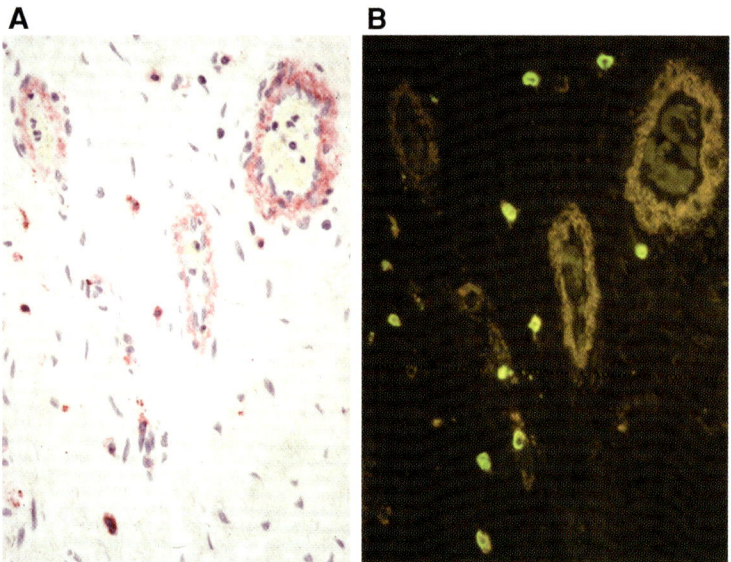

Fig. 1. Double immunohistostain of bFGF and MCs in human synovial tissue. A tissue section is first labeled with anti-bFGF by ABC-AP method using Fast Red as the chromogen. The section is subsequently labeled with anti-tryptase by SABC-FITC. **(A)** shows positive stain for bFGF in red (Fast Red) under light microscope. **(B)** shows positive stain for tryptase in green fluorescence in MCs and positive stain for bFGF in orange autofluorescence (Fast Red) under fluorescent microscope. Note the co-localization of two antigens (bFGF and tryptase) in the MCs and absence of tryptase stain in the bFGF-positive vascular walls. Original magnification, ×200.

tivity can be increased several folds by the enhancement (*[23]* and personal experience). In contrast, Fast Red has an unsurpassed feature of permanent orange-red fluorescence at excitation wavelength suitable for FITC with negligible interference with the emission color of FITC under a fluorescent microscope.This feature makes Fast Red an ideal chromogen, together with FITC, for double immunostaining of macromolecules co-localized subcellularly (**Fig. 1**). This is particular useful to identify GF/cytokine-positive MCs by double immunostaining *(25)*.

4. Notes

1. It is highly recommended to use heparin-adsorbed sera. Run the serum or sera through Affi-Gel® Heparin Gel column (Bio-Rad; cat. no. 153-6173) at a flow rate of 1 mL/min to eliminate intrinsic heparin-binding GFs. Alternatively, commercially available serum-free protein block (DakoCytomation, cat. no. X0909) should be used. Avoid using nonproteolytic enzymes for antigen-retrieval before GF stain. These two measures effectively minimize falsely specific positive stain caused by GF contamination. Diluent containing NaN_3 or thimerosal does not seem to affect enzyme activity when used for biotinylated secondary antibody in ABC method.

2. Soaking in a buffer may attenuate antigen retrieval by enzymatic digestion because the buffer can change the pH required for enzyme activity.

3. Proteins K (DakoCytomation) can also be used. But it is a proteolytic enzyme and may lead to deterioration of cytological detail and the quality of the 1st stain.

4. Use Heparin-adsorbed serum for blocking solution to eliminate all heparin-binding protein (GFs). Alternatively, use serum-free protein block (DakoCytomation).

5. Conventionally, endogenous peroxidase quenching is conducted before incubation with the blocking solution. Because serum and other proteins used in blocking solution and antibody diluent also contain peroxidase, it makes more sense and gives better results to perform the quenching step right before incubation with ABC–HRP. Although theoretically methanol may be ideal for H_2O_2 activity, it may also alter the tissue macromolecule conformation, especially after antigen retrieval. Replacing methanol with PBS is more practical and results in no perceivable change in inhibition of endogenous peroxidase.

6. H_2O_2 and NaN_3 irreversibly inhibit peroxidase enzyme activity and it is therefore very important to have a thorough wash before the incubation with ABC–HRP.

7. Use TBS-0.1% Tween-20 at pH 8.5 to eliminate nonspecific binding to MC granules if necessary. ABC–HRP also may be used. Streptavidin does not contain a carbohydrate moiety and, thus, possesses an acidic isoelectric point near 7.0. As a result, streptavidin has a lower nonspecific binding characteristic than that of avidin.

8. Imidazole prevents rapid color development, which often results in background. $NiCl_2$ imparts a purple–black color to DAB. More importantly, it allows subsequent enhancement of the stain when it becomes necessary *(37)*.

9. Fast Red is soluble in organic solvent (i.e., alcohol and xylene). Make sure that the hematoxylin is alcohol-free.

10. Adding streptavidin–biotin blocking solution (Vector Laboratories, cat. no. SA-5001) of equal volume to the serum-BSA blocking solution is highly recommended.

11. TBS at pH 8.5 helps retard FITC fading and intensify the existing nuclear couterstain by hematoxylin.

Acknowledgments

The author would like to thank Michael Covinsky, MD, PhD, in the Department of Pathology and Laboratory Medicine at the University of Texas Health Science Center at Houston for critical review of this chapter.

References

1. Kjellen, L. and Lindahl, U. (1991) Proteoglycans: structures and interactions. *Annu. Rev. Biochem.* **60,** 443–475.
2. Schiltz, P. M., Lieber, J., Giorno, R. C., and Claman, H. N. (1993) Mast cell immunohistochemistry: non-immunological immunostaining mediated by non-specific F(ab')2-mast cell secretory granule interaction. *Histochem. J.* **25,** 642–647.
3. Haynes, L. W. (1988) Fibroblast (heparin-binding) growing factors in neuronal development and repair. *Mol. Neurobiol.* **2,** 263–289.
4. Burgess, W. H. and Maciag, T. (1989) The heparin-binding (fibroblast) growth factor family of proteins. *Annu. Rev. Biochem.* **58,** 575–606.
5. Fritz, P., Muller, J., Reiser, H., et al. (1986) Avidin-peroxidase. A new mast cell staining method. *Acta. Histochem. Suppl.* **32,** 235–239.
6. Tharp, M. D., Seelig, L. L., Jr., Tigelaar, R. E., and Bergstresser, P. R. (1985) Conjugated avidin binds to mast cell granules. *J. Histochem. Cytochem.* **33,** 27–32.
7. Bergstresser, P. R., Tigelaar, R. E., and Tharp, M. D. (1984) Conjugated avidin identifies cutaneous rodent and human mast cells. *J. Invest. Dermatol.* **83,** 214–218.
8. Bussolati, G. and Gugliotta, P. (1983) Nonspecific staining of mast cells by avidin–biotin-peroxidase complexes (ABC). *J. Histochem. Cytochem.* **31,** 1419–1421.
9. Kreuger, J., Salmivirta, M., Sturiale, L., Gimenez-Gallego, G., and Lindahl, U. (2001) Sequence analysis of heparan sulfate epitopes with graded affinities for fibroblast growth factors 1 and 2. *J. Biol. Chem.* **276,** 30,744–30,752.
10. Roche, W. R. (1985) Mast cells and tumour angiogenesis: the tumor-mediated release of an endothelial growth factor from mast cells. *Int. J. Cancer* **36,** 721–728.
11. Grutzkau, A., Kruger-Krasagakes, S., Baumeister, H., et al. (1998) Synthesis, storage, and release of vascular endothelial growth factor/vascular permeability factor (VEGF/VPF) by human mast cells: implications for the biological significance of VEGF206. *Mol. Biol. Cell* **9,** 875–884.
12. Ueno, N., Baird, A., Esch, F., Ling, N., and Guillemin, R. (1987) Isolation and partial characterization of basic fibroblast growth factor from bovine testis. *Mol. Cell. Endocrinol.* **49,** 189–194.
13. Rahmanian, M. and Heldin, P. (2002) Testicular hyaluronidase induces tubular structures of endothelial cells grown in three-dimensional collagen gel through a CD44-mediated mechanism. *Int. J. Cancer* **97,** 601–607.
14. Bokemeyer, C., Kuczyk, M. A., Dunn, T., et al. (1996) Expression of stem-cell factor and its receptor c-kit protein in normal testicular tissue and malignant germ-cell tumours. *J. Cancer Res. Clin. Oncol.* **122,** 301–306.
15. Sandlow, J. I., Feng, H. L., Cohen, M. B., and Sandra, A. (1996) Expression of c-KIT and its ligand, stem cell factor, in normal and subfertile human testicular tissue. *J. Androl.* **17,** 403–408.

16. Ergun, S., Luttmer, W., Fiedler, W., and Holstein, A. F. (1998) Functional expression and localization of vascular endothelial growth factor and its receptors in the human epididymis. *Biol. Reprod.* **58,** 160–168.

17. Hammadeh, M. E., Fischer-Hammadeh, C., Hoffmeister, H., Herrmann, W., Rosenbaum, P., and Schmidt, W. (2004) Relationship between cytokine concentrations (FGF, sICAM-1 and SCF) in serum, follicular fluid and ICSI outcome. *Am. J. Reprod. Immunol.* **51,** 81–85.

18. Jones, A., Fujiyama, C., Turner, K., et al. (2000) Elevated serum vascular endothelial growth factor in patients with hormone-escaped prostate cancer. *BJU Int.* **85,** 276–280.

19. Eckenstein, F., Woodward, W. R., and Nishi, R. (1991) Differential localization and possible functions of aFGF and bFGF in the central and peripheral nervous systems. *Ann. N. Y. Acad. Sci.* **638,** 348–360.

20. Collins, R. A. and Grounds, M. D. (2001) The role of tumor necrosis factor-alpha (TNF-alpha) in skeletal muscle regeneration. Studies in TNF-alpha(–/–) and TNF-alpha(-/-)/LT-alpha(-/-) mice. *J. Histochem. Cytochem.* **49,** 989–1001.

21. Aoki, M., Pawankar, R., Niimi, Y., and Kawana, S. (2003) Mast cells in basal cell carcinoma express VEGF, IL-8 and RANTES. *Int. Arch. Allergy Immunol.* **130,** 216–223.

22. Kibe, Y., Takenaka, H., and Kishimoto, S. (2000) Spatial and temporal expression of basic fibroblast growth factor protein during wound healing of rat skin. *Br. J. Dermatol.* **143,** 720–727.

23. Wei, P., Yu, F. Q., Chen, X. L., Tao, S. X., Han, C. S., and Liu, Y. X. (2004) VEGF, bFGF and their receptors at the fetal-maternal interface of the rhesus monkey. *Placenta* **25,** 184–196.

24. Baek, J. Y., Tefferi, A., Pardanani, A., and Li, C. Y. (2002) Immunohistochemical studies of c-kit, transforming growth factor-beta, and basic fibroblast growth factor in mast cell disease. *Leuk. Res.* **26,** 83–90.

25. Reed, J. A., Albino, A. P., and McNutt, N. S. (1995) Human cutaneous mast cells express basic fibroblast growth factor. *Lab. Invest.* **72,** 215–222.

26. Reed, J. A., McNutt, N. S., Bogdany, J. K., and Albino, A. P. (1996) Expression of the mast cell growth factor interleukin-3 in melanocytic lesions correlates with an increased number of mast cells in the perilesional stroma: implications for melanoma progression. *J. Cutan. Pathol.* **23,** 495–505.

27. Walker, K. F., Lappin, D. F., Takahashi, K., Hope, J., Macdonald, D. G., and Kinane, D. F. (2000) Cytokine expression in periapical granulation tissue as assessed by immunohistochemistry. *Eur. J. Oral. Sci.* **108,** 195–201.

28. Qu, Z., Picou, M., Dang, T. T., et al. (1994) Immunolocalization of basic fibroblast growth factor and platelet-derived growth factor-A during adjuvant arthritis in the Lewis rat. *Am. J. Pathol.* **145,** 1127–1139.

29. Ceponis, A., Konttinen, Y. T., Takagi, M., et al. (1998) Expression of stem cell factor (SCF) and SCF receptor (c-kit) in synovial membrane in arthritis: correlation with synovial mast cell hyperplasia and inflammation. *J. Rheumatol.* **25,** 2304–2314.

30. Simak, R., Capodieci, P., Cohen, D. W., et al. (2000) Expression of c-kit and kit-ligand in benign and malignant prostatic tissues. *Histol. Histopathol.* **15,** 365–374.

31. Calabrese, F., Valente, M., Giacometti, C., et al. (2003) Parenchymal transforming growth factor beta-1: its type II receptor and Smad signaling pathway correlate with inflammation and fibrosis in chronic liver disease of viral etiology. *J. Gastroenterol. Hepatol.* **18,** 1302–1308.

32. Young, A., Thomson, A. J., Ledingham, M., Jordan, F., Greer, I. A., and Norman, J. E. (2002) Immunolocalization of proinflammatory cytokines in myometrium, cervix, and fetal membranes during human parturition at term. *Biol. Reprod.* **66,** 445–449.

33. Fenhalls, G., Stevens, L., Bezuidenhout, J., et al. (2002) Distribution of IFN-gamma, IL-4 and TNF-alpha protein and CD8 T cells producing IL-12p40 mRNA in human lung tuberculous granulomas. *Immunology* **105,** 325–335.

34. Stitt, A. W., Simpson, D. A., Boocock, C., Gardiner, T. A., Murphy, G. M., and Archer, D. B. (1998) Expression of vascular endothelial growth factor (VEGF) and its receptors is regulated in eyes with intra-ocular tumours. *J. Pathol.* **186,** 306–312.

35. Klein, M., Picard, E., Vignaud, J. M., et al. (1999) Vascular endothelial growth factor gene and protein: strong expression in thyroiditis and thyroid carcinoma. *J. Endocrinol.* **161,** 41–49.

36. Smith, B. D., Smith, G. L., Carter, D., Sasaki, C. T., and Haffty, B. G. (2000) Prognostic significance of vascular endothelial growth factor protein levels in oral and oropharyngeal squamous cell carcinoma. *J. Clin. Oncol.* **18,** 2046–2052.

37. Gallyas, F. and Merchenthaler, I. (1988) Copper-H2O2 oxidation strikingly improves silver intensification of the nickel-diaminobenzidine (Ni-DAB) end-product of the peroxidase reaction. *J. Histochem. Cytochem.* **36,** 807–810.

38. Green, N. M. (1975) Avidin. *Adv. Protein Chem.* **29,** 85–133.

VI

MAST CELL INTERACTIONS WITH OTHER CELL TYPES

21

Endothelial Cell Activation by Mast Cell Mediators

Kottarappat N. Dileepan and Daniel J. Stechschulte

Summary

Mast cells are important cells of the immune system, and their secretory products regulate many vascular functions. Although considerable interest is focused on the role of mast cells and infectious agents in atherosclerosis, whether or not mast cell mediators act in concert with bacterial agents to regulate endothelial activation is not known. Here, we have described experimental techniques and presented related results to demonstrate how mast cell granule (MCG) mediators and bacterial products synergize endothelial cell inflammatory responses (*see* **Note 1**). The described methods outline: (1) the collection of rat peritoneal mast cells; (2) preparation of MCGs; (3) co-culture of human endothelial cells with mast cell granules; (4) determination of the regulation of endothelial cell inflammatory responses; (5) demonstration of the role of MCG protease and histamine in the regulation of endothelial cell function; (6) amplification of lipopolysaccharide-induced signal transduction pathways by mast cell granules; (7) elucidation of histamine-induced amplification of endothelial cell responses to Gram-negative and Gram-positive bacterial cell wall components; and (8) determination of the expression of Toll-like receptor 2 and 4. We hope the techniques described here can be used for designing experiments focusing on the regulatory role of mast cell mediators on cell functions.

Key Words: Mast cell granules; endothelial cells; histamine; proteases; bacterial components; interleukin-6; interleukin-8; Toll-like receptors; calcium; MAP kinase; nuclear factor-κB; electron microscopy.

1. Introduction

Mast cells are normal constituents of the vessel wall and are primarily located in the connective tissue matrices. Upon activation, mast cells release many inflammatory mediators, including histamine, proteases, heparin, prostaglandins, leukotrienes, and a variety of cytokines *(1–5)*. These mast cell products are well recognized for their regulatory actions on vascular endothelium, and many reports have documented the role for mast cells in the development of atherosclerosis *(6–12)*. We have shown that mast cell granule (MCG)-

From: *Methods in Molecular Biology, vol. 315: Mast Cells: Methods and Protocols*
Edited by: G. Krishnaswamy and D. S. Chi © Humana Press Inc., Totowa, NJ

derived serine proteases and histamine induce inflammatory responses in endothelial cells *(13–17)*. These results emphasize the importance of mast cell-derived serine proteases and histamine in vascular inflammation and atherogenesis.

The activation of endothelial cells with resultant syntheses of proinflammatory mediators and the expression of cell adhesion molecules is critical for immune surveillance. However, uncontrolled and persistent inflammation can initiate atherogenesis. In recent years, increasing attention has focused on the role of infectious agents in atherosclerosis *(18–20)*. The first line of immune defense to invading microbes is the recognition of pathogen-associated molecular patterns that evoke an inflammatory response *(21)*. The innate recognition of microbial pathogens by mammalian cells is mediated through Toll-like receptors (TLRs). Mammalian cells express at least 10 TLRs and, among these, TLR4 mediates responses to Gram-negative bacterial lipopolysaccharide (LPS *[22,23]*), and TLR2 recognizes a number of components associated with Gram-positive bacteria *(24–26)*. Human endothelial cells constitutively express low levels of TLR2 and TLR4 and are activated by Gram-positive and Gram-negative bacterial components *(17,27,28)*. Further evidence for the possible involvement of innate immune system in coronary disease is the substantial increase in TLR2 and TLR4 message in the endothelium of human atherosclerotic lesions *(29)* and the reduced incidence of atherosclerosis in patients with TLR4 polymorphism *(30)*.

Reports from our laboratory have shown that Gram-negative bacterial cell wall component, LPS, and Gram-positive bacterial components, lipoteichoic acid (LTA) and peptidoglycan (PGN), stimulate human endothelial cells to produce interleukin (IL)-6 and IL-8, which is greatly enhanced by the presence of histamine *(15,17)*. These results suggest that the co-operative action between histamine and bacterial components lead to amplified inflammatory responses in vascular endothelium. We have further demonstrated that histamine amplifies endothelial cell responsiveness to both Gram-negative and Gram-positive cell wall components via enhanced expression of TLR2 and TLR4 *(17)*. In this chapter, we describe methods to demonstrate the mast cell/endothelial cell interaction and how cooperation between these two cell types amplifies inflammatory responses. Furthermore, using histamine as an activating molecule, we have illustrated how this mast cell mediator could amplify endothelial cell sensitivity to bacterial pathogens.

2. Materials

1. Human coronary artery endothelial cells (HCAECs; Cambrex, San Diego, CA).
2. Endothelial growth media (EGM-2; Cambrex).

3. Minimum essential medium with Eagle's salts (HMEM): minimum essential medium (Hyclone, Hogan, UT) containing 15 mM N-2-hydroxyethylpiperazine-N'-ethanesulfonic acid (HEPES), 100 U/mL penicillin, 100 µg streptomycin, 10% fetal bovine serum (FBS), and 5 U/mL heparin (Sigma, St. Louis, MO).
4. Low-endotoxin FBS (Hyclone, Hogan, UT).
5. Metrizamide (Sigma).
6. HEPES (Sigma).
7. EGM-2MV containing 1 µg/mL hydrocortisone acetate, 50 ng/mL gentamycin, 50 µg/mL amphotericin B, and the recommended concentrations of hEGF, VEGF, hFGF-B, R3IGF, ascorbic acid, and 5% FBS (all from Cambrex).
8. IL-6 and IL-8 enzyme-linked immunosorbent assay (ELISA) kits (R&D, Minneapolis, MN).
9. *Escherichia coli* (0111:B4) lipopolysaccharide (Sigma).
10. Phenylmethylsulfonyl fluoride (PMSF; Sigma).
11. 100 mM Tris-HCl, pH 7.5.
12. Histamine hydrochloride (Sigma).
13. Diphenhydramine (histamine receptor-1 antagonist).
14. Famotidine (histamine receptor-2 antagonist).
15. Oligonucleotide primers (Invitrogen, Carlsbad, CA).
16. Trypsin-ethylene diamine tetraacetic acid (EDTA; Cambrex).
17. Trypsin neutralizing solution (Cambrex).
18. Lipoteichoic acid (Sigma).
19. Peptidoglycan (Sigma).
20. Triton Lysis Buffer: 20 mM Tris (pH 7.4), 137 mM NaCl, 10% (v/v) glycerol, 1% (v/v) Triton X-100, 2 mM EDTA, 25 mM β-glycerol phosphate, 2 mM sodium pyrophosphate, 1% (v/v) protease inhibitor cocktail, and 0.5 mM dithiothreitol.
21. Polymyxin B (Sigma).
22. TLR2 (N-17, H-175) and TLR4 (H-180) antibodies (Santa Cruz Biotechnology, Santa Cruz, CA).
23. Cy3 goat anti-mouse and normal goat serum (Jackson Immunoresearch Laboratories, West Grove, PA).
24. Buffer I for nuclear factor (NF)-κB: 10 mM HEPES-KOH, 10 mM KCl, and 1.5 mM MgCl$_2$, pH 7.9.
25. Buffer II for NF-κB: 20 mM HEPES, 420 mM NaCl, 1.5 mM MgCl$_2$, 0.2 mM EDTA, and 25% glycerol, pH 7.9.
26. Dilution buffer for NF-κB: 20 mM HEPES, 50 mM KCl, 0.2 mM EDTA, and 20% glycerol, pH 7.9.
27. Electrophoretic mobility shift assay (EMSA) buffer for NF-κB: 10 mM Tris-HCl, pH 7.5, containing 40 mM NaCl, 1 mM EDTA, 1 mM β-mercaptoethanol, 4% glycerol, 0.1% Nonidet-P40, and 1 µg/µL bovine serum albumin.
28. TRIzol Reagent (Life Technologies, Rockville, MD).
29. RNAse–free DNAse1 (Life Technologies).
30. Superscript^{TM}II RNase H$^-$ Reverse Transcriptase system (Life Technologies,).
31. Taq Polymerase (Life Technologies).

32. The gene-specific primers used in reverse transcription polymerase chain reaction (RT-PCR; Invitrogen Life Technologies).
33. Nuclear and cytoplasmic protein extraction reagents (NE-PER™; Pierce-Endogen, Rockford, IL).
34. Poly dI-dC (Pharmacia).
35. Enzyme immuno-competition assay kit for histamine (Beckman-Coulter).
36. Calcium Crimson and Fluo-4 (Molecular Probes, Eugene, OR).
37. ERK1/ERK2 assay reagents and antibodies (Santa Cruz Biotechnology).
38. Blocking solution: phosphate-buffered saline containing 1% bovine serum albumin, 5% normal goat serum, and 0.3% Triton X-100.
39. TBST: 20 m*M* Tris-HCl, 150 m*M* NaCl, 0.1% Tween-20.

3. Methods

The methods described in **Subheadings 3.1.–3.8.** outline: (1) the collection of rat peritoneal mast cells; (2) preparation of MCGs; (3) co-culture of human endothelial cells with MCGs; (4) determination of the regulation of endothelial cell inflammatory responses; (5) demonstration of the role of MCG protease and histamine in the regulation of endothelial cell function; (6) amplification of LPS-induced signal transduction pathways by MCGs; (7) elucidation of histamine-induced amplification of endothelial cell responses to Gram-negative and Gram-positive bacterial cell wall components; and (8) determination of the expression of Toll-like receptor 2 and 4.

3.1. Collection and Isolation of Mast Cells

Three- to four-month-old Sprague–Dawley rats (350–400 g) are used as the source of peritoneal mast cells. The methods employed for the isolation of mast cells have been previously described *(13,14,16)*.

1. The peritoneal cavity of each rat is lavaged under sterile conditions with minimum essential medium containing 15 m*M* HEPES, 100 U/mL penicillin, 100 μg of streptomycin, 10% FBS (HMEM), and 5 U/mL heparin.
2. The peritoneal cells are then pooled, centrifuged at 250*g* for 10 min at room temperature, and washed twice with HMEM.
3. Two-milliliter aliquots of the cell suspension (6–8 × 10^7 cells) are layered on 4-mL columns of 22.5% (w/v) metrizamide (density 1.125 g/mL) in HMEM and centrifuged at 200*g* for 15 min.
4. Macrophages are collected at the gradient interface and mast cells are sedimented at the bottom.
5. The mast cells are collected, washed twice, and resuspended in HMEM. Mast cells collected by this procedure usually exceed 95% in purity and viability when tested by trypan blue exclusion.
6. One to two million peritoneal mast cells can be collected from one 300-g rat. A scanning electron micrograph of an enriched preparation of rat peritoneal mast cells is presented in **Fig. 1**. The transmission electron micrograph depicts a mast cell filled with electron-dense granules **(Fig. 2)**.

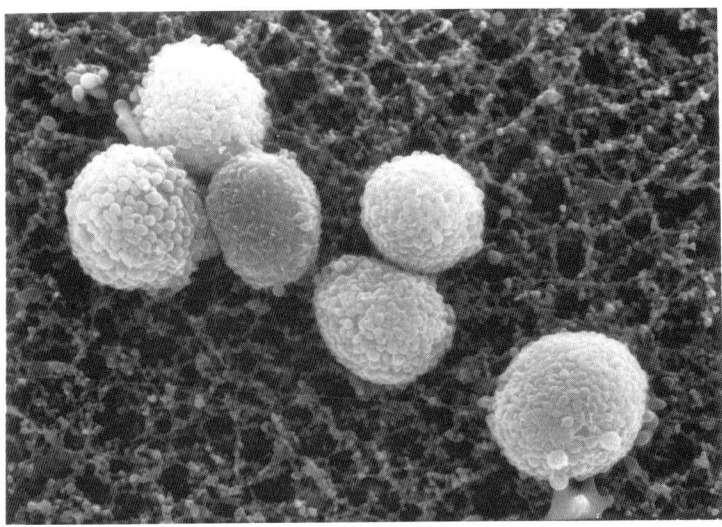

Fig. 1. Scanning electron micrograph of a typical rat peritoneal mast cell preparation.

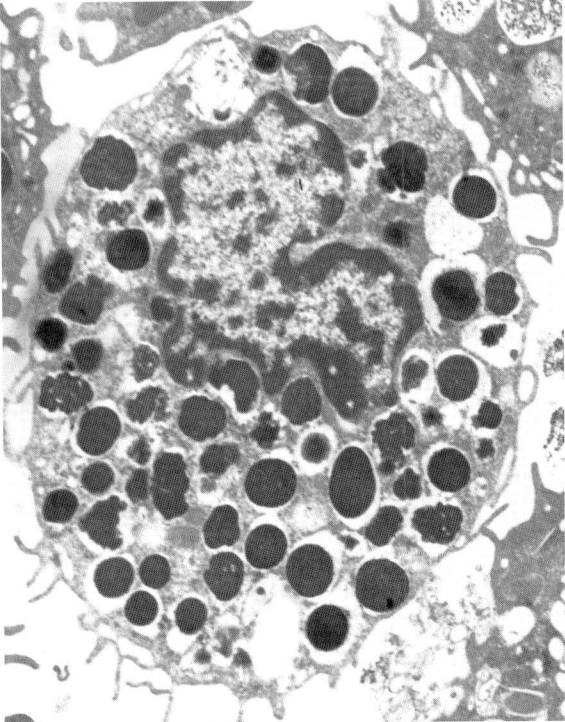

Fig. 2. Transmission electron micrograph of a rat peritoneal mast cell depicting the presence of many electron-dense granules.

3.2. Preparation of MCGs

Under sterile conditions at 0–4°C, MCGs are prepared from metrizamide-purified mast cells by controlled sonication and sucrose gradient centrifugation (*13,14,16*).

1. The purified mast cells are suspended in 2 mL of HMEM and sonicated twice for 15 s at a power setting of 2.5 with a microtip sonicator (Sonifier Cell Disrupter, model W140).
2. The disrupted cells and MCG are incubated at 30°C for 15 min and mixed vigorously for 1 min.
3. The cell suspension is then layered over 2 mL of 0.34 *M* sterile sucrose and centrifuged at 50*g* for 10 min at 4°C.
4. The MCG fraction at the interface is aspirated and the pellet containing cellular debris is discarded.
5. The MCG fraction is centrifuged at 1800*g* for 20 min at 4°C. The resulting homogeneous preparation of sedimented MCG is washed twice and resuspended in the appropriate tissue culture medium.
6. On the basis of the histamine content of the starting number of mast cells, the recovery of MCG ranged from 50 to 70%. The quantity of MCG used in each experiment can be expressed as the equivalent of the starting mast cell number. Transmission electron micrograph of a typical MCG preparation is given (**Fig. 3**; *see* **Notes 2–4**).

3.3. Endothelial Cell Culture

1. HCAECs (Cambrex) are grown in EGM-2MV.
2. At confluence, the cells are detached from the culture flasks using trypsin–EDTA, washed twice, and resuspended in EGM-2MV. The cells are studied between three and six passages.
3. Human umbilical vein endothelial cells (HUVECs) also can be maintained in the same culture media and can be used to demonstrate inflammatory responses to MCG proteases and histamine (*see* **Note 5**).

3.4. Electron Microscopic Analysis of Mast Cell–Endothelial Cell Interaction

The interaction of mast cells with endothelial cells and the fate of MCG can be documented by scanning and transmission electron microscopy.

1. HCAECs are cultured on sterile cover slips inserted in six-well culture plates for 24 h in the presence or absence of purified mast cells at a mast cell:endothelial cell ratio of 1:2.
2. After 24 h, the cells are washed twice with phosphate-buffered saline. The cells are then fixed in 2% glutaraldehyde, and processed for scanning electron microscopy (**Fig. 4**).

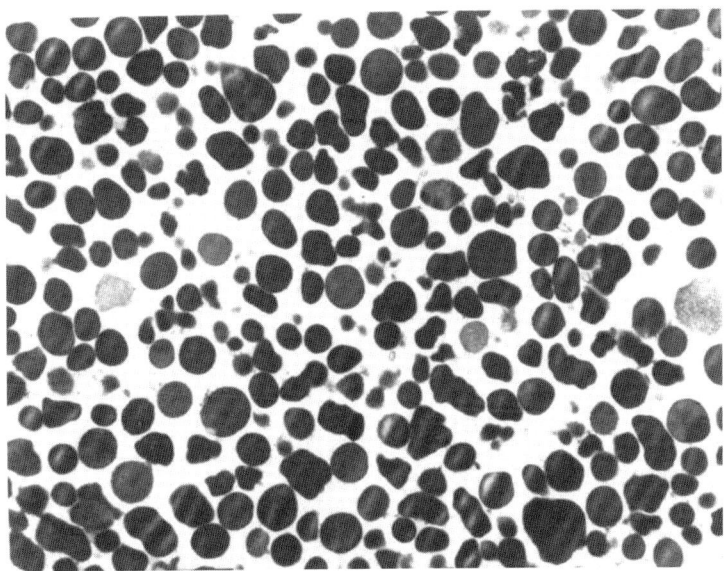

Fig. 3. Transmission electron micrograph of a typical rat peritoneal MCG preparation.

3. **Figure 4A** depicts the typical features of an unactivated HCAECs, and **Fig. 4B** illustrates the interaction of a degranulating mast cell with the endothelial cell in culture *(14)*.

4. Transmission electron microscopic analyses can be carried out to demonstrate the uptake of MCG by endothelial cells in vitro.

5. Endothelial cells are co-cultured with MCGs at a mast cell:endothelial cell ratio of 1:2.

6. After incubating for 24 h, the cells are washed twice with fresh medium to remove free MCG.

7. The cells are then detached from the flasks using trypsin–EDTA, washed, fixed in 2% glutaraldehyde, and processed for transmission electron microscopy.

8. **Figure 5** demonstrates that MCGs are internalized by endothelial cells and remain morphologically intact even after 24 h in culture (*see* **Note 6** *[13]*).

3.5. Determination of the Direct and Regulatory Effects of MCG on Endothelial Cell Inflammatory Responses

1. HCAECs ($2–4 \times 10^4$) are added to each well of a 96-well flat-bottom microtiter plate and allowed to adhere for 24 h in EGM complete medium.

2. After the adherence, MCG, LPS, MCG + LPS, or medium is added to HCAEC monolayers and the final volume adjusted to 0.2 mL with the complete EGM.

3. Routinely all incubations are carried out for 24 h at 37°C under the atmosphere of 5% CO_2. The 24-h incubation period is chosen after conducting time-kinetic studies.

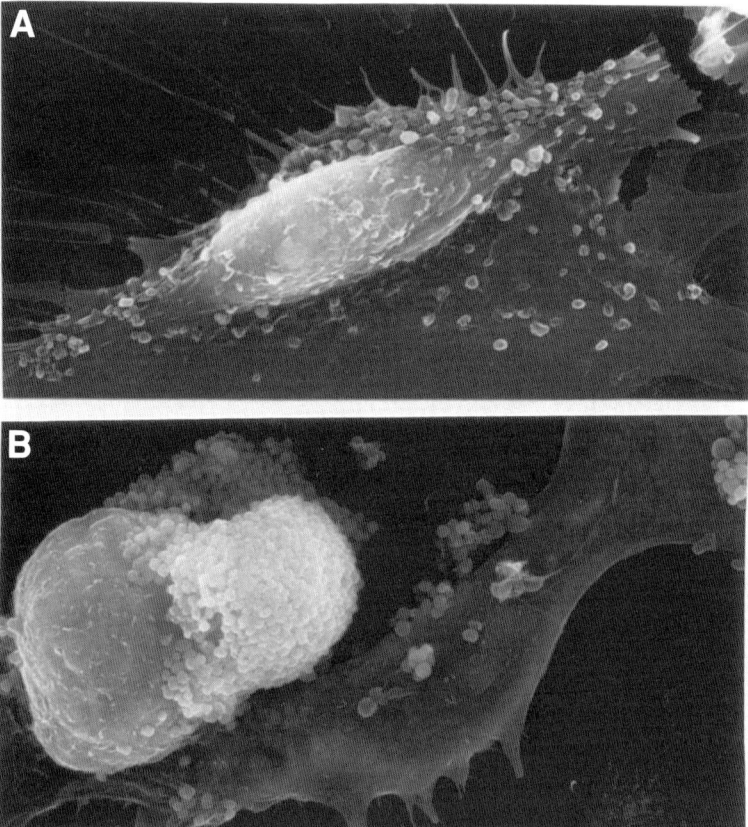

Fig. 4. Scanning electron micrographs of human coronary artery endothelial cells cultured for 24 h with medium alone (**A**) or with mast cells (**B**). Photomicrograph in (**B**) demonstrates the interaction between a degranualating mast cell and an endothelial cell in co-culture. (Reproduced with permission from **ref. *14*.**)

4. After the incubation, aliquots of the culture supernatants are collected, appropriately diluted, and assayed for IL-6 and IL-8 according to the instructions provided by the ELISA kit manufacturers. The cytokine levels are quantified by comparison with a standard curve generated concurrently, utilizing recombinant human IL-6 and IL-8.
5. The effects of MCG on IL-6 and IL-8 production by resting or LPS-activated HCAEC are shown in **Fig. 6**. Resting HCAECs do not produce detectable amounts of IL-6 or IL-8. However, LPS stimulates the production of cytokines in a dose-dependent manner. Both IL-6 and IL-8 production by HCAECs reach a plateau at LPS doses of 50–100 ng/mL. The simultaneous addition of MCG and LPS to HCAEC monolayers causes marked potentiation of IL-6 and IL-8 pro-

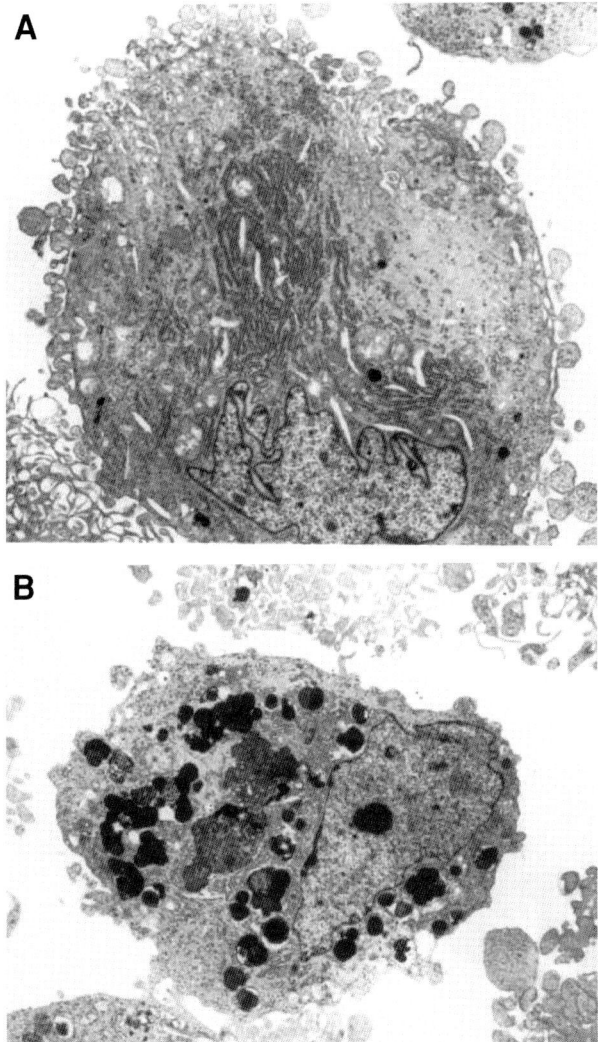

Fig. 5. Transmission electron micrograph of HUVECs cultured for 24 h with medium alone (**A**) or with MCGs (**B**). The ratio of mast cell equivalent MCG:HUVECs was 1:2. Numerous endocytosed MCGs can be seen in HUVECs after a 24 h co-culture with MCGs. (Reproduced with permission from **ref.** *13*.)

duction at all doses of LPS tested. The amplification of LPS-induced cytokine production by MCG is evident even at the maximal stimulatory dose of LPS. Increased levels of these cytokines are not derived from MCG because equal amounts of MCG cultured alone or in the presence of LPS do not possess detectable amounts of IL-6 or IL-8 *(14)*.

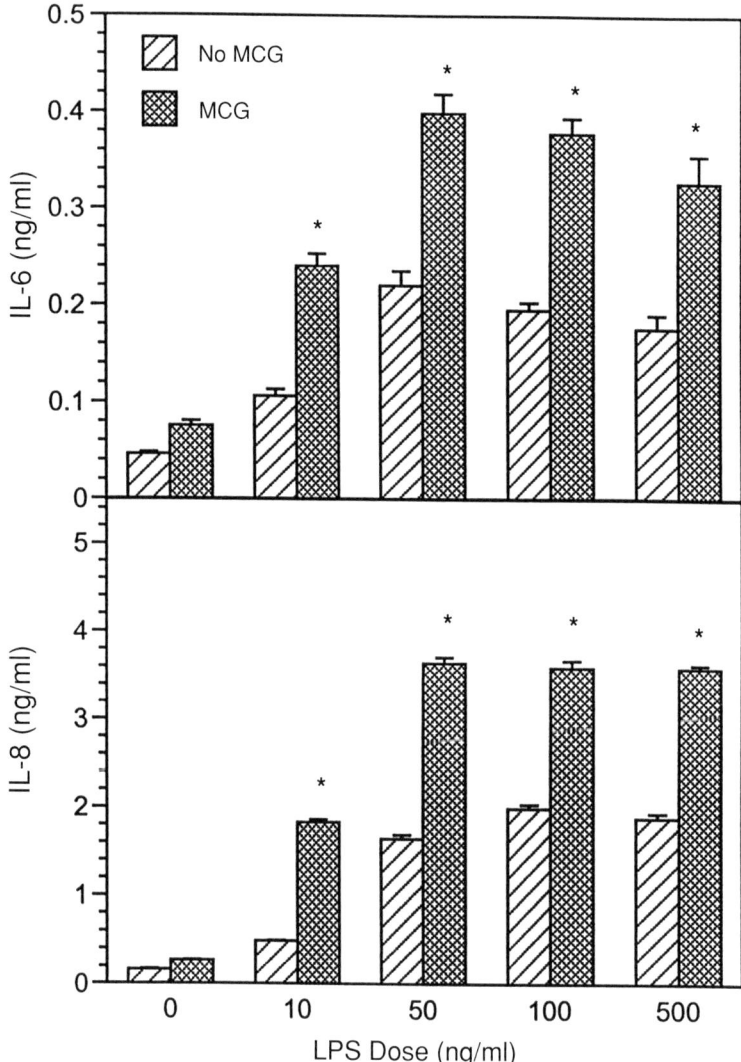

Fig. 6. Effect of MCG on IL-6 **(top panel)** and IL-8 **(bottom panel)** production by LPS-activated HCAECs. HCAEC monolayers (10,000) were cultured with the indicated doses of LPS for 24 h in the presence or absence of MCGs (5000 mast cell equivalent). The IL-6 and IL-8 concentrations in the culture media were assayed by ELISA. Each value is the mean ± SEM of quadruplicate culture wells, and the results are representative of three separate experiments. *Statistically significant effect of MCG + LPS at $p < 0.05$ when compared with the corresponding dose of LPS alone. (Reproduced with permission from **ref. 14**.)

3.5.1. The Role of MCG-Derived Serine Protease and Histamine in the Amplification of LPS Effect

Mast cell granules contain serine proteases and histamine and a variety of other inflammatory mediators. The role of serine proteases can be evaluated by inhibiting the enzyme activity by treating MCG preparations with the serine protease inhibitor, phenylmethylsulfonyl fluoride (PMSF). Dialysis of PMSF-treated MCG is required to remove unbound PMSF (*see* Note 7). Dialysis will also remove more than 99% of histamine as well as other soluble low molecular weight components of MCG. However, dialysis of untreated MCG will remove only histamine and soluble substances without affecting protease activity. To achieve this objective, MCG preparations are treated with medium or PMSF (1 m*M*) for 12 h at 4°C and dialyzed against 100 m*M* of Tris-HCl (pH 7.5) for 4 h with three changes of buffer. Using untreated MCG, PMSF-treated/dialyzed MCG, and dialyzed MCG (without PMSF treatment) we can demonstrate the relative contributions of MCG proteases and histamine in amplifying LPS responsiveness.

The results depicted in **Fig. 7** demonstrate the effects of MCG on LPS-activated HUVECs. The production of IL-6 by HUVECs could be detected as early as 2 h after incubation with MCG. IL-6 production gradually increased and plateaued by 8 h and remained unchanged throughout the remaining 48 h. In the presence of MCG, production of IL-6 induced by LPS was greatly amplified during the 48-h incubation period. Dialysis of MCG, which removed more than 99% of histamine, decreased endothelial cell IL-6 production by 40–60%. Inhibition of serine protease activity in MCG by treatment with PMSF and depletion of histamine completely abolished the direct and modulating effect of MCG (*16*).

3.5.2. Measurement of Proteases and Histamine Levels in MCGs

It is important to show that PMSF treatment inhibits MCG protease activity and dialysis removes histamine. The serine protease activity (chymase) in the preparation of MCGs can be assayed spectrophotometrically at 405 n*M* by monitoring the hydrolysis of succinyl-phenylalanyl-leucyl-phenylanyl-*p*-nitroanalide (*see* Chapter 15 *[1]*). The reaction is condcuted at 37°C in 150 m*M* Tris-HCl (pH 7.6) in the presence of 1 m*M* substrate and a MCG preparation (equivalent to 0.5 million mast cells) in a final volume of 1 mL. The enzyme activity is continuously monitored and the rate of reaction was calculated using the extinction coefficient of 8800 M^{-1} cm^{-1} for *p*-nitroanalide. Histamine content in MCGs can be quantified using an enzyme-immuno-competition assay using monoclonal antibody-based kit (Beckman-Coulter; *see* Chapter 16).

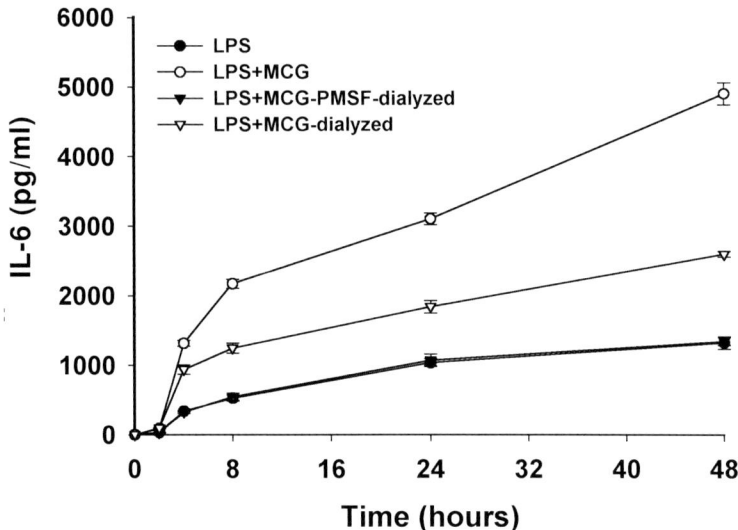

Fig. 7. Kinetics of IL-6 production by LPS- and MCG-activated HUVECs. HUVEC monolayers (10,000 cells) were cultured with PMSF-treated and dialyzed MCG, dialyzed MCG, or intact MCG (5000 mast cell equivalents) in the presence of 100 ng/mL of LPS for the time intervals indicated. Dialysis depleted more than 99% histamine and PMSF treatment inhibited all serine protease activity in MCG. IL-6 concentrations in the culture media were assayed by ELISA. Values are the mean ± SEM of quadruplicate culture wells. (Reproduced with permission from **ref. 16**.)

3.6. Signal Transduction Pathways Altered by MCG Protease and Histamine

Assays of changes in intracellular calcium, mitogen-activated protein kinase activation, and NF-κB translocation are described in the following sections to demonstrate typical signal transduction pathways that are involved in MCG-mediated inflammatory responses in endothelial cells.

3.6.1. Changes in Intracellular Calcium

1. Endothelial cells are plated on glass cover slips and allowed to grow to confluence within 48 h.
2. Aliquots equivalent to 3×10^5 mast cells are added to cover slips on which monolayers of HUVEC (6×10^5) are grown.
3. Cells were incubated with the Ca^{2+}-sensing fluorophore, Fluo-4 ($1 \ \mu M$) for 45 min at 37°C in 5% CO_2.
4. Cover slips are placed in a Fluorochamber on an Olympus Fluoview 300 Confocal Microscope. Cells are illuminated with an argon laser at 488 nm and emitted light was detected at 510 nm. Images are captured every 6 s during a 10-min period.

5. In additional experiments, the cells are imaged on an inverted Nikon microscope with a SPOT fluorescence sensing camera. In this case, cells are loaded with the Ca^{2+} indicator, Calcium Crimson. Background images are collected from each field and digitally subtracted from the regions of interest. Images are analyzed with the Fluoview and Photoshop software, allowing mean fluorescence values to be obtained from individual cells over time. To normalize for variations in dye loading, the initial three fluorescence values for each cell are averaged to determine the basal fluorescence level. This value is referred to as Fo. Each subsequent fluorescence value (F) is divided by Fo, and F/Fo ratio provides a clear illustration of changes in Ca^{2+} over the course of time.

6. **Figure 8** depicts the peak transient changes in Ca^{2+} for each of the agonists calculated from a kinetic study on the effect of various agonists. In this experiment, F/Fo values for control cells bathed in media during the course of 6 min were 0.87 ± 0.04 ($n = 53$ cells), demonstrating the level of photobleaching that the fluorophore underwent with normal laser illumination. LPS (100 ng/mL) induced a rapid increase in fluorescence indicating rising Ca^{2+} levels (F/Fo = 1.47 ± 0.07; $n = 78$). MCG caused a greater transient peaking at 2.21 ± 0.18; $n = 66$. Dialysis of MCG, which removed histamine, blunted the MCG response to 1.19 ± 0.14; $n = 24$. Inhibition of serine protease activity by treatment with PMSF and subsequent dialysis completely abrogated the effect of MCG (0.84 ± 0.03; $n = 16$). The combined application of MCG and LPS caused a peak transient change that was only slightly greater than MCG alone (F/Fo = 2.33 ± 0.13; $n = 41$).

3.6.2. Assay of ERK1/2 Activity

1. Confluent monolayers are incubated with indicated concentrations of untreated MCG, PMSF-treated/dialyzed MCG, or dialyzed MCG.
2. After incubation, the cells are lysed with Triton Lysis Buffer at 4°C for 30 min.
3. Cell debris is removed by centrifugation at 13,000g for 10 min. The protein content in the supernatants is measured and subjected to extracellular signal-regulated kinase (ERK) 1/2 activity assay (*see* Chapter 12).
4. Mast cell granules depleted of both active protease and histamine failed to induce ERK1/2 activation where as those devoid of histamine alone (dialyzed only) retained partial capacity (**Fig. 9**). Histamine-induced ERK1/2 activation is completely abrogated by histamine receptor-1 antagonist, diphenhydramine (25 μmol/L), whereas MCG-induced effects is only partially inhibited (data not shown). These results further demonstrate that both the serine protease and histamine present in MCG are capable of independently activating ERK1/2 *(16)*.

3.6.3. NF-κB Activation Assay

1. To evaluate the role of NF-κB in MCG- and LPS-mediated activation of endothelial cells, the nuclear NF-κB proteins are analyzed by EMSA (*see* Chapter 11).
2. Confluent endothelial cell monolayers are treated with MCG, LPS, or the combination of the MCG and LPS for the indicated time intervals at 37°C. Preparation of nuclear extracts is performed as described previously. Nuclear protein extracts are prepared by the method described previously (*see* Chapter 11 *[31,32]*).

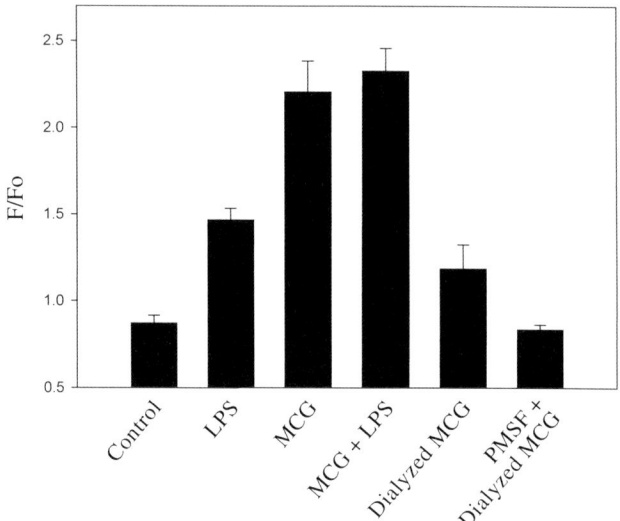

Fig. 8. MCG- and LPS-induced peak transient changes in intracellular calcium levels. Fluo-4-labeled HUVECs (6×10^5) were monitored with confocal microscopy during stimulation with LPS (100 ng/mL), MCG (3×10^5 mast cell equivalents), and a combination of both agonists. The data are plotted as F/Fo as described in the methods section. The fluorescence values (indicating free intracellular calcium) increased after the addition of each agonist. The changes in calcium were followed for a 5-min period. Peak calcium transient changes for each treatment (obtained within 2–4 min) were plotted. The data are plotted as F/Fo as described in the methods section. The results presented are from one of three similar experiments using two different fluorophores (calcium crimson and Fluo-4) on both a confocal microscope and a SPOT fluorescence microscope. In total, over 150 cells were analyzed for each condition except for dialyzed MCG. Each bar represents the mean ± SEM. (Reproduced with permission from **ref. *16*.)

3. The exposure of endothelial cells to MCG in the presence of LPS for 3 h substantially increased translocation of NF-κB proteins to the nuclei (**Fig. 10**). MCG alone caused an increase in NF-κB protein levels in the nuclei, which is of lesser magnitude than that induced by LPS. Both the MCG- and LPS-induced NF-κB translocation returned to baseline by 8–16 h *(16)*. The augmented levels of nuclear NF-κB proteins in HUVECs treated with the combination of MCG and LPS decreased with time but remained elevated throughout the 24-h period *(16)*.

3.6.4. Effect of Histamine on the Expression of TLR2, TLR4, MD2, and MyD88

Gram-positive and Gram-negative bacterial cell wall components are recognized by TLR2 and TLR4, respectively. Therefore, determining the expres-

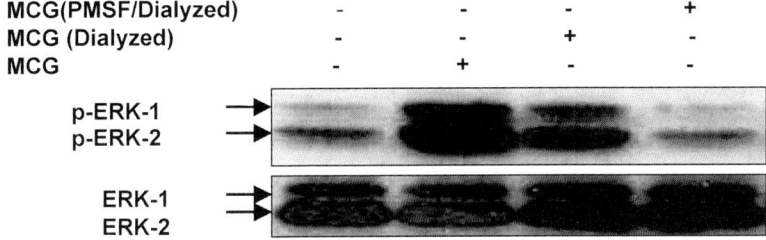

Fig. 9. The involvement of serine protease and histamine in MCG-induced activation of MAP kinase, ERK1/2. Confluent HUVECs (5×10^6) were incubated with MCG, dialyzed MCG, PMSF-pretreated, and dialyzed MCG (2.5×10^6 mast cell equivalents). After a 30-min treatment, cells were washed and cell lysates prepared and subjected to SDS-PAGE followed by immunoblotting with phospho-specific ERK1/2 monoclonal antibody. Protein loads were monitored by Western blot using ERK1/2 antibodies. Similar results were obtained in three experiments. (Reproduced with permission from **ref. *16*.**)

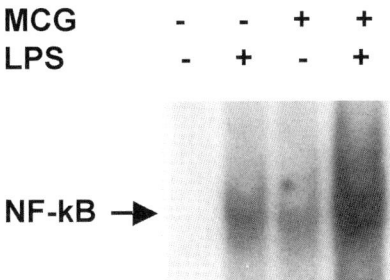

Fig. 10. Electrophoretic mobility shift assay of nuclear NF-κB translocation in HUVECs treated with MCG and LPS. Confluent monolayers of HUVECs (5×10^6) were incubated with MCG (2.5×10^6 mast cell equivalents) in the presence or absence of LPS (100 ng/mL) at 37°C for 3 h. The nuclear proteins extracted from the cells were incubated with g-[^{32}P]-labeled oligonucleotide containing NF-κB binding sites. The samples were subjected to electrophoresis on polyacrylamide gels, and the bands were identified by autoradiogragh. The amplification of LPS-induced NF-κB translocation by MCG was also noted in three other experiments. (Reproduced with permission from **ref. *16*.**)

sion of TLR2 and TLR4 will provide insight into the mechanism of histamine-induced sensitivity of endothelial cells to bacterial products. Similarly the assessment of the expression of TLR-associated accessory molecules, MD-2 and MyD88 also will be useful for understanding the role of histamine-induced synergy of endothelial cell activation by bacterial components.

1. Total ribonucleic acid (RNA) is isolated from endothelial cells treated with medium or histamine (10 μM), or appropriate activators, using TRIzol Reagent and treated with RNAse–free DNAse.
2. For reverse transcription reaction, Superscript™II RNase H⁻ Reverse Transcriptase system is used.
3. PCR amplification is performed with Taq polymerase for 32 cycles at 95°C for 45 s, 54°C for 45 s, and 72°C for 1 min (for TLR2, TLR4, and GAPDH); 95°C for 45 s, 60°C for 45 s, and 72°C for 1 min (for IL-6); 95°C for 30 s, 52°C for 45 s, and 72°C for 45 s (for MD-2); and 94°C for 30 s, 60°C for 40 s, and 70°C for 2 min (for MyD88).
4. PCR products are electrophorosed on 2% agarose gel. The oligonucleotide primers used for RT-PCR are given in **Table 1**.

3.6.5. Immunofluorescent and Western Blot Analyses of TLR2 and TLR4 Proteins

Immunofluorescence and Western blot analyses can be conducted to determine whether histamine-induced TLR2 and TLR4 mRNA expression is associated with increased expression of proteins.

3.6.5.1. IMMUNOFLUORESCENT ANALYSIS OF TLR2 AND TLR4 PROTEINS

1. Endothelial cells (20,000/well) grown on chamber slides are incubated either with medium or histamine for 3, 6, 14, and 24 h.
2. The cells are then fixed with 4% paraformaldehyde, washed and blocked with blocking solution and stained with mouse anti-human TLR2 or TLR4.
3. After overnight staining, the cells are washed, and incubated for 1 h with the secondary antibody (Cy3 goat anti-mouse).
4. The slides are then viewed under a fluorescence microscope and imaged.

3.6.5.2. WESTERN BLOT ANALYSIS OF TLR2 AND TLR4 PROTEINS

1. Confluent HUVEC monolayers are incubated with histamine (10 μM) for 16 h at 37°C.
2. The cells are then lysed in Triton Lysis Buffer at 4°C for 30 min.
3. Cell debris is removed by centrifugation of the lysate at 13,000g for 10 min.
4. Aliquots of supernatants normalized for protein concentrations were mixed with equal volumes of 2X SDS sample buffer and heated to 100°C for 5 min.
5. Samples are resolved on 10% sodium dodecyl sulfate polyacrylamide gel electrophoresis gel and transferred onto a nitrocellulose membrane.
6. After blocking for 2 h in TBST containing 5% nonfat milk, membranes are washed thrice in TBST and probed for 1 h at 4°C with anti-TLR4 (H-80, Santa Cruz) and for 18 h at 4°C for TLR2 using anti-TLR2 antibody (N-17, Santa Cruz).
7. After washing three times, membranes are incubated with horseradish peroxidase-conjugated secondary antibodies and washed five times and bands are detected using ECL reagents (Bio-Rad).

Table 1
Gene-Specific Primers Used in RT-PCR

Gene	Primer sequence (5'–3')	PCR product (Size, bp)
IL-6	ATGAACTCCTTCTCCACAAGCGC	620
	GAAGAGCCCTCAGGCTGGACTG	
TLR-2	GCCAAAGTCTTGATTGATTGG	347
	TTGAAGTTCTCCAGCTCCTG	
TLR-4	TGGATACGTTTCCTTATAAG	548
	GAAATGGAGGCACCCCTTC	
MD-2	GAAGCTCAGAAGCAGTATTGGGTC	422
	GGTTGGTGTAGGATGACAAACTCC	
MyD88	TAAGAAGGACCAGCAGAGCC	200
	CATGTAGTCCAGCAACAGCC	
GAPDH	TGATGACATCAAGAAGGTGGTGAAG	240
	TCCTTGGAGGCCATGTGGGCCAT	

4. Notes

1. By MCG we refer to mast cell granules, which contain specific serine proteases and histamine.

2. The methods described here deal with interaction between rat mast cells and human endothelial cells. Rat mast cells are selected because of their availability, richness in granules, and the convenience in MCG preparation. We recognize the importance of using a human mast cell/human endothelial cell system. However, the difficulty in obtaining sufficient amounts of human mast cells has made such a study impossible. Using histamine, purified human tryptase, and protease-activated receptor activating peptides, we have shown that these agonists mimic the effects of MCG in amplifying infection-associated inflammatory responses in endothelial cells. Therefore, the use of rat MCG is a reasonable approach to study the mast cell/endothelial cell interaction.

3. With the recent development of cell culture conditions, human mast cells can be grown from peripheral blood CD34[+]/c-kit[+]/CD13[+] progenitor cells (*33*). Many investigators have also used human mast cell line-1 for a variety of in vitro experiments (*34*).

4. Preparation of MCG requires sonication of the mast cell preparation. This should be conducted with caution because excessive disruption will damage the granules with resultant discharge of its components.

5. We have used both human umbilical vein endothelial cells and human coronary artery endothelial cells in our experiments to demonstrate mast cell mediator-induced modulation of inflammatory responses to LPS and tumor necrosis factor-α. Although we noted similar responses and regulatory effects in both venous and arterial endothelial cells, it should be emphasized that phenotypic differences exist between endothelial cells depending on their in vivo microenvironment (*35*).

6. Some investigators may be concerned with the possible heterogeneity of commercially available primary endothelial cells. The homogeneity can be tested by monitoring the expression of von Willebrand factor (an endothelial cell marker) by flow cytometry or immunofluorescence analyses. In our experience, 100% of HCAECs and HUVECs maintained in culture expressed von Willebrand factor, which argues against the possible contamination of other cell types.

7. After treating MCGs with PMSF, the free inhibitor should be removed by extensive dialysis. If PMSF is carried over to the cell culture, it will inhibit several signal transduction pathways including NF-κB activation.

Acknowledgments

The authors are grateful to Drs. Yuai Li, Alexander Jehle, Luqi Chi, Mohammad Kabir, and Jaya Talreja for their work, which contributed significantly to our understanding of the role of mast cell mediators on endothelial cell activation. This study was supported by the American Heart Association, and the Joseph and Elizabeth Carey Arthritis Funds, Hinman Fund, and Jones Fund from the Kansas University Endowment Association, and by the Lied Endowed Basic Science Research Fund from the University of Kansas Medical Center Research Institute.

References

1. Schwartz, L. B., Irani, A. A., Roller, K., Castells, M. C., and Schechter, N. M. (1987) Quantitation of histamine, tryptase and chymase in dispersed human T and TC mast cells. *J. Immunol.* **138,** 2611–2615.

2. Galli, S. J. (1993) New concepts about the mast cell. *N. Engl. J. Med.* **328,** 257–265.

3. Reynolds, D. S., Gurley, D. S., Stevens, R. L., Sugarbaker, D. J., Austen, K. F., and Serafin, W. E. (1989) Cloning of cDNAs that encode human mast cell carboxypeptidase A, and comparison of the protein with mouse mast cell carboxypeptidase A and rat pancreatic carboxypeptidases. *Proc. Natl. Acad. Sci. USA* **86,** 9480–9484.

4. Vanderslice, P., Ballinger, S. M., Tam, E. K., Goldstein, S. M., Craik, C. S., and Caughey, G. H. (1990) Human mast cell tryptase: multiple cDNAs and genes reveal a multigene serine protease family. *Proc. Natl. Acad. Sci. USA* **87,** 3811–3815.

5. Urata, H., Kinoshita, A., Misono, K. S., Bumpus, P. M., and Husain, A. (1990) Identification of a highly specific chymase as major angiotensin II forming enzyme in human heart. *J. Biol. Chem.* **265,** 22,348–22,357.

6. Kokkonen, J. O., Vartianen, M., and Kovanen, P. T. (1986) Low density lipoprotein degradation by secretory granules of rat serosal mast cells. *J. Biol. Chem.* **261,** 16,067–16,072.

7. Lindstedt, K. A. (1993) Inhibition of macrophage-mediated low-density lipoprotein oxidation by stimulated rat serosal mast cells. *J. Biol. Chem.* **268,** 7741–7746.

8. Atkinson, J. B., Harlan, C. W., Harlan, G. C., and Viramani, R. (1994) The association of mast cells and atherosclerosis. A morphologic study of early lesions in young people. *Hum. Pathol.* **25,** 154–159.

9. Jeziorska, M., McCollum, C., and Wooley, D. E. (1997) Mast cell distribution, activation, and phenotype in atherosclerotic lesions of human carotid arteries. *J. Pathol.* **182,** 115–122.

10. Kalsner, S. and Richards, R. (1984) Coronary arteries of cardiac patients are hyper reactive and contain stores of amines: a mechanism for coronary spasm. *Science* **223,** l435–1437.

11. Forman, M. B., Oates, J. A., Robertson, D., Robertson, R. M., Roberts. L. J., and Virmani R. (1985) Increased adventitial mast cells in a patient with coronary spasm. *N. Engl. J. Med.* **313,** 1138–1141.

12. Jeziorska, M., McCollum, C., and Wooley, D. E. (1998) Calcification in athero-sclerotic plaque of human carotid arteries: associations with mast cells and mac-rophages. *J. Pathol.* **185,** 10–17.

13. Li, Y., Stechschulte, A. C., Smith, D. D., Lindsley, H. B., Stechschulte, D. J., and Dileepan, K. N. (1997) Mast cell granules potentiate endotoxin-induced IL-6 pro-duction by endothelial cells. *J. Leukoc. Biol.* **62,** 210–216.

14. Jehle, A. B., Li, Y., Stechschulte, A. C., Stechschulte, D. J., and Dileepan, K. N. (2000) Endotoxin and MCG proteases synergistically activate human coronary artery endothelial cells to generate interleukin -6 and interleukin-8. *J. Interferon Cytokine Res.* **20,** 361–368.

15. Li, Y., Chi, Y., Stechschulte, D. J., and Dileepan, K. N. (2001) Histamine-induced production of interleukin-6 and interleukin-8 by human coronary artery endothelial cells is enhanced by endotoxin and tumor necrosis factor-α. *Microvasc. Res.* **61,** 253–262.

16. Chi, L., Stehno-Bittel, L., Smirnova, I., Stechschulte, D. J., and Dileepan, K. N. (2003) Signal transduction pathways in MCG-mediated endothelial cell activa-tion. *Med. Inflamm.* **12,** 79–87.

17. Talreja, J., Kabir, M. H., Filla, M. B., Stechschulte, D. J., and Dileepan, K. N. (2004) Histamine induces Toll-loke receptor 2 and 4 expression in endothelial cells and enhances sensitivity to Gram-positive and Gram-negative bacterial cell wall components. *Immunology* **113,** 224–233.

18. Grayston, J. T., Campbell, L. A., Kuo, C. C., et al. (1990) A new respiratory tract pathogen. *Chlamydia pneumoniae* strain TWAR. *J. Infect. Dis.* **161,** 618–625.

19. Stille W., Dittman R., and Just-Nubling G. (1997) Atherosclerosis due to chronic arteritis caused by Chlamydia Pneumoniae: a tentative hypothesis. *Infection* **25,** 281–285.

20. Hansson, G. K., Libby, P., Schonbeck U., and Yan Z. Q. (2002) Innate and adap-tive immunity in the pathogenesis of atherosclerosis. *Circ. Res.* **91,** 281–291.

21. Medzhitov, R. and Janeway C., Jr (2002) Decoding the patterns of self and non-self by the innate immune system. *Science* **296,** 298–300.

22. Takeuchi, O., Hoshino, K., Kawai, T., et al. (1999) Differential roles of TLR2 and TLR4 in recognition of Gram-negative and Gram-positive bacterial cell wall com-ponents. *Immunity* **11,** 443–451.

23. Beutler, B. (2202) Toll-like receptors: how they work and what they do. *Curr. Opin. Hematol.* **9,** 2–10.

24. Hirschfeld, M., Kirschning, C. J., Schwandner, R., et al. (1999) Cutting edge: inflammatory signaling by *Borrelia burgdorferi* lipoproteins is mediated by toll-like receptor 2. *J. Immunol.* **163**, 2382–2386.

25. Brightbill, H. D., Libraty, D. H., Krutzik, S. R., et al. (1999) Host defense mechanisms triggered by microbial lipoproteins through toll-like receptors. *Science* **285**, 732–736.

26. Hertz, C. J., Kiertscher, S. M., Godowski, P. J., et al. (2001) Microbial lipopeptides stimulate dendritic cell maturation via Toll-like receptor 2. *J. Immunol.* **166**, 444–450.

27. Faure, E., Equils, O., Sieling, P. A., et al. (2000) Bacterial lipopolysaccharide activates NF-κB through Toll-like receptor-4 in cultured human dermal endothelial cells. *J. Biol. Chem.* **275**, 11,058–11,063.

28. Zeuke, S., Ulmer, A., Kusumoto, S., Katus, H. A., and Heine, H. (2002) TLR4-mediated inflammatory activation of human coronary artery endothelial cells by LPS. *Cardiovasc. Res.* **56**, 126–134.

29. Edfeldt, K., Swedenberg, J., Hansson, G. K., and Yan, C-Q. (2002) Expression of Toll-like receptors in human atherosclerotic lesions. A possible pathway for plaque activation. *Circulation* **105**, 1158–1161.

30. Kiechl, S., Lorenz, E., Reindl, M., et al. (2002) Toll-like receptor 4 polymorphism and atherogenesis. *N. Engl. J. Med.* **347**, 185–192.

31. Muroi, M., Muroi, Y., Yamamoto, K., and Suzuki, T. (1993) Influence of 3' half-site sequence of NF-κB motifs on binding of lipopolysaccharide-activatable macrophage NF-κB proteins. *J. Biol. Chem.* **268**, 19,534–19,539.

32. Ito, N., Li, Y., Suzuki, T., Stechschulte, D. J., and Dileepan, K. N. (1998) Transient degradation of NF-κB proteins in macrophages after interaction with mast cell granules. *Med. Inflamm.* **7**, 397–407.

33. Krishenbaum, A. S., Goff, J. P., Semere, T., Foster, B., Scott, L. M., and Metcalfe, D. D. (1999) Demonstration that human mast cells arise from progenitor cell population that is CD34+, c-kit+, and express aminopeptidase N (CD13). *Blood* **94**, 2333–2342.

34. Butterfield, J. H., Weiler, D. A., Dewald, G., and Gleigh, G. J. (1988) Establishment of an immature mast cell line from a patient with mast cell leukemia. *Leuk. Res.* **12**, 345–355.

35. Chi, J. T., Chang, H. Y., Haraldsen, G., et al. (2003) Endothelial cell diversity revealed by global expression profiling. *Proc. Natl. Acad. Sci. USA.* **100**, 10,623–10,628.

22

Co-Culture of Mast Cells With Fibroblasts

A Tool to Study Their Crosstalk

Ido Bachelet, Ariel Munitz, and Francesca Levi-Schaffer

Summary

Mast cell development, function, and survival are likely to be regulated by a complex interplay of cellular signaling. Usually, these signals derive from the cellular milieu associated with the specific mast cell environment in health or disease conditions. A major methodological issue in studying in vitro mast cells, as well as any other tissue dwelling cell, is the essential lack of all the tissue-derived signals. Because some of the signals can be unknown, the in vivo system they form is virtually impossible to mimic completely in vitro. The mast cell–fibroblast co-culture system partially overcomes this problem and is the main topic of this chapter. The experimental importance of mast cell–fibroblast co-culture for the mast cells derives mainly from two reasons: first, fibroblasts constitute a major cellular scaffold of the tissues where mast cells dwell in the body, and as such are one of the fundamental cells participating in mast cell regulation in vivo and, second, there is an analogy with the traditional model of allergic inflammation, where the late, chronic phase is characterized by mast cell–structural cell crosstalk and eventual fibrotic outcome. Therefore, the co-culture system can be viewed as a suitable tool to investigate mast cell–fibroblast crosstalk.

Key Words: Mast cells; fibroblasts; co-culture; 3T3; cord blood-derived mast cell (CBDMC); rat peritoneal mast cell (RPMC); primary cultures; cell lines; activation; mediator assays.

1. Introduction

Mast cell development, function, and survival are likely to be regulated by a complex interplay of cellular signaling. A wide body of evidence has accumulated in the past years concerning signaling molecules and pathways controlling mast cells during maturation, survival, and degranulation. Usually, these signals derive from the cellular milieu associated with the specific mast cell environment in health or disease conditions. A major methodological issue in

From: *Methods in Molecular Biology, vol. 315: Mast Cells: Methods and Protocols*
Edited by: G. Krishnaswamy and D. S. Chi © Humana Press Inc., Totowa, NJ

studying in vitro mast cells, as well as any other tissue dwelling cell, is the essential lack of all the tissue-derived signals, either cell-borne or secreted under these conditions. Because some of the signals can be unknown, the in vivo system they form is virtually impossible to mimic completely in vitro. In addition, there is the quest to simplify the in vitro conditions to better dissect and analyze the system.

The idea of mixed cell culture systems for in vitro studies was described as early as the 1970s for various purposes *(1–4)*, such as virus–host and tumor–lymphocyte interactions. Numerous co-culture systems have been developed throughout the years using almost any cell type, using both cell lines and primary cells derived from tissues. Mixed cultures involving mast cells have been studied, mostly with the mast cells serving as effector cells or a stimulus targeting another cell type *(5,6)*.

The first defined co-culture system of primary mast cells, both of human and of rodent origin with 3T3 fibroblasts, was introduced by Levi-Schaffer et al. (**Fig. 1** *[7–12]*). The purpose was to prolong mast cell survival for long-term studies. Later on, characteristics such as mast cell mediator content and activity were studied once it was realized that mast cells could actually mature and change phenotype in this system. The co-culture system led, for example, to the discovery of the importance of stem cell factor (SCF) as a unique human mast cell growth factor *(13)*.

The experimental importance of mast cell-/fibroblast co-culture for the mast cells derives mainly from two reasons: first, fibroblasts constitute a major cellular scaffold of the tissues where mast cells dwell in the body (e.g., skin, lungs, intestines), and as such are one of the fundamental cells participating in mast cell regulation in vivo both in health and disease, and second, there is an essential analogy with the traditional model of allergic inflammation, where the late, chronic phase is characterized by mast cell–structural cell crosstalk and eventual fibrotic outcome. Moreover, in this system the effects of the mast cells on fibroblasts have been extensively studied. Therefore, the co-culture can be viewed as a suitable tool to investigate mast cell–fibroblast crosstalk.

This chapter will describe in detail major techniques for the co-culture of human mast cells with fibroblasts of human or rodent origin to study the mast cells. We shall discuss mast cell maintenance, separation and selection techniques, activation assays, and protein detection adapted to the co-culture system and also the methodological and technical problems of this system.

2. Materials

1. Culture media: *see* **Table 1**. All the reagents were supplied from Biological Industries, Beth Haemek, Israel.
2. Cytokines, growth factors, antibodies: *see* **Table 2**.

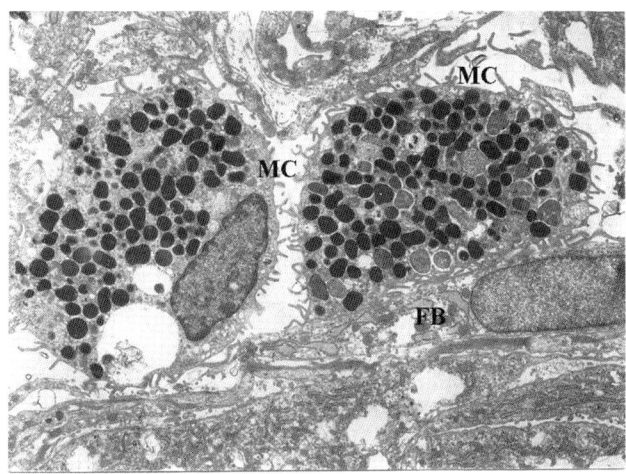

Fig. 1. Electron micrograph of rat peritoneal mast cells (MC) co-cultured with Swiss Albino 3T3 fibroblasts (FB) for 8 d *(11)*.

Table 1
Culture Media

Culture media	Supplements required
DMEM (4.5 g/L glucose)	10% v/v, FCS (heat inactivated)
	100 U/mL penicillin
	100 µg/mL streptomycin
	2 mM L-glutamine
MEM-alpha (1 g/L glucose + L-glutamine)	10% v/v, FCS (heat inactivated)
	100 U/mL penicillin
	100 µg/mL streptomycin
	10 µg/mL ribonucleosides/ deoxyribonucleosides
FCS	Obtained from Biological Industries, Beit Haemek, Israel
Trypsin–EDTA	Obtained from Biological Industries, Beit Haemek, Israel

3. Buffers: *see* **Table 3**.
4. Sensitive reagents: *see* **Table 4**. After the preparation of working solutions from these reagents, maintain them on ice in a foil-wrapped or blackened vessel. Whenever possible, prepare the working solution exactly in the required amount. The chromogenic substrates usually decompose with time. They should be stored at −70°C for longer periods, but it is preferable to prepare them fresh whenever possible.

Table 2
Cytokines, Growth Factors, Antibodies

Growth Factor/Antibody	Source[a]	Clone	Cat. No.
SCF	Amgen	*(A generous gift)*	AA1580–00
Anti-human, C. D.117 (*c-kit*)	Pharmingen	YB5.B8	33651A
Chimeric IgE Anti-NP	Serotec	JW8/1	MCA333B
Goat anti-mouse λ-chain	SouthernBiotech	Purified	1060–01
Anti-human, SCF neutralizing antibody	R&D	Purified	AF-255-NA

[a]These were the sources for the reagents that were used to obtain most of the data described in this chapter.

Table 3
Buffers and Solutions

Buffer	Content
PBS	137 mM NaCl, 2 mM KCl, 10 mM Na$_2$HPO$_4$, 1mM KH$_2$PO$_4$, pH 7.4
Hank's Balanced Salt Solution (HBSS)	1X and 10X obtained from Biological Industries, Beth Haemek, Israel
Tyrode's buffer	137 mM NaCl, 12 mM NaHCO$_3$, 5.5 mM L-glucose, 2 mM KCl, 0.3 mM Na$_2$HPO$_4$
TG (Tyrode's gelatin buffer)	0.1% w/v gelatin in Tyrode's buffer
TG++ (Tyrode's gelatin buffer, supplemented)	1.8mM CaCl$_2$, 0.9 mM MgCl$_2$ in, TG buffer
HBA (HBSS, BSA, Azide)	0.1% w/v bovine serum albumine, 0.01% sodium azide in HBSS
Permeabilization/Blocking buffer for IF	0.1% w/v saponin, 10% w/v bovine serum albumine, 0.1% v/v human serum, 10 mM HEPES in HBA
Washing buffer for IF	0.1% w/v saponin, 10 mM HEPES in HBA
Citrate/phosphate buffer for β-hexosaminidase	0.12 M citric acid, 0.14 M Na$_2$HPO$_4$, pH 4.5

5. Cellular stains: *see* **Table 5**.
6. β-Hexosaminidase substrate: dissolve 20 mg of substrate (p-NP N-acetyl β-D-glucosaminide) in 4.5 mL of deionized water and 3 mL of substrate buffer (0.12 M citric acid, 0.14 M Na$_2$HPO$_4$, pH 4.5), mix well. This yields an 8 mM substrate solution. Keep foil-wrapped at 4°C.

Table 4
Sensitive Reagents

Sensitive reagents	Source[a]	Cat. No.
Metrizamide	Sigma	M-3383
Compound 48/80	Sigma	C-2313
β-hexosaminidase chromogenic substrate		
(*p*-nitrophenyl-*N*-acetyl-β-D-glucosaminide)	Sigma	N-9376
Tryptase chromogenic substrate		
(*N*-*p*-tosyl-gly-pro-lys-*p*-nitroanilide)	Sigma	T-6140
Cathpesin G chromogenic substrate		
(*N*-succinyl-ala-ala-pro-phe-*p*-nitroanilide)	Sigma	S-7388
OPT	Sigma	P-0657
Percoll	Sigma	P-1644
Collagenase	Sigma	C-0130
Hyaluronidase	Sigma	H-3506
DNase	Sigma	D-5025
NH₄OH (ammonium hydroxide)	Frutatom, Israel	
Trichloroacetic acid	Frutarom, Israel	
NaOH (sodium hydroxide)	BDH	5553510
DMSO	Sigma	D-5879

[a]These are the sources for the reagents that were used to obtain most of the data described in this chapter.

Table 5
Cellular Stains

Stain	Content
Toluidine blue	0.07% w/v toluidine blue in 60% ethanol pH 3.5
Kimura's stain	0.03% w/v toluidine blue, 0.001% w/v light green, 1.4% w/v saponin dissolved in 137 mM NaCl, 2.7 mM KCl, pH 7.4
Methylene blue	1% w/v methylene blue in 0.1 N boric acid, pH 8.5
Trypan blue	Commercially obtained from Sigma, cat. no. T-8154

7. Tryptase substrate: dissolve 10 mg of substrate (*N*-*p*-Tosyl-Gly-Pro-Lys *p*-NA) in 630 µL of dimethyl sulfoxide (DMSO), which will yield a substrate solution of 25 mM. Keep aluminum foil-wrapped in −20°C.

8. Cathepsin-G substrate: dissolve 5 mg of substrate (*N*-Succinyl-Ala-Ala-Pro-Phe *p*-NA) in 200 µL of 0.1 M NH₄OH. This yields a stock substrate solution of 40 mM. Keep aluminium foil-wrapped in −20°C.

Table 6
Several Sources of Mast Cells

Mast cell type	Source	Subheading/Chapter	Ref.
RPMC	Rat peritoneum	3.1.1	*14*
BMDMC	Mouse bone marrow		*8*
HMC-1 (line)	Human mast cell leukemia	Chapter 15	*15*
CBDMC	Human umbilical cord blood	Chapters 7,8,15	*16*
HLMC	Human lung	3.1.2	*21*
HSMC	Human skin	3.1.2	*18*
HIMC	Human intestines	3.1.2	*20*
HCMC	Human heart	3.1.2	*17*
HUMC	Human uterus	3.1.2	*19*

9. 10% trichloroacetic acid.
10. OPT solution: dissolve 5 mg of *o*-phthalaldehyde (OPT) in 0.5 mL of methanol, yielding a 10 mg/mL solution. Keep foil-wrapped in −20°C.

3. Methods

3.1. Co-Culture Setup

Although this volume mainly focuses on human mast cells, it also is important to describe the protocols for the purification of mast cells from the peritoneal cavity of a rodent because historically these cells were the first mast cells in co-culture with fibroblasts and are still useful counterparts of human connective tissue type mast cells (especially of human dermal mast cells).

3.1.1. Mast Cells

The conditions of maintenance of a co-culture system greatly depend on the source of mast cells. There are several sources to be considered, although they are not equally easy to obtain and culture. In **Table 6**, we have listed some of the more commonly used sources of mast cells *(14–21)*. It is important to mention that any tissue that can be enzymatically digested or any cavity that can be lavaged is a potential source of mast cells.

Different mast cells behave differently in vitro. For example, rat peritoneal cells do not proliferate in co-culture, whereas human mast cell (HMC)-1, being a transformed line, and bone marrow-derived mast cells (i.e., BMDMCs), in the presence of interleukin (IL)-3, do. It is important to take this into account because it determines the number of cells that are to be added to the co-culture during its setup. When the mast cells proliferate, they create overcrowding, depletion of nutrients, and finally damage of the fibroblast monolayer. Thereafter, the culture starts an in vitro wound healing process. During this process, activated fibroblasts in turn can activate mast cells, and the co-culture behaves as if it was stimulated by an exogenous stimulus, even though it has not.

3.1.2. Fibroblasts

Unlike mast cells, fibroblasts can be chosen from an enormous selection of lines and primary sources. In addition, there are many commercial sources for animal and human fibroblasts. Primary fibroblasts can be obtained easily from any tissue that is surgically removed both from normal and pathological samples according to the aim of the co-culture.

An important point to consider is whether the fibroblast of choice is contact-inhibited. Contact inhibition occurs in all primary cultures but also in some lines, such as the 3T3 line.

Although it seems more logical to assemble the co-culture using fibroblasts and mast cells from the same species and anatomical location, the best support for human mast cells is given by the 3T3 fibroblast cell line *(12,22)*. It is also important to check the type of each line, for instance, the Swiss Albino 3T3 is different from the NIH 3T3 and is usually the preferred one for co-cultures.

3.1.2.1. RAT/MOUSE PERITONEAL MAST CELLS (*SEE* **NOTE 1**)

1. Use rats (250–300 g) or mice (2–3 mo), preferably males.
2. Euthanize animals using ether-soaked cotton wool inside a closed compartment or a dessicator.
3. Lie the animal down on its back, spray 70% ethanol over the abdomen, and perform a midline vertical cut. Expose the abdominal fascia just underneath the fur.
4. Wash the peritoneal cavity with Tyrode's gelatin (TG) buffer by injecting 50 mL for rats and 5 mL for mice in the appropriate syringe with a 23-gage needle, taking care not to puncture the intestines.
5. Gently massage the abdomen.
6. Aspirate (using the same syringe) at least 40 mL (for rats) or 4 mL (for mice) of fluid from the buffer. For mice, pool together lavage fluids from three or four animals.
7. Spin the lavage at 400g for 7 min at room temperature.
8. Resuspend cell pellet in 1 mL of TG buffer and load 1 mL of metrizamide (22.5% for rats, 22% for mice, in TG buffer).
8. Centrifuge 350g for 20 min at 20°C without breaks. Aspirate the supernatant using vacuum.
9. Resuspend cell pellet containing the mast cells in medium, and assess their purity by toluidine blue staining (50% v/v) and viability by trypan blue (50% v/v). Examine immediately under microscope upon staining.

3.1.2.2. HUMAN TISSUE-DERIVED MAST CELLS (*SEE* **NOTE 2**)

1. Place the obtained tissue in a Petri dish. Add 5 mL of ice-cold medium to maintain the tissue and prevent it from drying. Cut with scissors or with a scalpel to pieces of maximum 2–3 mm.
2. Transfer the pieces to a 50-mL tube, complete to 50 mL with medium (*see* **Note 3**), and centrifuge at 600g for 7 min.
3. Prepare enzymatic digestion cocktail:

    a. Calculate enzymatic digestion final volume: 4 mL/g of tissue.

    b. To one fifth of this volume, add the following enzymes (per milliliter of final volume):

       i. Collagenase (1.5 mg/mL).

      ii. Hyaluronidase (0.75 mg/mL).

     iii. Dnase (0.01 mg/mL).

    c. Dissolve by vortex, followed by a short sonication on ice until no solid particles are visible. The mixture should be clear and tea-colored.

4. Add the digestion cocktail to the tissue pellet. Complete with medium to the *final* digestion volume.

5. Shake in a bath at 37°C, at least at 100 Hz, for 60 min (*see* **Note 4**).

6. Complete to 50 mL with medium. Centrifuge at 600g for 5 min to get rid of undigested, gross tissue parts.

7. Filter the supernatant through a filter or gauze (maximum, 0.3 mm) into a 100-mL beaker. Constantly pour medium through the filter along with the supernatant to a final filtrate volume of 100 mL.

8. Centrifuge at 600g for 5 min at 4°C and resuspend the pellet in 5 mL of medium.

9. Stain a 10-µL sample with toluidine blue. It is recommended to continue the procedure upon the presence of sufficient mast cells in the tissue. Assume a yield of 30–40% at the end of the process.

10. Prepare Percoll gradient as follows:

    a. Dissolve 1 mg of Dnase in 5 mL of Hank's solution containing 25 mM HEPES.

    b. Mix well 3.4 mL of the Dnase solution with 2.2 mL of 10X Hank's solution and 19.5 mL of Percoll in a 50-mL tube. Mix by flipping the tube four to five times.

11. Load cells on the gradient and centrifuge at 2000g for 20 min at 20°C without breaks (*see* **Note 5**).

12. Collect the middle phase very carefully using a Pasteur pipet and transfer it into a 50-mL tube.

13. Centrifuge 600g for 5 min, resuspend with Hank's-FCS (Hank's solution containing 2% FCS), and spin again the same way.

14. Resuspend cells in 1 mL of Hank's-FCS and add to it an anti-*c-kit* antibody (YB5.B8, 5 ng/mL). Shake on ice for 1 h.

15. Wash with Hank's-FCS as in **step 13**.

16. Incubate cells with anti-mouse immunomagnetic beads (Miltenyi, Dynal) and perform a positive selection using magnetic column (MACS) according to the manufacturer's instructions.

17. Culture cells with RPMI or minimum essential medium (MEM) containing 10% fetal calf serum (FCS). Check purity and viability of mast cells (*see* **Note 6**).

3.1.2.3. PRIMARY FIBROBLASTS (*SEE* **NOTE 7**)

1. Place the tissue in Dulbecco's modified Eagle's medium (DMEM; 2% FCS) and cut it using scissors or scalpel to obtain 2- to 3-mm pieces.

2. Carve several scratches horizontally and vertically on the vessel's floor (preferably 12- or 24-well plate), creating a 3 × 3 mm "net."

Table 7
Trypsin Volumes for Plating/Passaging

Type of culture vessel	Trypsin–EDTA volume	Ice lift volume
200-mL bottle	3–5 mL	10 mL
75-mL bottle	1–2 mL	5 mL
35-mm dish	0.5–1 mL	2 mL
24-well plate	200 μL	0.5 mL

3. With forceps put a piece of tissue (2–3 mm) directly in the center of the net.
4. Using a pincers' edge gently spread it once or twice over the scratches.
5. Pour 100–200 μL of DMEM (10% FCS) on the tissue, just enough to cover the piece but taking care not to lift it.
6. Incubate at 37°C for 2–3 h, and then add more DMEM 10% FCS.
7. Incubate at 37°C for several days until cells start to sprout along the scratches (usually between 5 and 7 d).
8. Using forceps, remove the large piece and change medium.
9. When cells are confluent, passage by trypsinization.

3.1.2.4. PLATING/PASSAGING FIBROBLAST CULTURES IN MONOLAYERS (*SEE* **NOTE 8**)

1. Filter and warm trypsin–ethylene diamine tetraacetic acid (EDTA; amount according to **Table 7**) to 37°C in a bath.
2. Gently draw all medium from the vessel, avoid perturbing the floor.
3. Pour trypsin–EDTA, shake on a flat surface and incubate for 1–5 min at 37°C (consult **Table 7** for specific volume settings).
4. Once cells are detached and therefore floating as single cells or cell aggregates, mix well using a pipet to obtain a more homogeneous cell suspension, and add DMEM twice the volume of trypsin.
5. Centrifuge at 400*g* for 7 min.
6. Vigorously resuspend the cell pellet in DMEM at the desired volume (*see* **Note 9**).
7. Count cells, seed in new vessels at the desired concentration, and return to incubation (*see* **Note 9**).

3.1.2.5. FIBROBLAST LINES

A wide selection of fibroblast lines is available for us. For mast cells, from both rodent and human origin, the preferred line is the 3T3 Swiss Albino from ATCC, Rockville, MD (cat. no. CCL-92)

3.2. MC/FB Long-Term Co-Culture (Monolayer)

Co-culture can be performed in monolayers or in a 3D system. This system has been described by Eckes et al. *(23)* to study the influence of the mast cells on the fibroblasts. We provide the most common one both for mast cell and for fibroblast studies, the monolayer co-culture system. This system can be set up

Table 8
Fibroblast Concentrations

Type of culture vessel	No. of cells for seeding
200-mL culture bottle	1×10^5
75-mL culture bottle	5×10^4
35-mm dish	2×10^4
24-well plate	5×10^3
96-well plate	1×10^3

Table 9
Mast Cell Concentrations

Type of culture vessel	Mast cell concentration
35-mm dish	$0.8–1 \times 10^5/2$ mL
12-well plate	$0.4–0.5 \times 10^5/1$ mL
24-well plate	$2–4 \times 10^4/0.5$ mL
96-well plate	$5 \times 10^3/0.2$ mL

using virtually any type of mast cells, such as CBDMC *(12)*, lung *(24)*, or skin *(25,26)* mast cells.

1. Seed fibroblasts (either freshly purified or passaged) on a culture vessel selected for this purpose (flask, dish, multiwell, and so on) and culture in DMEM. Consult **Table 8** for cell concentrations (*see* **Note 10**).
2. Seed freshly purified mast cells on a fibroblast monolayer at full confluency, as observed under an inverted microscope, when the cells are after P6-P7 at most (but preferably as early as possible). Consult **Table 9** for mast cell concentrations (*see* **Note 11**).
3. After 24 h, carefully draw out medium by using a low-power vacuum, preferably tipped thinly (using a 200 μL-pipet tip). This first medium replacement will dispose of all nonadherent mast cells, which might be either dead or other cell types that may have contaminated the initial mast cell population.
4. Replace culture medium every 2 d (*see* **Notes 12** and **13**).

3.3. Activation of Mast Cells in Co-Culture

This section will discuss in detail the ways to activate mast cells in co-culture and the methodological adjustments to this system.

3.3.1. Planning the System

The success of any experiment conducted in co-culture depends on one's ability to point out the effects caused by mast cells alone (**Fig. 2**). This is diffi-

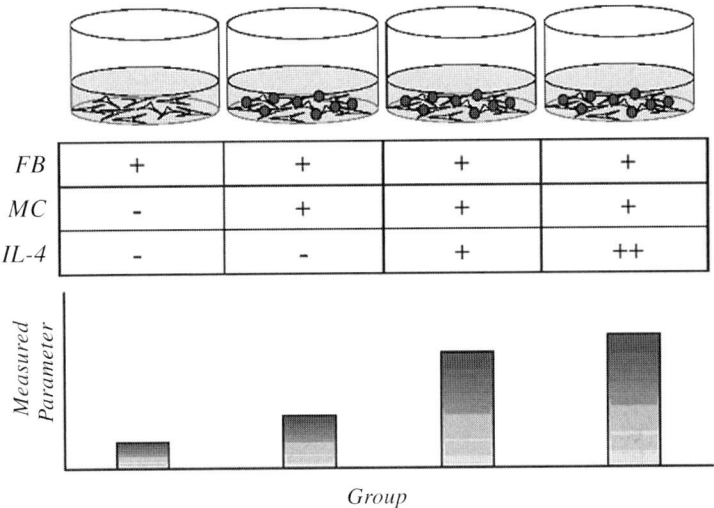

Fig. 2. An exemplary experiment planned for the co-culture system. A control group containing only fibroblasts (left) defines the system's background. IL-4 and the measured parameters are arbitrary in this example. FB, fibroblasts; MC, mast cells.

cult for several reasons. First, fibroblasts usually outnumber the mast cells in the system and therefore that the level of background they give is always high. Second, the fibroblasts (and especially the cell lines) are usually more active in protein synthesis. Third, and most importantly, fibroblasts might contain or produce mediators that originate also from mast cells, for example, prostaglandin E_2, cytokines, and chemokines. The latter point will be discussed in **Subheading 3.3.2.1.**

To overcome these difficulties, a co-culture should always include one control group composed only of fibroblasts. This group should undergo any treatment, exactly as if it contained mast cells. Eventually, this group will define the background level of the system (*see* **Note 14**).

3.3.1.1. KINETIC STUDY FOR EVALUATION OF OPTIMAL MAST CELL ACTIVATION PERIOD

1. Set up the desired co-culture: set up a group for time zero and for each day (at least for 7 d) and an additional parallel group for each time point, composed only of fibroblasts as control.
2. Once the mast cells have attached, perform activation for time zero group.
3. Maintain the co-culture as usual while performing activation each day for the appropriate group.
4. Plot the response magnitude as a function of the activation day and extrapolate the optimal time (*see* **Note 15**).

3.3.2. Activation

Although mast cells can undergo activation when in their culture medium, a stronger response is usually achieved in buffers. For IgE-dependent activation, Tyrode's gelatin buffer supplemented with 1.8 mM CaCl$_2$ and 0.9 mM MgCl$_2$ (termed TG++ buffer) usually gives the best response. However, for IgE-independent activations, phosphate-buffered saline (PBS) supplemented with 137 mM NaCl, 2.7 mM KCl, 8.1 mM Na$_2$HPO4, 1.5 mM KH$_2$PO$_4$, 5.55 mM dextrose, 0.9 mM CaCl$_2$, and 0.05% essential fatty acid free bovine serum albumin is better.

The use of buffer also allows for spectrometric and fluorometric assays such as β-hexosaminidase or fluorometric histamine without color interference, as media often contain phenol red that disturbs such assays.

1. Carefully wash the culture once with warm TG++ buffer. Add the new buffer very slowly and from the side of the vessel. Avoid adding it directly at the center of the dish (*see* **Note 16**).
2. Add TG++ buffer at the desired volume for activation. Consider sufficient volume for each assay to be performed afterwards, keeping in mind that large volumes dilute the mediators that we want to detect. This is also determined by the assay's sensitivity.
3. Add the activatory stimulus.
4. Shake gently and incubate as needed.
5. Gently collect the supernatant, and centrifuge to get rid of possible cell contamination that might alter true mediator content release (*see* **Note 17**).

3.3.2.1. MEDIATOR ASSAYS

The main problem in quantitating released mediators in co-culture is that there are two possible sources of mediators. If it is certain that fibroblasts do not express the molecule of interest (e.g., histamine and tryptase), or mediators that might interfere with the detection method, it is generally safe to assume that mast cells are the sole source of it. However, fibroblasts may secrete cytokines, enzymes and alike or more upon mast cell activation, so the selection of release assays should be carefully done.

Assaying histamine is most reliable because fibroblasts do not contain it and mast cells release large amounts of it. However, the common sensitive laboratory method is radioactive, expensive, and relatively time-consuming. The commercially available radioimmunoassay is expensive and mainly used for evaluating histamine in serum/plasma and urine (*see* Chapter 16). Assays based on chromogenic reactions generally are quick and simple; however, they require careful calibration before their use.

Described next are three mediator assays based on chromogenic substrates that detect enzymes released by activated mast cells. Even though these substrates are not specific (for instance, tryptase substrate is also cleaved by plasmin), the signal-to-noise ratio for co-cultures with fibroblasts generally is low. Theoretically, any enzyme can be similarly detected given the proper peptidyl substrate.

A peptidyl chromogenic substrate has generally three portions: 1) chromophore, 2) quencher, and 3) cleavable bridge, generally made of a short sequence recognized by the target enzyme. The chromophore continuously emits at a certain wavelength, but because of the fluorescence resonance energy transfer (i.e., FRET) phenomenon, the quencher in proximity captures the emission energy. Once the bridge is enzymatically cleaved, the chromophore is released and the emission is visible. Some chromophores (e.g., the β-hexosaminidase substrate) are unstable at first and need to be stabilized for the emission to show.

In coming to calibrate such a protocol, one has to keep in mind the following parameters: 1) the reaction buffer must be at a pH in which the target enzyme will work. Most mast cell enzymes operate at acidic pH, but are also functional at pH 7.0–8.0 range. 2) When the substrate is present at a too large concentration, intermolecular FRET will occur, meaning that a chromophore from one molecule will be quenched by another molecule's quencher. Therefore, substrate concentration also should be calibrated and should fall between 1 and 10 mM.

As a general rule, standard curves are most desirable, and should be included whenever possible. When purified form of the mediator exists (e.g., in the case of histamine and tryptase) a standard calibration performed first to fit the assay's sensitivity to a good standard range, should be done. When no such purified mediator exists, the results should be presented either semi-quantitatively as a percentage of release (*see* **Subheading 3.3.2.1.1.**) or as fold-over-basal or simply as an, optical density (OD) count at a specific absorbance.

To obtain a percentage of release, in addition to the supernatant total cells should be harvested and disrupted by sonication. Collection and sonication of the cells should be done very quickly (*see* protocol in **Subheading 3.3.1.1.**).

3.3.2.1.1. Collection and Lysis of Cells to Yield % Release.

1. Add an equal volume of buffer (same as the activation buffer) to each group (*see* **Note 18**).
2. Scrape cells using a Teflon policeman (scraper) or a tip of a Pasteur pipet, as to the vessel's size.
3. Transfer to tubes. Make sure you collect all cells by repeated pipetting inside the vessel.
4. Transfer cells to a tube and lyse by sonicating 1 min on ice.
5. Assay the specific mediator in the lysate. Make sure to multiply at the proper dilution factor, if any.

Express the % release as follows:

$$\%R = Sup / (Sup + Lys)$$

Where *Sup* is the supernatant mediator content and *Lys* is the lysate mediator content.

3.3.2.1.2. Histamine Enzyme Immunoassay (see Chapter 16).

3.3.2.1.3. β-Hexosaminidase Assay.

This protocol is adapted for small volumes and is of high sensitivity *(27)*.

1. In a flat-bottom 96-well plate, prepare 42 μL/well of β-hexosaminidase substrate solution in as many wells as there are samples, plus wells for a blank control. It is recommended to perform this assay at least in triplicates.
2. To each well, add 18 μL of supernatant to be assayed and mix well. To the blank wells, add 18 μL of TG++ buffer.
4. Incubate for 2 h at 37°C, gently shaking the plate every 20 min (*see* **Note 19**).
5. Stop the reaction: to each well add 120 mL of ice-cold glycine (0.2 *M*, pH 10.7). The presence of β-hexosaminidase is revealed by the appearance of yellow color. Immediately read OD at 410 nm absorbance.

3.3.2.1.4. Tryptase Assay.

This assay can be performed also in real time *(28)*.

1. In a flat-bottom 96-well plate mix in each well 96 μL of supernatant and 4 μL of tryptase substrate (*see* **Note 20**).
2. Incubate at 37°C for approx 1 h or until a yellow color starts to appear.
3. Immediately read OD at 410 nm absorbance.

3.3.2.1.5. Cathepsin-G Assay.

This assay also can be performed in real time.

1. Mix 52 μL of the supernatant with 4 μL of the Cathepsin-G substrate solution in a flat-bottom 96-well plate (final concentration 3 m*M*/well).
2. Incubate at 37°C for 30–60 min or until yellow color starts to appear.
3. Immediately read OD at 410 nm absorbance.

3.3.2.1.6. Fluorometric Histamine Assay (see **Note 21 [29]**).

1. Mix 20 μL of supernatant with 20 μL of 10% trichloroacetic acid and centrifuge at 2000*g* for 2 min at 4°C. Transfer the supernatant to a fresh tube to continue.
2. In a flat-bottom 96-well plate, mix in each well 8 μL of 3 *M* NaOH with 37 μL supernatant (if not performing the TCA precipitation, add the supernatant undiluted)
3. Add 2 μL of OPT solution (10 mg/mL) and mix well.
4. Incubate at room temperature for 5–8 min. Faint yellow color should appear where high histamine content is present.
5. Add ice-cold 6 *M* HCl and shake well. The yellow should turn into faint pink.
6. Immediately read OD at 440 nm.

3.3.2.1.7. Arachidonic Acid Metabolites.

Arachidonic acid metabolites, such as prostaglandins (PGs) and leukotrienes (LTs), are newly-synthesized mediators produced and released upon IgE-mediated mast cells stimulation. PGs and LTs have a wide array of effects, e.g., leukocyte chemotaxis, endothelium activation, smooth muscle contraction, and proliferation and so on. Importantly, these mediators are markely short lived. However, supernatants may be kept for further analysis of these mediators under nitrogen atmosphere to prevent their oxidation (especially for the leukotriens). The common way to assay these mediators is by specific enzyme-linked immunosorbent (ELISA), and the most abundant mediators are usually PGD_2 and LTC_4. However, as mentioned previously, it should be taken into account that fibroblasts are able to synthesize eicosanoid products given certain stimuli; moreover, ELISA for PGs and LTs are not always very specific.

3.3.2.1.8. Cytokines/Chemokines.

In principle, ELISA systems are commercially available targeting almost every cytokine or chemokine secreted by mast cells. However, because fibroblasts also strongly produce and secrete such molecules, the background levels of these assays are relatively high.

3.3.3. Mast Cell-Specific Studies

The co-culture system presents a major challenge when coming to perform studies on the mast cells as an isolated population. Separating mast cells from the fibroblasts constitutes a problem of its own, and it will be discussed in the next section.

By means of their physical parameters, mast cells and fibroblasts are difficult to distinguish after trypsinization. Metrizamide gradients varying from 22 to 24.5% do not yield mast cells efficiently. When using fluorescence-activated cell sorting (FACS), the analysis of forward scatter (FSC) vs side scatter (SSC) parameters of a mast cell–fibroblast co-culture does not clearly distinguish between these two populations. Nevertheless, focusing on mast cells in FACS is feasible by first gating all FcεRI[(+)] cells, presumably mast cells.

Several methods exist for extracting mast cells from the fibroblast monolayer. One must take in account that by using a trypsin digestion method, there is a chance that the surface molecules will degrade, depending on the specific molecule. Consult **Table 10** for recommended lifting volumes.

3.3.3.1. TRYPSIN DIGESTION

1. Gently aspirate, using vacuum, the buffer or culture medium from the vessel.
2. Filter the desired amount of trypsin and warm to 37°C (*see* **Note 22**).
3. Pour the trypsin over the surface. Shake a few times to cover the vessel thoroughly, and incubate at 37°C for 1–5 min.

Table 10
Trypsin and Buffer Volumes for Mast Cell Separation

Type of culture vessel	Trypsin volume	Ice lift volume
200-mL flask	3–5 mL	10 mL
75-mL flask	1–2 mL	5 mL
35-mm dish	0.5–1 mL	2 mL
24-well plate	200 μL	0.5 mL

4. Every other minute, examine under the inverted microscope whether the cells have detached.
5. To stop the trypsin, add cold medium (10% FCS) at twice the trypsin volume.
6. Draw medium, centrifuge at 700*g* for 5 min, and resuspend as desired.

3.3.3.2. "ICY LIFT BUFFER" METHOD

1. Gently aspirate the buffer or culture medium from the vessel.
2. Place vessel on ice.
3. Gently pour ice-cold lift buffer (1 m*M* ethylene diamine tetraacetic acid in PBS) and vigorously pipet up and down four or five times. Avoid touching the monolayer or perturbing the vessel floor.
4. Collect buffer, centrifuge at 700*g* for 5 min, and resuspend as desired (*see* **Note 23**).

3.3.3.3. TRYPSIN/ICE LIFT COMBINATION

1. Gently draw buffer or culture medium from the vessel.
2. Filter trypsin and warm to 37°C.
3. Pour the trypsin and incubate at 37°C for 1 min.
4. Transfer the vessel to ice. Gently pour ice-cold lift buffer (1 m*M* EDTA in PBS), and continue as in the "icy lift" method (*see* **Note 24**).

3.3.4. Co-Culture Studies

Much information can be obtained by observing the co-culture as a whole, that is, without separating it to its cellular elements. This usually is accomplished by sheer visual techniques, mainly immunocytochemistry (ICC) or immunofluorescence (IF) in combination with microscopy, either light, confocal, or electron.

An extremely useful approach for these studies is the use of sterile glass cover slips, on which the monolayer is first grown and which mast cells are later added. Such cover slips allow for convenient manipulation of the co-culture for ICC/IF. A more modern method makes use of culture plates whose bottom itself serves as slides for ICC/IF. However, the method described in the following steps is much cheaper (*see* **Note 25**).

1. Seed fibroblasts on sterile 12-mm round glass cover slips within a 24-well plate
2. Add mast cells and co-culture for additional 3–4 d (*see* **Note 26**).
3. Fix co-cultures by formaldehyde 2% or *p*-formaldehyde 4% in cold PBS for 10 min on ice.
4. Wash twice with cold PBS (aspiration of existing buffers and addition of new buffers should be performed very carefully).
5. Permeabilize co-cultures by incubating for 10 min with permeabilization and blocking buffer.
6. Wash twice with cold washing buffer.
7. Incubate with primary antibody, diluted properly in washing buffer, for 1 h at room temperature.
8. Wash twice with washing buffer.
9. Incubate with secondary antibody, diluted properly in washing buffer, 1 h at room temperature (*see* **Note 27**).
10. Wash twice with PBS.
11. Apply a drop of mounting medium on a glass slide.
12. Place the cover slip *upside-down* on the glass slide where the drop was applied, and keep in a wrapped tray at −20°C (*see* **Note 28**).

3.4. Advanced Applications in Co-Culture

This section will discuss certain variations on the traditional co-culture system, as solutions or adaptations for specific biological questions or technologies that are unapplicable otherwise.

3.4.1. Transwell Co-Culture

Among the signals that mediate mast cell–fibroblast crosstalk in co-culture, some are secreted and some are contact-transmitted. Distinguishing between the two might help to define the a mechanism underlying a phenomenon.

In a transwell co-culture, mast cells and fibroblasts are grown on the opposing sides of a polycarbonate membrane, allowing free flow of medium between the two compartments, but not allowing the cells to physically interact. Therefore, it is possible to detect secreted signals.

3.4.2. Knockout Fibroblasts

To establish the involvement of a specific signal molecule, one would want to observe the co-culture in the absence of that molecule. In co-culture systems, several approaches are feasible:

1. A special fibroblast line, devoid of the molecule by genetic means (if such a line exists).
2. Purification of primary fibroblasts from a knock out mouse (such as in the case of *Sl/Sl*[d] mice, devoid of the membrane bound form of SCF *[11]*).

3. Anti-sense treatment of the fibroblasts before initiation of the co-culture. This method is described in **Subheading 3.4.3.**

3.4.3. Antisense Treatment for Fibroblasts

This method is used to silence a specific ribonucleic acid (RNA) species and thus to abolish the expression of a target protein. A set of oligomeres (a sense as control, and anti-sense as a blocking agent) should be designed (*see* **Note 29**).

1. Prepare working solutions of the desired oligomeres: dilute in *serum-free* medium to a concentration of 20 μ*M*.
2. Assuming a 1-mL volume, mix 175 μL of medium with 15 μL of *Oligofectamine*™, and leave for 5 min at room temperature to equilibrate.
3. Add to the mixture 10 μL of oligomeres 20 μ*M* and incubate 20 min at RT.
4. Resuspend the desired amount of cells in 800 μL of medium.
5. Mix the 200 μL oligomere/*Oligofectamine* mixture with the 800 μL cell mixture, and incubate for 24–48 h at 37°C.
6. After 24 h, add oligomere/*Oligofectamine* to compensate for lost material

3.4.4. Membrane SCF-Neutralized Fibroblasts

1. Incubate a monolayer of confluent fibroblasts for 24 h with an anti-human SCF neutralizing antibody in the proper concentration for neutralizing.
2. Wash the fibroblasts twice in medium.
3. Add mast cells and continue as described.

4. Notes

1. The yield varies according to animal type. For Sabra rats, an outbred strain of the Hebrew University of Jerusalem, in the following weight, the expected yield is approx 3×10^5 mast cells per animal. Sprague–Dawley rats usually yield approx 8×10^5 cells or more. Mice usually yield approx 10^4 mast cells per animal.
2. a. This protocol is a general protocol for obtaining mast cells from human tissues, such as lungs, intestines, skin, heart, and uterus. If a certain tissue contains some special component, such as mucus in nasal polyps, enzymatic activity can be strengthened by adding a specific enzyme or increasing the concentration of an existing enzyme. In any case, it is not recommended to increase the digestion time because a larger fraction of the cells might either die or "spontaneously" degranulate, increasing the baseline level of any following experiment.
   b. After digestion, the cells should be kept on ice to avoid spontaneous degranulation.
   c. The medium used, unless otherwise stated, is DMEM as described previously, with 2% instead of 10% v/v FCS.
3. Most tissues may be kept at 4°C before this stage for as long as 12–18 h in DMEM with 200 mg/mL streptomycin and 200 μ/mL penecillin, without substantial loss of mast cell viability.

4. Avoid using magnetic stirrers, which might damage the cells.
5. After the spin down, three phases will become apparent. The mast cells are retained in the middle phase.
6. The approximate yield for 1g human tissue is 2×10^5; the actual yield may vary depending upon the tissue source and disease.
7. The source of tissue for this protocol is practically any tissue that has been surgically removed from an organism. The DMEM used here is supplemented with 2 or 10% FCS. As for the mast cells, you can store the tissue at 4°C for as long as 24 h without any substantial loss of mast cell viability as stated.
8. Fibroblasts are usually cultured and propagated in flasks. Plating is required to maintain the fibroblasts in an ongoing state of growth without contact-dependent growth arrest, providing culture continuity. Perform the plating once every several days, depending on fibroblast type and conditions, always before they reach full confluency. Avoid using fibroblasts after the seventh passage.
9. Choose the volume of resuspension medium according to the intended new vessels.
10. The concentration of fibroblasts can be calculated directly to form a confluent monolayer once they attach, even though it is recommended to calculate the concentration for 70% confluency, and then wait 2–3 d until full confluency. Consult **Table 9** to determine the fibroblast concentration. Fibroblasts attach to plastic substrate within minutes. However, it is recommended to wait at least overnight before adding mast cells, to let the system stabilize.
11. Within less than an hour, mast cells become attached to the fibroblasts and medium replacement can be done. Avoid flicking the vessel against the bench or other objects, as the mast cells might detach. Rat peritoneal mast cells (RPMCs) adhere stronger to the fibroblast monolayer than BMDMCs and CBDMCs.
12. Although while in co-culture mast cells apparently receive almost every signal needed for their long-term survival and maturation, it is important to ensure optimal conditions. Therefore, the medium replaced should include all growth factors, such as SCF for human mast cells, IL-3 for murine mast cells, and so on. However, not all cells require these factors. For example, RPMCs and human lung mast cells (HLMCs) do not need any **(Table 6)**. Adjust the factors added to the specific cell type.
13. a. Once set up, a co-culture can be maintained for time periods of more than 4 wk given that the medium is properly replaced and the fibroblast monolayer is not wounded by mistake when changing the medium.
    b. After a certain period, depending on the system's composition, the mast cells reach an optimal state for activation where their responses are stronger. For CBDMC/3T3 this period starts at around d 3–4. For RPMCs/3T3, it starts at 24 h. The optimal period can be determined by a kinetic experiment (*see* **Subheading 3.3.1.1.**).
14. It is important to stabilize the co-culture system before adding priming factors or agonists by waiting at least 24 h before this addition.

15. This experiment should be first done using the simplest activatory stimulus, e.g., compound 48/80. After this has been calibrated, one can move on to optimum time with primed co-culture(s).

16. All washings in this protocol are performed by gentle vacuum aspiration, since cells are adherent. Use a thin pipet, and always draw from the side, not from the middle.

17. Some activators, such as calcium ionophores, kinins, are not specific to mast cells but also will activate fibroblasts; However, fibroblasts can release mediators that activate or prime mast cells, e.g., SCF, nerve growth factor, and PGE_2. The specific stimulus also should be considered regarding the particular fibroblast source, that is, 3T3, human lung, and human skin. In fact, different cells can produce mediators that vary quantitatively and qualitatively.

18. The volume may vary but it is recommended to add the same volume as the activation volume. In case bigger volumes are added, remember the dilution factor for the final analysis.

19. The incubation time is largely dependent on cell number. The base of 2 h is sufficient to quantify b-hex release from approx 10^5 cells/100 mL. If this number changes, adjust the time accordingly (e.g., 1 h for 2×10^5 cells, 3–4 h for 5×10^4 cells).

20. If performing a real time assay, mix 4 mL of substrate with 96 mL of PBS or Hank's solution per sample and use this as the reaction buffer, that is, after the wash, add this buffer and then the activating stimulus.

21. This assay is based on a phthalic condensation of histamine to yield a fluorescent product. Although histamine is the major reagent for this reaction in activated mast cell supernatants, amine groups from other proteins also might react with the substrate and interfere with the true reading. The assay therefore cannot be performed in TG++ buffer, because the gelatin enhances the background. It is recommended to perform this assay in Tyrode's buffer supplemented with 1.8 mM $CaCl_2$ and 0.9 mM $MgCl_2$, without gelatin. The assay includes a preparative stage in which most proteins are precipitated using trichloroacetic acid, but this stage is mostly necessary with protein-rich environments.

22. Do not exceed an amount sufficient to cover the entire vessel surface with 1–2 mm-high liquid. In addition, consider that trypsin self-digests at 37°C. Do not leave it too long at this temperature.

23. It is important for the entire process to be executed quickly and on ice, using ice-cold buffer. This method yields a lower number of cells but at high purity. If a FACS staining is to follow, resuspend cells in cold HBA buffer.

24. The method to be used should be chosen and calibrated specifically to every co-culture type, and depending on the eventual desired process.

25. This protocol is adapted for detection of an intracellular molecule. For a surface molecule, omit **step 5** and perform all washes and incubations with PBS.

26. Perform next stages while glasses are still inside the plate wells.

27. If the secondary antibody is fluorescent, this incubation should be made in a dark chamber or foil-wrapped vessels. If secondary antibody is biotinylated, repeat this stage for the third avidin-conjugated antibody.

28. One slide is large enough to contain two 12-mm cover slips conveniently. This makes better use of the slide and simplifies the storage and analysis.
29. In this protocol, nucleic acid transfection is achieved by using the *Oligofectamine* reagent, by Invitrogen; however, any other method would do according to the manufacturer's instructions.

References

1. Bausher, J. C. and Smith, R. T. (1973) Studies of the Epstein-Barr virus-host relationship: autochthonous and allogeneic lymphocyte stimulation by lymphoblast cell lines in mixed cell culture. *Clin. Immunol. Immunopathol.* **1,** 270–281.
2. Nagel, G. A. and Holland, J. F. (1970) The mixed lymphocyte tumor cell culture and the fluorescein diacetate cytotoxicity test: two useful methods for the demonstration of cell mediated tumor specific immunity in man. *Acta. Haematol.* **44,** 129–141.
3. Subrahmanyan, T. P., Blaskovic, P., Wilson, I. J., and Labzoffsky, N. A. (1974) The development of double-seeded and mixed cell culture systems for use in diagnostic virology. *Arch. Gesamte. Virusforsch.* **44,** 291–297.
4. Hellmann, A., Th'ng, K. H., and Goldman, J. M. (1980) Production of colony stimulating activity in mixed mononuclear cell culture. *Br. J. Haematol.* **45,** 245–249.
5. Medvedev, A. E. (1988) Humoral mechanisms of in vitro inhibition of mouse lymphocyte immunoreactivity by mastocytoma P815 cells. *Biull. Eksp. Biol. Med.* **105,** 701–703.
6. Khan, M. M., Strober, S., and Melmon, K. L. (1986) Regulatory effects of mast cells on lymphoid cells: the role of histamine type 1 receptors in the interaction between mast cells, helper T cells and natural suppressor cells. *Cell. Immunol.* **103,** 41–53.
7. Levi-Schaffer, F., Austen, K. F., Caulfield, J. P., Hein, A., Gravallese, P. M., and Stevens, R. L. (1987) Co-culture of human lung-derived mast cells with mouse 3T3 fibroblasts: morphology and IgE-mediated release of histamine, prostaglandin D2, and leukotrienes. *J. Immunol.* **139,** 494–500.
8. Levi-Schaffer, F., Dayton, E. T., Austen, K. F., et al. (1987) Mouse bone marrow-derived mast cells cocultured with fibroblasts. Morphology and stimulation-induced release of histamine, leukotriene B4, leukotriene C4, and prostaglandin D2. *J. Immunol.* **139,** 3431–3441.
9. Katz, H. R., Dayton, E. T., Levi-Schaffer, F., Benson, A. C., Austen, K. F., and Stevens, R. L. (1988) Coculture of mouse, I. L.-3-dependent mast cells with 3T3 fibroblasts stimulates synthesis of globopentaosylceramide (Forssman glycolipid) by fibroblasts and surface expression on both populations. *J. Immunol.* **140,** 3090–3097.
10. Dayton, E. T., Pharr, P., Ogawa, M., et al. (1988) 3T3 fibroblasts induce cloned interleukin 3-dependent mouse mast cells to resemble connective tissue mast cells in granular constituency. *Proc. Natl. Acad. Sci. USA* **85,** 569–572.
11. Levi-Schaffer, F. (1995) Mast cell/fibroblast interactions in health and disease. *Chem. Immunol.* **61,** 161–185.

12. Piliponsky, A. M., Gleich, G. J., Nagler, A., Bar, I., and Levi-Schaffer, F. (2003) Non-IgE-dependent activation of human lung- and cord blood-derived mast cells is induced by eosinophil major basic protein and modulated by the membrane form of stem cell factor. *Blood* **101,** 1898–1904.

13. Hogaboam, C., Kunkel, S. L., Strieter, R. M., et al. (1998) Novel role of transmembrane, S. C.F for mast cell activation and eotaxin production in mast cell-fibroblast interactions. *J. Immunol.* **160,** 6166–6171.

14. Yurt, R. W., Leid, R. W., and Austen, K. F. (1977) Native heparin from rat peritoneal mast cells. *J. Biol. Chem.* **252,** 518–521.

15. Nilsson, G., Blom, T., Kusche-Gullberg, M., et al. (1994) Phenotypic characterization of the human mast-cell line, H. M.C-1. *Scand. J. Immunol.* **39,** 489–498.

16. Saito, H., Ebisawa, M., Sakaguchi, N., et al. (1995) Characterization of cord-blood-derived human mast cells cultured in the presence of Steel factor and interleukin-6. *Int. Arch. Allergy Immunol.* **107,** 63–65.

17. Sperr, W. R., Bankl, H. C., Mundigler, G., et al. (1994) The human cardiac mast cell: localization, isolation, phenotype, and functional characterization. *Blood* **84,** 3876–3884.

18. Church, M. K. and Clough, G. F. (1999) Human skin mast cells: in vitro and in vivo studies. *Ann. Allergy Asthma. Immunol.* **83,** 471–475.

19. Massey, W. A., Guo, C. B., Dvorak, A. M., et al. (1991) Human uterine mast cells. Isolation, purification, characterization, ultrastructure, and pharmacology. *J. Immunol.* **147,** 1621–1627.

20. Fox, C. C., Dvorak, A. M., Peters, S. P., Kagey-Sobotka, A., and Lichtenstein, L. M. (1985) Isolation and characterization of human intestinal mucosal mast cells. *J. Immunol.* **135,** 483–91.

21. Salari, H., Takei, F., Miller, R., and Chan-Yeung, M. (1987) Novel technique for isolation of human lung mast cells. *J. Immunol. Methods* **100,** 91–97.

22. Irani, A. A., Craig, S. S., Nilsson, G., Ishizaka, T., and Schwartz, L. B. (1992) Characterization of human mast cells developed in vitro from fetal liver cells cocultured with murine 3T3 fibroblasts. *Immunology* **77,** 136–143.

23. Eckes, B., Hunzelmann, N., Ziegler-Heitbrock, H. W., et al. (1992) Interleukin-6 expression by fibroblasts grown in three-dimensional gel cultures. *FEBS Lett.* **298,** 229–232.

24. Kambe, N., Kambe, M., Kochan, J. P., and Schwartz, L. B. (2001) Human skin-derived mast cells can proliferate while retaining their characteristic functional and protease phenotypes. *Blood* **97,** 2045–2052.

25. Levi-Schaffer, F., Kelav-Appelbaum, R., and Rubinchik, E. (1995) Human foreskin mast cell viability and functional activity is maintained ex vivo by coculture with fibroblasts. *Cell Immunol.* **162,** 211–216.

26. Dvorak, A. M., Furitsu, T., Estrella, P., and Ishizaka, T. (1991) Human lung-derived mature mast cells cultured alone or with mouse 3T3 fibroblasts maintain an ultrastructural phenotype different from that of human mast cells that develop from human cord blood cells cultured with 3T3 fibroblasts. *Am. J. Pathol.* **139,** 1309–1318.

27. Schwartz, L. B., Austen, K. F., and Wasserman, S. I. (1979) Immunologic release of beta-hexosaminidase and beta-glucuronidase from purified rat serosal mast cells. *J. Immunol.* **123,** 1445–1450.

28. Greenfeder, S., Gilchrest, H., Cheewatrakoolpong, B., et al. (2003) Real-time assay of tryptase release from human umbilical cord blood-derived mast cells. *Biotechniques* **34,** 910–912, 914.

29. Siraganian, R. P. (1975) Refinements in the automated fluorometric histamine analysis system. *J. Immunol. Methods* **7,** 283–290.

23

Detection of ε Class Switching and IgE Synthesis in Human B Cells

Jérôme Pène, Florence Guilhot, Isabelle Cognet,
Paul Guglielmi, Angélique Guay-Giroux, Jean-Yves Bonnefoy,
Greg C. Elson, Hans Yssel, and Jean-François Gauchat

Summary

We observed that mast cells, as other cells expressing the CD40 ligand CD154, can trigger IgE synthesis in B cells in the presence of interleukin (IL)-4. Numerous complementary techniques can be used to follow the succession of molecular events leading to IgE synthesis. This chapter will illustrate how human B cells (naïve or memory) can be purified, stored, and cultivated in medium that is permissive for IgE synthesis and stimulated with IL-4 or IL-13 and CD40 activation, the latter being induced by soluble CD154, anti-CD40 antibodies, or CD154-expressing cells. All these molecules are expressed by mast cells. The quantification of the ε-sterile transcript synthesis by polymerase chain reaction or Northern blot, the ε excision circles produced during immunoglobulin heavy chain locus rearrangement by polymerase chain reaction, and the IgE production by enzyme-linked immunosorbent assay will be described.

Key Words: IgE; ε sterile transcript; germline ε transcript; mast cells; interleukin-4; interleukin-13; CD154; CD40; CD40 ligand; CD27; B cells; mast cells; isotype class switching; ε excision circles.

1. Introduction

The mechanisms controlling the induction of class switch recombination and production of IgE by switched B cells have been studied extensively (reviewed recently in **ref. 1**). In vitro, the production of IgE by human B cells, specifically induced by interleukin (IL)-4 or IL-13 and signalling via the CD154 cell surface molecule, can be monitored at various levels of the ε class switching process, including during the induction of the sterile ε transcript, which precedes Ig heavy chain locus rearrangement by reverse transcription polymerase chain reaction (RT-PCR) or Northern blot assay *(2,3)*, the detec-

From: *Methods in Molecular Biology, vol. 315: Mast Cells: Methods and Protocols*
Edited by: G. Krishnaswamy and D. S. Chi © Humana Press Inc., Totowa, NJ

tion of production of ε excision circles during the Ig heavy chain locus rearrangement by PCR *(4,5)* and the detection of production of IgE by isotype-specific enzyme-linked immunosorbent assay (ELISA *[6–8]*).

2. Materials

1. Human peripheral or cord blood (*see* **Note 1**).
2. Human spleen or tonsil samples (*see* **Note 1**).
3. Human erythrocytes (RBCs).
4. Phosphate-buffered saline (PBS).
5. Histopaque® (Sigma, St. Louis, MO).
6. Fetal calf serum (FCS; *see* **Note 2**).
7. Bovine serum albumin (BSA; fraction V, Sigma, cat. no. A2153).
8. Petri dishes (10-cm diameter, BD biosciences, San Jose, CA).
9. Centrifuge tubes (15 or 50 mL: BD biosciences).
10. CD19 Microbeads (Miltenyi Biotec; Auburn, CA, cat. no. 130–050–301).
11. 25 MS Separation Columns (Miltenyi Biotec, cat. no. 130–041–301).
12. *VarioMACS*™ (Miltenyi Biotec).
13. RosetteSep® antibody cocktail (StemCell Technologies; Seattle, WA, cat. no. 15064).
14. Anti-CD27-FITC conjugated monoclonal antibody (MAb) (BD Biosciences/Pharmingen, San Diego, CA, cat. no. 555440).
15. FACSvantage® (BD Biosciences) or equivalent.
16. Tissue culture medium (Yssel's medium or equivalent).
17. RPMI-1640 (Invitrogen, Carlsbad, CA).
18. Dimethyl sulfoxide (DMSO, Sigma, cat. no. D5879).
19. Recombinant IL-4 and IL-13 (Peprotech, Rocky Hill, NJ).
20. Anti CD40 MAb, clone 89 (Schering-Plough Corp. Kenilworth, NJ).
21. Anti-CD154 MAb.
22. Mouse fibroblasts, transfected with CD154 or soluble CD154.
23. Tissue culture plates (24 or 96 wells: Nunc, Roskilde, Denmark).
24. Trizol® (Invitrogen).
25. Agarose gel and electrotransfer equipment.
26. Stratalinker (Stratagene, La Jolla, CA).
27. Proteinase K.
28. Phenol-chlorophorm isoamyl alcohol, 50:50:1.
29. SEVAG: chlorophorm isoamyl alcohol, 50:2.
30. Nuclease free water.
31. pBS⁺ (Stratagene).
32. T3 polymerase (Stratagene).
33. α-^{32}P-UTP (3000 Ci/mmoles).
34. Northern blot hybridisation buffer: 50% formamide (molecular biology grade); 50 mM Na citrate, pH 7.0, 25 mM phosphate buffer, pH 6.5, 0.75 M NaCl, 1 mM ethylene diamine tetraacetic acid (EDTA), pH 7.0, 10% polyethylene glycol,

0.1% Na pyrophosphate, 1% sodium dodecyl sulphate (SDS), 20 µg/mL poly A (Amersham Biosciences Piscataway, NJ), 20 µg/mL poly C (Amersham Biosciences), 100 µg/mL yeast ribonucleic acid (RNA; Sigma), 10X Denhardt's solution.
35. Hybridization oven.
36. Thermocycler.
37. Spectrophotometer DU640 (Beckman Coulter, Fullerton, CA).
38. Sandard IgE serum (Pharmacia Diagnostics, total IgE control LMH, cat. no. 10–9267–01).
39. Rabbit anti-human IgE polyclonal antibody (Dako, Glostrup Denmark, cat. no. A0094).
40. Goat anti-mouse IgG-alkaline phosphatase (Dako, cat. no. D0486).
41. Substrate solution (Sigma 104, Sigma).
42. 1 *M* Diethanolamine/HCl buffer, pH 9.8.
43. Nunc Maxisorp™ 96-well plate (eBioscience, San Diego, CA).
44. Microplate reader (Molecular Devices, Menlo Park, CA).

3. Methods

3.1. Isolation of Total, Naïve, or Memory B Cells From Human Spleen, Tonsil, Peripheral Blood, or Cord Blood

B cells constitute approx 30% of human splenocytes, as much as 50% of tonsilar lymphocytes, between 5 and 10% of peripheral and cord blood mononuclear cells, and can be isolated by positive or negative selection. Positive selection, based on the expression of the CD19 cell surface antigen, can be conducted with a specific MAb coated onto paramagnetic beads as described in **Subheading 3.1.1.** Negative selection can be achieved rapidly and efficiently using the RosetteSep procedure, provided that the samples contain RBC: a cocktail of bifunctional antibodies is used, recognizing the undesired leukocyte subsets and the RBC-specific glycophorin (*see* **Subheading 3.1.2.**).

Naive or memory B cells can be isolated from purified CD19+ B cells by FACS™ sorting based on the absence or the presence of the CD27 cell surface antigen *(9,10)*.

Cord blood is an excellent source of naïve (CD27-) B cells.

3.1.1. Isolation of Human Spleen or Tonsillar B Cells by Positive Selection With Paramagnetic Beads

1. Transfer spleen or tonsil fragments into a 10-cm Petri dish, add PBS supplemented with 2% FCS, and mince using two scalpels (*see* **Note 1**).
2. Gently push minced samples through a fine metal mesh using a syringe plunger and transfer the cell suspension to a 50-mL centrifuge tube.
3. Sediment the remaining fragments and transfer the cell suspension to a new tube.
4. Repeat mincing on the sedimented fragments in PBS/2% FCS.

5. Isolate mononuclear cells by centrifugation over a Histopaque (Sigma) cushion ($850g$; 20 min; $\leq 10^8$ cells per 50-mL centrifuge tube).
6. Collect mononuclear cells at the interface.
7. Resuspend at a concentration of 1.25×10^8 cells/mL in PBS, supplemented with 0.5% BSA and 2 m*M* EDTA (PBS/BSA/EDTA) in a 5-mL round-bottom sterile FACS tube (BD Biosciences).
8. Incubate for 30 min at 4°C under constant rotation with 2 μL of CD19 Microbeads per 10^6 cells.
9. Filter cells over a 100-μm grid and dilute to 1.3 10^6/mL in 600-μL aliquots.
10. For each 600-μL aliquot, use a 25 MS Separation Column.
11. Wash the separation columns on a *VarioMACS™* magnet with 1.2 mL of ice-cold PBS/BSA/EDTA.
12. Load columns with 600 μL of cell suspension.
13. Wash 4X with 600 μL of PBS/BSA/EDTA.
14. Remove the columns from the magnet and add 1.2 mL of PBS/BSA/EDTA to recover the CD19$^+$ cells.
15. Spin the purified cells for 5 min at $320g$ in 15-mL tubes and resuspend in culture medium.

3.1.2. Isolation of B Cells by Negative Selection From Cord or Peripheral Blood Samples

1. Add 50 μL of CD19$^+$ RosetteSep antibody cocktail (StemCell Technologies) per milliliter of heparinated cord or peripheral blood and incubate for 20 min at 20°C in 50-mL conical tubes.
2. Mix very gently with an equal volume of PBS, underlay the cell suspension with Histopaque, and centrifuge ($850g$ for 20 min).
3. Collect B cells at the interface, transfer to 50-mL centrifuge tubes, and add an equal volume of PBS/2% FCS.
4. Spin the cells ($320g$ for 7 min) and wash once with PBS/2% FCS.
5. Resuspend cells in culture medium.

3.1.3. Isolation of B Cells by Negative Selection From Spleen or Tonsil

Mononuclear cells isolated from spleen or tonsil samples as described in **Subheading 3.1.1.** no longer contain RBCs. To purify B cells from these samples with the RosetteSep procedure, human RBCs have to be added.

1. Spin whole blood ($1700g$ for 10 min).
2. Wash the RBCs once with cold PBS ($1700g$ for 10 min) and keep at 4°C in Alsever medium until use (RBCs can be stored at 4°C for several weeks).
3. Before use, wash RBCs and resuspend at 30×10^8 RBCs/mL in PBS, 20% FCS.
4. Spin the tonsil or spleen cell suspension ($320g$ for 10 min) and add RBCs to the cell pellet at a ratio of 100:1 RBCs per mononuclear cell.
5. Add 1 μL per 10^6 mononuclear cells of CD19$^+$ RosetteSep antibody cocktail and incubate for 20 min at 20°C in 50-mL centrifuge tubes.

Pursue procedure as described in **Subheading 3.1.2.**

3.1.4. Storage of the Purified B Cells: Freezing

1. Spin cells at 320*g* for 7 min and resuspend in RPMI-1640, supplemented with 10% serum, and put on ice.
2. Dilute DMSO in cold RPMI-1640/10% FCS to a final concentration of 20%. Because adding DMSO results in an increase in temperature, cool on ice for 5 min.
3. Add an equal volume of the 20% DMSO solution in a dropwise fashion to the cell suspension while gently shaking.
4. Transfer 1 mL of the cell suspension to a cryovial, freeze in cryocontainers at −80°C overnight, and subsequently transfer the vials to liquid nitrogen. Use 10^6 to 10^8 cells per vial.

3.1.5. Storage of the Purified B Cells: Thawing

1. Thaw the vial quickly in a 37°C water bath, transfer the cells to a 15-mL tube, and put on ice.
2. Add 2 mL of cold PBS dropwise, at first very slowly, while gently shaking, during a time period of approx 2–3 min.
3. Using a 2-mL pipet, add 2 mL of human serum or FCS under the cell suspension layer.
4. Spin the cells at 320*g* for 5 min.
5. Wash cells once with culture medium.

3.1.6. Isolation of Naïve and Memory B Cells

CD19$^+$CD27$^-$ (naïve) and CD27$^+$ (memory) B cells can be further purified by FACS sorting.

1. Incubate purified B cells for 30 min at 4°C with an anti-CD27-FITC conjugated MAb or an isotype matched IgG-FITC.
2. Wash three times with PBS supplemented with 30% FCS and resuspend at a concentration of 3×10^6 cells/mL in PBS/30%FCS.
3. Sort the cell population with a flow cytometer.
4. Collect the CD27$^+$ and CD27$^-$ cells in 5-mL FACS tubes, containing 0.5 mL of FCS.
5. Pool the FACS-sorted populations in 15-mL centrifuge tubes, spin (320*g* for 7 min) and resuspend in culture medium.

3.2. Activation of B Cells With Anti-CD40MAb or With CD154-Expressing Cells

The production of IgE by memory B cells, as a result of class switch recombination to the ε constant region, requires IL-4 or IL-13, as well as activation through the CD40 receptor *(1)*. The latter is provided by agonistic anti-CD40 MAbs, soluble CD154, or CD154-expressing cells, such as activated mast cells.

1. Resuspend B cells in Yssel's modified IMDM medium *(11)* or equivalent *(12)* supplemented with 10% FCS (*see* **Note 2**).
2. Culture B cells (5×10^5 cells/mL) with IL-4 (20 ng/mL) or IL-13 (10 ng/mL) and

either anti-CD40 MAb (MAb 89 *[13]*; 1 μg/mL) or CD154. The latter can be provided by an irradiated (40 Gy) mouse fibroblast cell line transfected with CD154 cDNA and expressing CD154 at the cell surface (2.5×10^4 cells/mL) or soluble CD154 (2 μg/mL; produced as described in *[14]*).

3. Alternatively, B cells (5×10^5/mL) can be cocultured with autologous T cells or c-kit ligand-activated (72 h; 10 ng/mL) mast cells and IL-4 or IL-13 both at a 1:1 ratio.
4. Incubate for 5–7 d (for analysis of sterile ε RNA and switch circular DNA, respectively) or for 12 d (for analysis of IgE synthesis; *see* **Note 3**).
5. Store cells or supernatants in aliquots at –80°C until analysis.

3.3. Detection of the Sterile ε Transcript and IgE Messenger RNA by Northern Blot Assay

3.3.1. Isolation of Total RNA

RNA is conveniently isolated using a chaotropic agent-phenol based procedure (e.g., Trizol *[15]*) or by cell lysis in guanidium–thyocyanate followed by ultracentrifugation on CsTFA in a micro-ultracentrifuge *(16)*. To improve the RNA stability of the Trizol-purified RNA, the protocol recommended by the manufacturer can be modified as follows.

1. An additional extraction with phenol:chlorophorm:isoamylalcohol (50:50:1) is performed before the isopropanol precipitation *(17)*. Glycogen (2–5 μg) is used as a carrier for the RNA precipitation *(18)*.
2. The glycogen-containing RNA pellets are dissolved in 20 mM Tris, pH 7.0; 1 mM EDTA; 150 mM NaCl; 1% SDS; and 1 mg/mL proteinase K and incubated for 1 h at 37°C.
3. Proteinase K-treated RNA is then successively extracted with phenol–chlorophorm isoamyl alcohol and chlorophorm isoamyl alcohol (SEVAG *[17]*), precipitated with 2 volumes of ethanol, and recovered by centrifugation for 30 min at 16,000g *(18)*.
4. The RNA is washed twice with 70% ethanol, dried at room temperature, and dissolved in nuclease free water on ice with periodic 2-min incubations at 65°C.
5. RNA is quantified by 260/280 nm optical density measurement *(18)* using a DU640 spectrophotometer and a 50-μL quarz cuvette.

3.3.2. Synthesis of ε Complementary RNA Probe for Northern Blot Analysis

To detect the ε RNAs by Northern blot using minimal amounts of total RNA (1–2 μg), a single-stranded complementary (cRNA) probe labeled to very high specific activity using α^{32}P-UTP *(2,19)* is used. The template for probe synthesis is a 241-bp *Sac*I-*Sma*I restriction fragment containing the CH_2–CH_3 junction of the human IgE cDNA (*[20]*; a kind gift from Dr. Honjo, Osaka University Medical School, Japan) cloned in the phagemid pBS$^+$ (Stratagene). To increase the hybridization signal, hybridization is performed in the presence of polyethyleneglycol as a volume excluder *(21)* and, during the washes, the membranes are treated with RNAse A to decrease nonspecific background *(21)*.

1. Linearize the plasmid template with the restriction enzyme *EcoR*I.
2. Purify the linearized plasmid by successive extractions with phenol;chlorophorm: isoamyalcohol and SEVAG followed by ethanol precipitation.
3. Wash with 70% ethanol, air dry, and dissolve in TE at a final concentration of 1 µg/mL.
4. Dry 125 µCi of α^{32}P UTP (3000 Ci/mmol) using a Speed Vac.
5. Transcribe 1 µg of the plasmid template for 3 h using 10 U of T3 polymerase in 10 µL of a standard T3 buffer containing 10 m*M* rATP, rCTP, and rGTP *(19)* and ^{32}P UTP.
6. Stop reaction by adding 40 µL of TE pH 7.0, 1% SDS, and 250 µg/mL transfer RNA.
7. Clean the ε riboprobe from free UTP by chromatography on a Sephadex G50 spin column. (*see* **Note 4**)

3.3.3. RNA Gel Electrophoresis and Transfer

1. RNA aliquots (1–2 µg) are subjected to formaldehyde–MOBS gel electrophoresis *(22,23)* in 10×15 cm 1% agarose gels.
2. Electrotransfer the RNA from the gel to a positively charged Nylon membrane using a Bio-Rad transfer chamber, or equivalent, in 10 m*M* phosphate buffer pH 6.5 for 1 h at 10 V and 2 h at 30 V *(24)*.
3. Fix RNA covalently on the Nylon membrane by ultraviolet irradiation (Stratalinker; default irradiation conditions *[24]*) and stain with methylene blue *(23)* to check for RNA integrity and transfer (*see* **Fig. 1**).

3.3.4. Northern Blot Assay

1. Prehybridize membranes 1–4 h at 57.5°C in hybridization buffer *(23)*.
2. Hybridize for 5–16 h at 57.5°C with the ε cRNA probe (10^6 cpm/mL).
3. Wash membrane 3X for 20–30 min in 0.1 standard saline citrate (SSC *[23]*) and 1% SDS at 65°C.
4. Rinse three times in 50 m*M* Tris-HCl, pH 7.0, and 300 m*M* NaCl at room temperature.
5. Incubate membranes for 30 min with 0.5 µg/mL RNase A (Sigma) in 50 m*M* Tris-HCl pH 7.0, 300 m*M* NaCl *(21)*.
6. Inactivate RNase by rinsing with 0.1 SSC and 1% SDS (*see* **Note 5**).
7. Wash for 20–30 min in 0.1 SSC and 1% SDS at 65°C.
8. Reveal the hybridization signal by autoradiography using an intensifying screen (*see* **Fig. 1** *[23]*).

3.4. Detection of the Sterile ε Transcript by RT-PCR

1. Use aliquots of RNA (1–2 µg) isolated as described in **Subheading 3.3.1.** as a template for cDNA synthesis using Superscript II (Invitrogen) reverse transcriptase, following the manufacturer's instructions. Prime reverse transcription with random hexamers.
2. Amplify the ε sterile transcript with the primers GAC GGG CCA CAC CAT CC and CGG AAG GTG GCA TTG GAG G using standard PCR conditions (25–35 cycles) and one tenth of the cDNA synthesized in **step 1**.

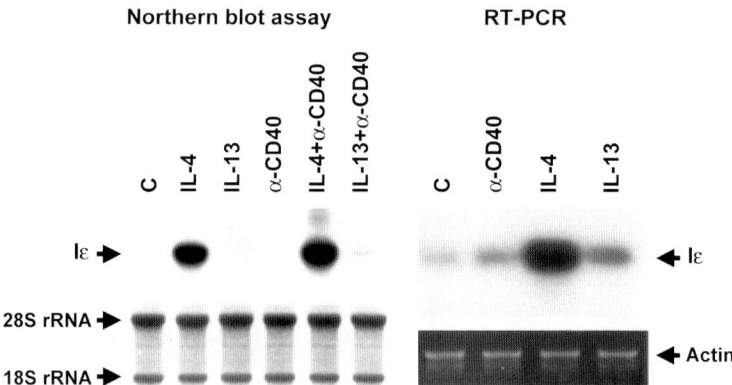

Fig 1. Detection of the sterile ε transcript by Northern blot or RT-PCR. Purified B cells were subjected to the indicated stimuli and harvested after 5 d of incubation. (**Left panels**) aliquots of RNA (2 µg) were subject to formaldehyde agarose gel electrophoresis and electrotransferred to nylon membranes. Membranes were stained with methylene blue to reveal ribosomal RNA (**lower left panel**) and hybridized with ε cRNA probes (**upper left panel**). (**Right panels**) cDNA was amplified with actin (**lower right panel**) or sterile ε transcript specific probes (**upper right panel**). PCR product was revealed by ethidium bromide staining (actin) or hybridization with a specific oligonucleotide probe (Iε) (*3*).

3. To increase sensitivity, the PCR product can be denatured (*23*), electrotransfered to a Nylon membrane, and detected by hybridization with a ^{32}P-labeled oligonucleotide probe (illustrated in **Fig. 1** *[2,3]*).

3.5. Detection of ε Excision Circles by PCR

Formation of DNA excision circles is a hallmark of ongoing class switch recombination (*4,25*). In a polyclonal B-cell population, they are heterogeneous in size, present only as single copy per cell and decay rapidly during cell expansion since they cannot replicate. It is often more convenient to detect spliced RNA transcribed from the sterile transcript (I) promoters present in DNA circles since they are homogeneous in size and present as several copies in cells after class switch recombination (*5*).

1. Use aliquots of RNA (5 µg) isolated as described in **Subheading 3.3.1.** as a template for cDNA synthesis using Superscript II (Invitrogen) reverse transcriptase, following the manufacturer's instructions. Prime reverse transcription with oligo dT.
2. Amplify the excision circle transcripts by PCR using Iε-Cµ sterile transcript detection primers: sense 5'-GACGGGCCACACATCCACAGGC-3 antisense 5'-AGGAAGTCCTGTGCGAGGCAG-3. PCR conditions: 32 cycles of 45 s at 94°C, 30 s at 55°C, and 1.5 min at 72°C. The PCR product should be 149 bp.

3.6. Measurement of IgE Production by Isotype-Specific ELISA

The concentration range of the IgE ELISA is 0.04–2.5 ng/mL. The samples should be diluted appropriately in PBS supplemented with 0.05% Tween-20 and 0.5% BSA (ELISA buffer). Use a standard IgE serum (Pharmacia Diagnostics) as the reference.

1. Coat microtitration plates (Nunc Maxisorp; eBioscience) with a rabbit anti-human IgE polyclonal antibody (Dako, cat. no. A0094) diluted in carbonate buffer pH 9.6 (indicative dilution: 1/8000) for 18 h at 4°C.
2. Wash plates three times with PBS, supplemented with 0.05% Tween-20.
3. Saturate with PBS, supplemented with 2% BSA (30 min at 20°C).
4. Add the diluted culture supernatants to the plates and incubate overnight at 4°C.
5. Wash three times and incubate for 2 h at 20°C with the detection MAb I-27 *(8)* or equivalent (G7–18, BD Biosciences/Pharmingen) at a final concentration of 0.25 µg/mL in ELISA buffer.
6. Wash three times and add goat anti-mouse IgG-alkaline phosphatase (Dako) diluted 1/2000 in ELISA buffer for 1 h at 20°C.
7. Wash three times, incubate with the substrate solution (Sigma 104) at 1 mg/mL in 1 M diethanolamine/HCl buffer, pH 9.8 for 30 min at 37°C.
8. Read the OD at 405–490 nm using a microplate reader.

4. Notes

1. Human clinical samples, blood and cells should be manipulated according to the biosafety guidelines of the NIH.
2. Not all FCS batches do not support IgE synthesis. Individual batches should be tested.
3. Because the analysis of IgE production by ELISA often yields highly variable results, it is recommended that cell cultures are performed in sextuplate (using 96-well culture plates) and that culture supernatants are analysed separately.
4. To maximize the sensitivity of the Northern blot assay, the specific activity of the riboprobe is increased using high specific activity α^{32}P-UTP. The drawback is that the riboprobe is very unstable and has to be used immediately.
5. The RNAse treatment strongly increases the signal to noise ratio. Unfortunately, it prevents the rehybridization of the membrane with a control probe specific for a housekeeping gene. One should rely on ribosomal RNA staining with methylene blue to control for the loading of the Northern blot gene and use a parallel membrane to be probed with a control probe.

Acknowledgments

We are grateful to Dr. Honjo, Osaka University Medical School, Japan, for the kind gift of the IgE cDNA. Our work is supported by grants from the Canadian Institute of Health Research and the Multiple Sclerosis Scientific Research Foundation. J.F.G. is a Canada Research Chair recipient.

References

1. Geha, R. S., Jabara, H. H., and Brodeur, S. R. (2003) The regulation of immuno-globulin E class-switch recombination. *Nat. Rev. Immunol.* **3,** 721–732.
2. Gauchat, J. F., Lebman, D. A., Coffman, R. L., Gascan, H., and de Vries, J. E. (1990) Structure and expression of germline epsilon transcripts in human B cells induced by interleukin 4 to switch to IgE production. *J. Exp. Med.* **172,** 463–473.
3. Gauchat, J. F., Aversa, G., Gascan, H., and de Vries, J. E. (1992) Modulation of IL-4 induced germline epsilon RNA synthesis in human B cells by tumor necrosis factor-alpha, anti-CD40 monoclonal antibodies or transforming growth factor-beta correlates with levels of IgE production. *Int. Immunol.* **4,** 397–406.
4. von Schwedler, U., Jack, H. M., and Wabl, M. (1990) Circular DNA is a product of the immunoglobulin class switch rearrangement. *Nature* **345,** 452–426.
5. Kinoshita, K., Harigai, M., Fagarasan, S., Muramatsu, M., and Honjo, T. (2001) A hallmark of active class switch recombination: transcripts directed by I promoters on looped-out circular DNAs. *Proc. Natl. Acad. Sci. USA* **98,** 12,620–12,623.
6. Gascan, H., Gauchat, J. F., Aversa, G., Van Vlasselaer, P., and de Vries, J. E. (1991) Anti-CD40 monoclonal antibodies or CD4+ T cell clones and IL-4 induce IgG4 and IgE switching in purified human B cells via different signaling pathways. *J. Immunol.* **147,** 8–13.
7. Gauchat, J. F., Henchoz, S., Mazzei, G., et al. (1993) Induction of human IgE synthesis in B cells by mast cells and basophils. *Nature* **365,** 340–343.
8. Pene, J., Rousset, F., Briere, F., et al. (1988) IgE production by normal human lymphocytes is induced by interleukin 4 and suppressed by interferons gamma and alpha and prostaglandin E2. *Proc. Natl. Acad. Sci. USA* **85,** 6880–6884.
9. Klein, U., Goossens, T., Fischer, M., et al. (1998) Somatic hypermutation in normal and transformed human B cells. *Immunol. Rev.* **162,** 261–280.
10. Nagumo, H., Agematsu, K., Kobayashi, N., et al. (2002) The different process of class switching and somatic hypermutation; a novel analysis by CD27(–) naive B cells. *Blood* **99,** 567–575.
11. Yssel, H., De Vries, J. E., Koken, M., Van Blitterswijk, W., and Spits, H. (1984) Serum-free medium for generation and propagation of functional human cytotoxic and helper T cell clones. *J. Immunol. Methods* **72,** 219–227.
12. Claassen, J. L., Levine, A. D., and Buckley, R. H. (1990) A cell culture system that enhances mononuclear cell IgE synthesis induced by recombinant human interleukin-4. *J. Immunol. Methods* **126,** 213–222.
13. Valle, A., Zuber, C. E., Defrance, T., Djossou, O., De Rie, M., and Banchereau, J. (1989) Activation of human B lymphocytes through CD40 and interleukin 4. *Eur. J. Immunol.* **19,** 1463–1467.
14. Mazzei, G. J., Edgerton, M. D., Losberger, C., et al. (1995) Recombinant soluble trimeric CD40 ligand is biologically active. *J. Biol. Chem.* **270,** 7025–7028.
15. Chomczynski, P. and Sacchi, N. (1987) Single-step method of RNA isolation by acid guanidinium thiocyanate-phenol-chloroform extraction. *Anal. Biochem.* **162,** 156–159.

16. Okayama, H., Kawaichi, M., Brownstein, M., Lee, F., Yokota, T., and Arai, K. (1987) High-efficiency cloning of full-length cDNA; construction and screening of cDNA expression libraries for mammalian cells. *Methods Enzymol.* **154,** 3–28.

17. Wallace, D. M. (1987) Large- and small-scale phenol extractions. *Methods Enzymol.* **152,** 33–41.

18. Wallace, D. M. (1987) Precipitation of nucleic acids. *Methods Enzymol.* **152,** 41–48.

19. Melton, D. A., Krieg, P. A., Rebagliati, M. R., Maniatis, T., Zinn, K., and Green, M. R. (1984) Efficient in vitro synthesis of biologically active RNA and RNA hybridization probes from plasmids containing a bacteriophage SP6 promoter. *Nucleic Acids Res.* **12,** 7035–7056.

20. Seno, M., Kurokawa, T., Ono, Y., et al. (1983) Molecular cloning and nucleotide sequencing of human immunoglobulin epsilon chain cDNA. *Nucleic Acids Res.* **11,** 719–726.

21. Wahl, G. M., Meinkoth, J. L., and Kimmel, A. R. (1987) Northern and Southern blots. *Methods Enzymol.* **152,** 572–581.

22. Lehrach, H., Diamond, D., Wozney, J. M., and Boedtker, H. (1977) RNA molecular weight determinations by gel electrophoresis under denaturing conditions, a critical reexamination. *Biochemistry* **16,** 4743–4751.

23. Sambrook, J., Fritsch,EF., and Maniatis, T. (1989) *Molecular Cloning. A Laboratory Manual. Second Edition*, Cold Spring Harbor Laboratory Press, Cold Spring Harbor, New York.

24. Khandjian, E. W. (1986) UV crosslinking of RNA to nylon membrane enhances hybridization signals. *Mol. Biol. Rep.* **11,** 107–115.

25. Iwasato, T., Shimizu, A., Honjo, T., and Yamagishi, H. (1990) Circular DNA is excised by immunoglobulin class switch recombination. *Cell* **62,** 143–149.

VII

Novel Aspects of Mast Cell Activation and Regulation

24

Gene Silencing Using Small Interference RNA in Mast Cells

Deling Yin and Charles A. Stuart

Summary

Small interfering RNA (siRNA) is a potent and specific method of inducing gene silencing through induction of RNA interference. siRNAs can be allowed for in vitro and in vivo applications. siRNAs have been successfully studied in vitro, but little is known about its efficacy in vivo. We have successfully applied the siRNA technique for silencing glucose transporter 3 in cultured L6 muscle cells. The siRNA technique has been used efficiently to silence RasGRP4 expression in mast cells.

Key Words: Small interfering RNA (siRNA); gene; transfection; mast cells; Western blot; reverse transcriptase polymerase chain reaction (RT-PCR).

1. Introduction

Small interfering RNA (siRNAs) are small RNA duplexes approx 21 nucleotides (nts) long *(1)*. siRNA includes two nucleotides (nt) 3' overhangs and a 5' phosphate group *(2)*. Fire et al. *(3)* identified double-stranded RNA (dsRNA) as a mediator for gene knock-down in *Caenorhabditis elegans* and referred to the term RNAi. siRNAs suppress gene expression through a highly regulated enzyme-mediated process called RNA interference. siRNAs serve as guides for enzyme complexes that degrade, inhibit, or modify the function of homologous nucleic acids *(4–13)*.

Although siRNAs have been studied successfully in vitro, little is known about their efficacy in vivo. Recently, a few groups have indicated siRNAs could be used directly as a therapeutic approach to inhibit gene expression in vivo in mice *(14–18)*. In this chapter, an in vitro model for silencing gene expression will be described.

2. Materials

2.1. Silencing siRNA Construction

All supplies are from Ambion the RNA Company (cat. no. 1620).

From: *Methods in Molecular Biology, vol. 315: Mast Cells: Methods and Protocols*
Edited by: G. Krishnaswamy and D. S. Chi © Humana Press Inc., Totowa, NJ

2.1.1. Template Preparation

1. DNA Hybridization buffer.
2. T7 Promoter primer.
3. 10X Klenow reaction buffer.
4. 10X dNTP Mix.
5. Exo-Klenow.

2.1.2. Transcription Reagents

1. T7 Enzyme mix.
2. 10X T7 Reaction buffer.
3. 2X NTP mix.

2.1.3. siRNA Purification

1. Digestion buffer.
2. DNase.
3. RNase.
4. siRNA binding buffer.
5. siRNA wash buffer.
6. Nuclease-free water.
7. Filter cartridges.
8. 2-mL tubes.

2.1.4. Other Reagents

1. siRNA oligonucleotide templates.

2.2. Silencing siRNA Transfection

All supplies from Ambion the RNA Company (cat. no. 1630).

1. Cell-culture materials.
2. Reagents for detecting gene knock-down, for example, antibody or PCR primers.
3. siPORT *Amine*.
4. siRNA GAPDH.
5. Negative control siRNA GAPDH.

3. Methods

3.1. Protocol for Silencing siRNA Construction

This subheading is modified from Ambion siRNA construction kit instruction.

3.1.1. siRNA Design

Elbashir et al. *(19)* indicate that the most siRNAs are affected by 21-nt dsRNAs with 3' overhanging dimers of uridine.

3.1.1.1. EXAMPLES OF siRNA OLIGONUCLEOTIDE TEMPLATE DESIGN

Example 1

Target mRNA sequence:
  5'- AACCCGCGGAGCUGCCUGCCU-3'
Antisense siRNA oligonucleotide template:
  5'- AACCCGCGGAGCTGCCTGCCTCCTGTCTC -3'
Sense siRNA oligonucleotide template:
  5'- AAAGGCAGGCAGCTCCGCGGGCCTGTCTC -3'

Example 2

Target mRNA sequence
  5'-AAGCGGCAGCGGGCACUGAUG-3'
Antisense siRNA oligonucleotide template:
  5'-AAGCGGCAGCGGGCACTGATGCCTGTCTC -3'
Sense siRNA oligonucleotide template:
  5'- AACATCAGTGCCCGCTGCCGCCCTGTCTC-3'

3.1.2. Preparation of siRNA Transcription Template

1. Dissolve the siRNA oligonucleotide template to 200 μM in nuclease-free water.
2. Check the siRNA oligonucleotide template concentration using A260.
3. Dilute a 100-μM solution of each siRNA oligo template.
4. Hybridize each siRNA oligo template to the T7 promoter primer.

   a. In separate tubes, mix each siRNA oligo template as the following:

      3 µL of T7 promoter primer;
      9 µL of DNA Hybridization buffer; and
      3 µL of either sense or antisense siRNA oligonucleotide template.

   b. Heat the mixture at 70°C for 5 min, then leave at room temperature for 6 min.

5. Fill in with Klenow DNA polymerase.

   a. Add the following regents to the hybridized oligonucleotides:

      3 µL of 10X Klenow reaction buffer;
      3 µL of 10X dNTP mix;
      6 µL of Nuclease-free water; and
      3 µL of Exo-Klenow (*see* **Note 1**).

   b. Mix gently by pipetting. Centrifuge briefly to collect the mixture at the bottom of the tube.
   c. Incubate at 37°C for 30 min.
   d. The siRNA templates can be used directly in the transcription reaction or kept at –20°C (until they are needed for transcription).

3.1.3. dsRNA Synthesis

1. To assemble the transcription reactions: mix for each transcription reaction according to following components in the order shown:

   > 3 µL of Antisense or sense siRNA template (*see* **Subheading 3.1.2., step 5d**)
   > 6 µL of Nuclease-free water;
   > 15 µL of 2x NTP Mix;
   > 3 µL of 10x T7 reaction buffer; and
   > 3 µL of T7 enzyme mix.

2. Mix gently by brief vortexing and then microfuge shortly to collect the reaction mixture at the bottom of the tube.
3. Incubate reactions at 37°C for 2 h (*see* **Note 2**).
4. Combine the antisense and sense transcription reaction and incubate at 37°C overnight.

3.1.4. Preparation and Purification for siRNA

1. Digest the siRNA using RNase and DNase
   a. Get the tube from **Subheading 3.1.3., step 4**, and add the following reagents:

      > 9 µL of Digestion buffer
      > 73 µL of Nuclease-free water
      > 4.5 µL of RNase
      > 3.8 µL of DNase

   b. Gently mix and incubate at 37°C for 2.5 h.

2. Add 600 µL of siRNA binding buffer and incubate at room temperature for 5 min (*see* **Note 3**).
3. Wash the filter cartridge using 2×700 µL of siRNA wash buffer. Apply wash buffer to the filter and spin at 9000g for 1.5 min.
4. Elute the siRNA with 150 µL of 75°C nuclease-free water. Spin the filter cartridge at 10,000g for 3 min. The purified siRNA will be in the eluate (in the 2-mL tube).
5. Keep siRNAs at −80°C until they are prepared for transfection.

3.1.5. siRNA Quantification

1. Determine siRNA concentration by A260.
   a. Dilute the siRNA 1:25 into TE (10 mM Tris-HCI, pH 8.0, 1 mM ethylene diamine tetraacetic acid) and read the absorbance 260 nm in a spectrophotometer.
   b. Example calculation: A 1:25 dilution of siRNA has an A260 = 0.5. The molar concentration is determined as follows:

      $$0.5 \times 1000 \text{ µg siRNA/mL per A260} = 500 \text{ µg/mL}$$

500 µg/mL divided by 14 µg of siRNA/nmol siRNA (21-mer dsRNA) = 35.7 µM siRNA

Table 1
Reagent Amounts in Each Well of a 96-Well Plate
for siRNA Transfection in Adherent Cells

Reagents	Volume (µL)
$2-3 \times 10^3$ cells/well	80
siPORT Amine	1.5
OPTI-MEM reduced serum medium	18
siRNA (stock solution at 20 µ*M*)	0.5

3.2. Silencing siRNA Transfection

siPORT Amine siRNA transfection protocol is used here. Please *see* **Table 1** to make approximate reagent amounts per 96 wells for transfection. We recommend performing this experiment in triplicate for each sample.

3.2.1. Transfection

1. At 24 h before transfection, plate cells in normal growth medium (e.g., Dulbecco's modified Eagle's medium with 10% fetal bovine serum) so that they will be around 40% confluent after 24 h.
2. Incubate overnight in normal cell culture conditions.
3. In a sterile, round bottom 96-well plate or in sterile polystyrene tubes, dilute 1.5 µL of siPORT Amine dropwise into 18 µL of OPTI-MEM-reduced serum medium (*see* **Note 4**).
4. Vortex thoroughly, incubate at room temperature for 20 min.
5. Add 0.5 µL of 20 µ*M* siRNA to diluted siPORT Amine transfection agent from **step 3** and mix by gently flicking the tube (*see* **Note 5**).
6. Incubate at room temperature for 20 min.
7. Adjust the volume of normal growth medium (e.g., Dulbecco's modified Eagle's medium, 10% fetal bovine serum) in each well containing cells to 80 µL.
8. Overlay the transfection agent/siRNA complex (from **step 6** of **Subheading 3.2.1.**) dropwise onto the cells.
9. Without swirling, gently rock the dish back and forth.
10. Incubate cells in normal cell culture conditions for 16 h.
11. Add 100 µL of fresh normal growth medium to each well after 16 h to prevent potential cytotoxicity.

3.2.2. Assay for Target Gene Activity
24, 48, and 72 Hours After Transfection

Expression of the cellular target gene at each time is tested (*see* **Note 6**). We have successfully applied siRNA technique for silencing glucose transporter 3 in myoblast L6 cells using the protocols stated above. Li et al. *(20)* indicated that RasGRP4 could be silenced by siRNA technique in RBL-2H3 mast cells.

4. Notes

1. The tube of Exo-Klenow should be kept at –20°C; do not vortex it.
2. Transcription reactions will be incubate at 37°C for 2 h, preferably in a cabinet incubator.
3. 100% ethanol should be added before using the siRNA binding and washing buffers for the first time and should be mixed thoroughly.
4. We recommend OPTI-MEM reduced serum medium (Gibco BRL) to dilute the siPORT Amine.
5. Vortex the siPORT Amine for 10 s before use.
6. Target gene can be tested either by Western blot (if antibody is available) or by reverse transcription polymerase chain reaction (if antibody is not available).

Acknowledgments

The authors thank Rhesa Dykes for technical assistance. This work was supported by Takeda Pharmaceuticals, ETSU grants 2–25453 and 2–25491.

References

1. Elbashir, S. M., Lendeckel, W., and Tuschi T. (2001) RNA interference is mediated by 21- and 22-nucleotide RNAs. *Gene Dev.* **15,** 188–200.
2. Elbashir S. M., Martinez, J., Patkaniowska, A., Lendeckel, W., and Tuschl, T. (2001) Functional anatomy of siRNAs for mediating efficient RNAi in *Drosophila melanogaster* embryo lysate. *EMBO J.* **20,** 6877–6888.
3. Fire, A., Xu, S., Montgomery, M. K., Kostas, S. A., Driver, S. E., and Mello, C. C. (1998) Potent and specific genetic interference by double-stranded RNA in Caenorhabditis elegans. *Nature* **391,** 806–811.
4. Paushkin, S. V., Patel, M., Furia, B.S., Peltz, S. W., and Trotta, C. R. (2004) Identification of a human endonuclease complex reveals a link between tRNA splicing and pre-mRNA 3' end formation. *Cell* **117,** 311–321.
5. Pham, J. W., Pellino, J. L., Lee, Y. S., Carthew, R. W., and Sontheimer, E. J. (2004) A Dicer-2-dependent 80s complex cleaves targeted mRNAs during RNAi in *Drosophila. Cell* **117,** 83–94.
6. Schütze, N. (2004) siRNA technology. *Mol. Cell. Endocrinol.* **213,** 115–119.
7. Amarzguioui, M. and Prydz, H. (2004) An algorithm for selection of functional siRNA sequences. *Biochem. Biophys. Res. Commun.* **316,** 1050–1058.
8. Schmitz, J. C., Chen, T. M., and Chu, E. (2004) Small interfering double-stranded RNAs as therapeutic molecules to restore chemosensitivity to thymidylate synthase inhibitor compounds. *Cancer Res.* **64,** 1431–1435.
9. Reynolds, A., Leake, D., Boese, Q., Scaringe, S., Marshall, W. S., and Khvorova, A. (2004) Rational siRNA design for RNA interference. *Nat. Biotechnol.* **22,** 326–330.

10. Mitchell, K. J., Tsuboi, T., and Rutter, G. A. (2004) Role for plasma membrane-related Ca2+-ATPase-1 (ATP2C1) in pancreatic beta-cell Ca2+ homeostasis revealed by RNA silencing. *Diabetes* **53,** 393–400.

11. Khvorova, A., Reynolds, A., and Jayasena, S. D. (2003) Functional siRNAs and miRNAs exhibit strand bias. *Cell* **115,** 209–216.

12. Mandelboim, M., Barth, S., Biton, M., Liang, X. H., and Michaeli, S. (2003) Silencing of Sm proteins in *Trypanosoma brucei* by RNA interference captured a novel cytoplasmic intermediate in spliced leader RNA biogenesis. *J. Biol. Chem.* **278,** 51,469–51,478.

13. McManus, M. T., Haines, B. B., Dillon, C. P., et al. (2002) Small interfering RNA-mediated gene silencing in T lymphocytes. *J. Immunol.* **169,** 5754–5760.

14. McCaffrey, A. P., Meuse, L., Pham, T. T., Conklin, D. S., Hannon, G. J., and Kay, M. A. (2002) RNA interference in adult mice. *Nature* **418,** 38–39.

15. Lewis, D. L., Hagstrom, J. E., Loomis, A. G., Wolff, J. A., and Herweijer, H. (2002) Efficient delivery of siRNA for inhibition of gene expression in postnatal mice. *Nat. Genet.* **32,** 107–108.

16. Xia, H., Mao, Q., Paulson, H. L., and Davidson, B. L. (2002) siRNA-mediated gene silencing in vitro and in vivo. *Nat. Biotechnol.* **20,** 1006–1010.

17. Kunath, T., Gish, G., Lickert, H., Jones, N., Pawson, T., and Rossant, J. (2003) Transgenic RNA interference in ES cell-derived embryos recapitulates a genetic null phenotype. *Nat. Biotechnol.* **21,** 559–561.

18. Tiscornia, G., Singer, O., Ikawa, M., and Verma, I. M. (2003) A general method for gene knockdown in mice by using lentiviral vectors expressing small interfering RNA. *Proc. Natl. Acad. Sci. USA* **100,** 1844–1848.

19. Elbashir, S. M., Harborth, J., Lendeckel, W., Yalcin, A., Weber, K., and Tuschl, T. (2001) Duplexes of 21-nucleotide RNAs mediate RNA interference in cultured mammalian cells. *Nature* **411,** 494–498.

20. Li, L., Yang, Y., and Stevens, R. L. (2003) RasGRP4 regulates the expression of prostaglandin D2 in human and rat mast cell lines. *J. Biol. Chem.* **278,** 4725–4729.

25

Mast Cell Activation by Lipoproteins

Jim Kelley, Gregory Hemontolor, Walid Younis, Chuanfu Li, Guha Krishnaswamy, and David S. Chi

Summary

Mast cells are activated by a number of agents that act independently from immunoglobulin E (IgE)-mediated hypersensitivity. One of these agents is oxidized low-density lipoprotein (oxLDL). OxLDL has been implicated in the pathogenesis of atherosclerosis and has been shown to induce microvascular dysfunction by the activation of mast cells. In this chapter, we describe the method for isolation of human LDL, oxidation of LDL, and demonstrate that oxLDL activates mast cells by measuring messenger ribonucleic acid (mRNA) levels and protein levels of interleukin (IL)-8 an inflammatory cytokine. IL-8 is a potent chemoattractant for neutrophils and monocytes, which would result in a chronic inflammatory response. IL-8 mRNA levels were measured by reverse-transcription polymerase chain reaction and protein levels by enzyme-linked immunoassay.

Key Words: HMC-1; mast cells; lipoproteins; cell culture; ELISA; interleukin-8; ultracentrifugation; mRNA.

1. Introduction

The ability of human mast cells to produce a variety of cytokines induced by multiple stimuli suggests that mast cells can participate in immunological processes other than immunoglobulin E (IgE)-mediated hypersensitivity reactions. In support of this view, several studies suggest a role for mast cells in vascular inflammation and arteriosclerosis (*1–4*), wound healing (*5*), and rheumatoid arthritis (*6*). Mast cells are activated to release histamine and cytokines by a number of agents, including anti-IgE, compound 48/80, calcium ionophore A23187, stem cell factor, and phorbol myristate acetate (PMA *[7,8]*). In this chapter, we use a unique activating agent, namely oxidized low-density lipoprotein (oxLDL). In this method, we describe the isolation and oxidation of human plasma LDL, culture of the human mast cell line HMC-1, the experimental design for activating mast cells using LDL and oxLDL, and verification

From: *Methods in Molecular Biology, vol. 315: Mast Cells: Methods and Protocols*
Edited by: G. Krishnaswamy and D. S. Chi © Humana Press Inc., Totowa, NJ

of activation by measuring interleukin (IL)-8 protein secretion by mast cells using enzyme-linked immunoassay (ELISA) and by changes in mRNA for IL-8 using reverse transcription-polymerase chain reaction (RT-PCR).

2. Materials

1. Fresh human plasma from normolipidemic subjects.
2. Density solution 1.006 g/mL: add 12.46 g of KBr to 5 mL of a 10% solution of ethylene diamine tetraacetic acid (EDTA) and bring volume to 1 L.
3. Density solution 1063 g/mL: add 91.98 g of potassium bromide (KBr) to 5 mL of a 10% solution of EDTA and adjust the volume to 1 L.
4. LDL dialysis buffer (phosphate-buffered saline [PBS]): 0.01 M sodium phosphate, 0.15 M NaCl, and 0.01% EDTA, pH 7.4.
5. Dialysis tubing: spectrapor membrane tubing, 10,000 MW cutoff (Spectrum, Los Angeles, CA).
6. BCA Protein Reagents: Pierce BCA Protein Assay Reagent Kit (Pierce, Rockford, IL).
7. Mast cell culture media: RPMI 1640 media, 5% heat inactivated fetal bovine serum, 0.01 M HEPES, 50 µg/mL gentamycin, 0.05 mM 2-mercaptoethanol, 5 µg/mL insulin transferrin solution and 2 mM L-glutamine.
8. Mast cell activator, PMA-ionomycin: 50 ng/mL PMA plus 5 µM Ionomycin.
9. Beckman Ultracentrifuge and Type 80 Ti rotor: Beckman Instruments, Palo Alto, CA.
10. Agarose gel electrophoresis equipment.
11. Thermal Cycler.
12. 96-well plate reader.

3. Methods

The methods described in **Subheadings 3.1.–3.3.** outline: (1) culture of the human mast cell line HMC-1; (2) isolation and oxidative modification of human plasma LDLs; and (3) activation of mast cells by oxLDLs.

3.1. Culture of the Human Mast Cell Line HMC-1

The human mast cell line HMC-1 (*[9]*; kindly provided by Dr. J. H. Butterfield, Mayo Clinic, Rochester, MN) was grown in mast cell culture media using standard sterile technique. Cells are counted and then seeded in culture flasks at a density of 20,000 cells/mL of media and recultured every 4 d. HMC-1 grow in suspension and their numbers double approximately every 24 h. Cell viability is measured using trypan blue exclusion and is usually greater than 95%. (*See* Chapter 16 for more information on the culture of HMC-1.)

3.2. Isolation and Oxidative Modification of Human Plasma LDL

Blood is collected from healthy fasting volunteers by venipuncture into tubes containing 1.5 mg of EDTA per milliliter of blood. Blood is centrifuged at

2000g for 10 min to separate the plasma from the cellular components of the blood. Lipoproteins are separated from plasma by sequential ultracentrifugal flotation as described in detail (*10*).

3.2.1. Isolation of LDL

1. Fill Beckman OptiSeal tubes with fresh human plasma and place the tubes into a Beckman Type 80 Ti rotor (*see* **Note 1**).
2. Centrifuge the plasma, which has a density of 1.006 g/mL, for 24 h at 14°C in a Beckman L5 75B ultracentrifuge, type 80 Ti rotor, at 112,000g to float the very low-density lipoproteins (VLDL) to the top of the tube (*see* **Note 2 [10]**).
3. Remove the VLDL from the top of the tube after the 24-h centrifugation using a Beckman tube slicing device (*see* **Note 3**). Discard the VLDL fraction.
4. Place the infranatant solution in a sterile plastic culture tube and adjust the density to 1.063 g/mL by adding KBr to float the LDL. Add 0.818 g of KBr for each milliliter of infranatant solution (*see* **Note 4**). Dissolve the KBr by gentle inversion of the tube. Fill the OptiSeal tubes with the solution at a density of 1.063 g/mL and centrifuge for 24 h at 14°C in a Beckman L5 75B ultracentrifuge at 112,000g to float the LDL to the top of the tube. Remove the LDL fraction (d = 1.006–1.063 g/mL) from the top of the tube using a Beckman tube slicing device and place into a sterile plastic culture tube. Dialyze the LDL at 4°C against 4 L of LDL dialysis buffer to remove high levels of salt. After dialysis, determine the protein content of LDL using the Pierce BCA protein assay (Pierce, Rockford, IL) with human serum albumin as the standard (*see* **Note 4**).

3.2.2. Oxidation of LDL

1. In preparation for oxidation, dialyze a portion of the LDL sample against 4 L of PBS at 4°C without EDTA, because the oxidation process will not work in the presence of EDTA which acts as an antioxidant.
2. Adjust the LDL solution (free of EDTA) to a protein concentration of 200 μg/mL, and then incubate overnight, with gentle stirring, at 37°C in the presence of 5 μM CuSO4 as the oxidizing agent (*see* **Note 5**).
3. Concentrate the LDL solution to less than 2 mL using a Centripep Concentrator (Centricon 30, Amicon, Beverly, MA). Verify the protein content of the oxLDL using the BCA protein assay. Confirm the oxidation of LDL by electrophoresis in an agarose gel using the Ciba-Corning Lipoprotein electrophoresis system following the manufacturer's instructions. Visualize the lipoproteins using fat Red 7B provided in the Ciba-Corning kit. OxLDL migrates three to four times faster in the agarose gel than native LDL (*see* **Note 6**; **Fig. 1**).

3.3. Activation of Mast Cells by oxLDL

3.3.1. Experimental Setup to Measure Activation of Mast Cells by oxLDL

1. Dispense the cultured HMC-1 into 60 × 15-mm culture dishes with a final concentration of 2 million cells in a total volume of 2 mL.

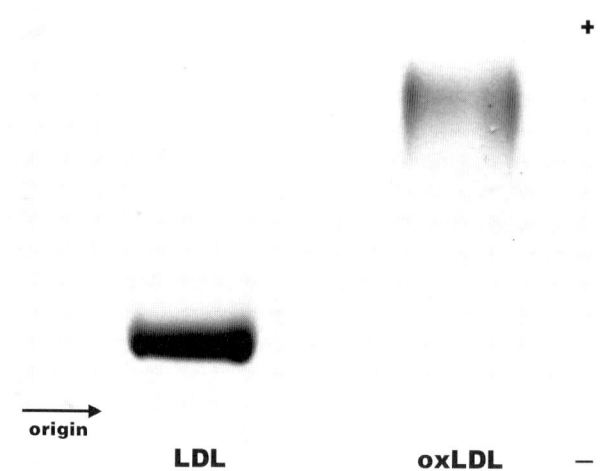

Fig. 1. Agarose electrophoresis of LDL and oxLDL. Lipoproteins were stained with Oil Red O. OxLDL migrates four times faster than LDL.

2. Incubate the cells for 24 h at 37°C in a humidified atmosphere of 5 % CO_2, with varying concentrations of native LDL (25, 50, and 100 μg /mL) and oxLDL (25, 50, 100, and 200 μg/mL) in triplicate. Activate HMC-1 using PMA-ionomycin as a positive control. Keep three dishes of HMC-1 in unsupplemented media as a negative control.

3. Harvest the cells after 24 h the cells by low speed centrifugation. Freeze the cell pellets in liquid nitrogen for safe storage. Freeze the culture media at –80°C. Assay the cell culture media for IL-8 protein levels by ELISA. Purify the cellular RNA from the frozen cell pellets and assay for IL-8 mRNA by RT-PCR.

3.3.2. Mast Cells Activated With oxLDL Express-Elevated Levels of IL-8 mRNA

Mast cell mRNA for IL-8 is measured, after treatment of cells with native and oxLDL, by RT-PCR (*see* Chapter 16). RNA was extracted and assessed for expression of IL-8 (Sense 5'ATG ACT TCC AAG CTG GCC GTG GCT 3' antisense 5' TCT CAG CCC TCT TCA AAA ACT TCT 3'; DNA synthesis Core Facility, John Hopkins University, Baltimore, MD) The RT-PCR is performed as previously described *(11)*. Briefly RT-PCR is performed with a GeneAmp kit from PerkinElmer (Branchburg, NJ) using a PerkinElmer thermal cycler. Cycles for RT consists of one cycle each of 42°C for 20 min, 99°C for 10 min and 5°C for 5 min. PCR consists of initial denaturation at 95°C for 2 min, denaturation at 94°C for 45 s, annealing at 60°C for 45 s, and extension

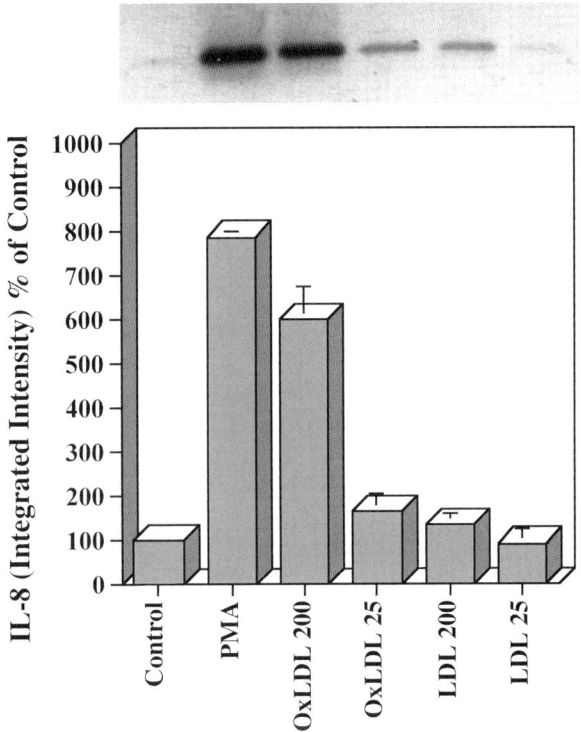

Fig. 2. Measurement of IL-8 mRNA by RT-PCR as a marker for activation of mast cells by lipoproteins. Mast cells were stimulated to express IL-8 mRNA after activation with PMA + ionomycin as a positive control and by oxLDL but not by native LDL. A representative agarose gel from RT-PCR for IL-8 is shown as an insert at the top of the figure. Integrated intensity was determined by scanning the gel. HMC-1 mast cells were incubated with 25 and 200 µg/mL of native LDL and 25 and 200 µg/ mL of oxLDL.

at 72°C for 90 s. Samples are run on agarose gels and photographs are scanned to measure the intensity of the bands. OxLDL treatment of mast cells results in a concentration-dependent increase in IL-8 mRNA (**Fig. 2**).

3.3.3 Mast Cells Activated With oxLDL Secrete IL-8 Protein Into the Media

Human IL-8 protein secreted into the media by mast cells was assayed using an ELISA kit developed by R & D Systems (Quantikine®, R&D Systems, Minneapolis, MN) according to the manufacturer's protocol (*see* Chapter 16). OxLDL treatment of mast cells results in a significant concentration-dependent increase in IL-8 protein as measured by ELISA (**Fig. 3**).

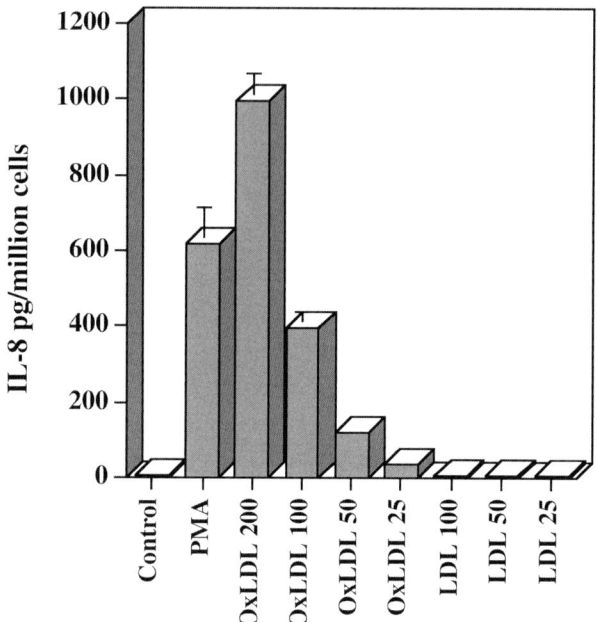

Fig. 3. Measurement of IL-8 protein by ELISA as a marker for activation of mast cells by lipoproteins. Mast cells were stimulated to secrete IL-8 into the media after exposure to PMA + ionomycin as a positive control and by increasing concentrations of oxLDL for 24 h. Native LDL did not stimulate secretion of IL-8. HMC-1 mast cells were incubated with 25, 50, and 100 µg/mL of native LDL and 25, 50, 100, and 200 µg/mL of oxLDL.

4. Notes

1. Other types of centrifuge tubes can be used, such as the Beckman QuickSeal tubes, but these tubes require a heat-sealing device, which is more difficult to use than the OptiSeal tubes. It is important that reagents and tubes that come in contact with the LDL are free of endotoxin because small amounts of endotoxin can activate mast cells.

2. Any ultracentrifuge or rotor combination may be used for this lipoprotein isolation method as long as they can achieve an average g-force of 112,000g. It is critically important to minimize vibration of the rotor containing the plasma during and after the centrifugation. All density solutions are prepared in pyrogen free water. For accuracy of the density solutions, the KBr is dried by heating at 100°C for 2 h then stored in a dessicator. Densities of all of the solutions is verified using a Mettler PAAR Density Meter.

3. If a tube-slicing device is not available, the lipoprotein fractions can be removed from the top of the tube using a syringe and a small bore needle. Aspirate slowly with the needle bevel in the down position.

4. At this step, it is important that the dialysis buffer contains EDTA to protect LDL from oxidation. LDL also should be protected from light and be used within 1 wk of preparation.
5. It is important not to be too vigorous in the stirring action during the oxidation step. Stirring too vigorously will cause the LDL to precipitate out of solution; the solution becomes very cloudy if this happens.
6. If the oxLDL does not migrate faster than the native LDL, the EDTA was not completely removed during dialysis. Repeat the dialysis and the oxidation steps.

Acknowledgments

The authors thank Dr. Butterfield for providing the HMC-1 cell line used in these studies. We also thank Karen Cantor her technical support. This work was supported by grants from East Tennessee State University RDC, Cardiovascular Research Institute and the Department of Internal Medicine.

References

1. Steinberg, D. (1997) Oxidative modification of LDL and atherogenesis. *Circulation* **95,** 1062–1071.
2. Liao, L. and Granger, D. N. (1996) Role of mast cells in oxidized low-density lipoprotein-induced microvascular dysfunction. *Am. J. Physiol.* **271,** H1795–H1800.
3. Laine, P., Kaartinen, M., Penttila, A., Panula, P., Paavonen, T., and Kovanen, P. T. (1999) Association between myocardial infarction and the mast cells in the adventitia of the infarct-related coronary artery. *Circulation* **99,** 361–369.
4. Kaartinen, M., Penttila, A., and Kovanen, P. T. (1994) Coronary heart disease/myocardial infarction: accumulation of activated mast cells in the shoulder region of human coronary atheroma, the predilection site of atheromatous rupture. *Circulation* **90,** 1669–1678.
5. Artuc, M., Hermes, B., Steckelings, U. M., Grutzkan, A., and Henz, B. M. (1999) Mast cells and their mediators in cutaneous wound healing-active participants or innocent bystanders. *Exp. Dermatol.* **8,** 1–16.
6. Woolley, D. E. and Tetlow, L. C. (2000) Mast cell activation and its relation to proinflammatory cytokine production in the rheumatoid lesion. *Arthritis Res.* **2,** 65–74.
7. Wierecky, J., Grabbe, J., Wolff, H. H., and Gibbs, B. F. (2000) Cytokine release from a human mast cell line (HMC-1) in response to stimulation with anti-IgE and other secretagogues. *Inflamm. Res.* **49,** 7–8.
8. Moller, A., Henz, B. M., Grutzkau, A., et al. (1998) Comparative Cytokine gene expression: regulation and release by human mast cells. *Immunology* **93,** 289–295.
9. Butterfield, J. H., Weiler, D., Dewald, G., and Gleich, G. J. (1988) Establishment of an immature mast cell line from a patient with mast cell leukemia. *Leukemia Res.* **12,** 345–355.
10. Kelley, J. L., Rozek, M. M., Suenram, C. A., and Schwartz, C. J. (1988) Activation of human peripheral blood monocytes by lipoproteins. *Am. J. Pathol.* **130,** 223–231.

11. Krishnaswamy, G., Lakshman, T., Miller, A. R., et al. (1997) Multifunctional cytokine expression by human mast cells: regulation by T cell membrane contact and glucocorticoids. *J. Interferon Cytokine Res.* **17,** 167–176.

26

Mast Cell Activation by Stress

Ann L. Baldwin

Summary

Mental or emotional stress has been shown to cause mast cell degranulation in several different tissues. Several lines of experimental evidence indicate that stress, working through the sympathetic nervous system, or the hypothalamus–pituitary–adrenal axis, stimulates peripheral nerves to release neuropeptides that bind to receptors on the mast cells, causing them to degranulate. In order to investigate the effects of stress on mast cell degranulation, it is necessary to first establish a reproducible animal model of stress (in this case, rat) and also to ensure that the control animals do not show any signs of stress. This procedure requires a great deal of care and attention because the methods used by many institutions to house laboratory rodents, do in fact cause them stress. This topic is addressed in this chapter. In addition, two histological techniques are described to visualize connective tissue and mucosal mast cells and to assess their degree of degranulation.

Key Words: Stress; rodent housing; noise, sympathetic nervous system; hypothalamus–pituitary–adrenal axis; mesenteric mast cells; connective tissue mast cells; mucosal mast cells; intestine; microscopy; Alcian blue; Safranin O; Toluidine blue; diaminobenzidine.

1. Introduction

Mental or emotional stress has been shown to cause degranulation of mast cells in the bladder (*1*), skin (*2–4*), dura (*5*), and the intestine (*6,7*). Several studies have shed light on possible mechanisms by which mast cells can be stimulated to degranulate by stress. Most of these investigations invoke release of neuropeptides or hormones from peripheral nerves (**Fig. 1**) because mast cells often are located adjacent to these nerve endings (*1,4,8*). In addition some of the mediators released from the nerves, such as substance P (*9*), neurotensin (*10*), and corticotrophin-releasing factor (CRF *[6]*), are known to cause mast cell degranulation. CRF is released by the hypothalamus in response to stress (*11*). In addition, CRF may be released from postganglionic sympathetic nerves

From: *Methods in Molecular Biology, vol. 315: Mast Cells: Methods and Protocols*
Edited by: G. Krishnaswamy and D. S. Chi © Humana Press Inc., Totowa, NJ

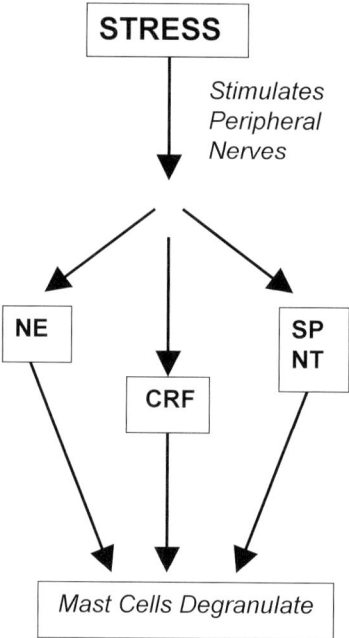

Fig. 1. Diagram to show possible mechanism for stress-induced mast cell degranulation. NE, norepinephrine; CRF, corticotrophin-releasing factor; SP, substance P; NT, neurotensin.

and/or peripheral sensory afferents *(4)*. Sympathetic nerves, in response to stress, also release norepinephrine, which can bind to α-receptors on mast cells and cause them to degranulate *(12)*.

A rat model of chronic stress will be described and two methods to demonstrate the degree of mast cell degranulation in the intestine will be presented. The first method will be applied to connective tissue mast cells in the mesentery, and the second method to mucosal mast cells in the intestinal mucosa.

2. Materials

1. Anesthetic: 5 mL of ketamine hydrochloride (100 mg/mL), 1 mL of acepromazine maleate (10 mg/mL), 2.5 mL of xylazine-20 (20 mg/mL); dose: 200 µL/100 g body weight
2. *N*-2-hydroxyethylpiperazine-*N'*-2-ethanesulfonic acid-buffer (HEPES) buffered saline, containing 0.5 g/100 mL bovine serum albumin Fraction V (Sigma, St. Louis, MO; pH 7.4).
3. Beuthanasia.
4. Formaldehyde: 3% in HEPES.

5. Alcian blue: 0.1% in 0.7 *M* HCl.
6. Safranin O: 0.5% in 0.125 *M* HCl.
7. Eosin: 0.1%.
8. Ethanol: 70%, 80%, 90%, 95%, 100%.
9. Xylene.
10. Mounting medium.
11. Karnovsky fixative, pH 7.4: gluteraldehyde (EM grade, 5 mL, 50%), formalde-hyde (12.5 mL, 16%), NaCl (0.3 g), $CaCl_2$ (0.015 g), sodium cacodylate (2.14 g), and distilled water to 100 mL.
12. Sodium cacodylate buffer (0.2 *M* and 0.15 *M*, pH 7.4).
13. Diaminobenzidine: 2% in 0.1 *M* monobasic phosphate.
14. Hydrogen peroxide.
15. Osmium tetroxide (2%).
16. Epoxy resin embedding medium (Spurr's).
17. Uranyl acetate.
18. Lead citrate.
19. Toluidine blue, pH 7.0.

3. Methods

The methods described in **Subheadings 3.1.–3.3.** outline: (1) the procedures required to reproducibly, chronically stress a rat and ensure that the control animals are unstressed; (2) the technique for staining connective tissue mast cells; and (3) the technique for preparing tissue for light and electron micros-copy for visualization of mucosal mast cells.

3.1. Animal Model for Chronic Stress

3.1.1. Pre-Experimental Treatment of Rats

On arrival in the animal facility, the rats should be placed two per cage (*see* **Note 1**). The animals should be divided into two groups and housed in two separate rooms with similar dimensions and furnishings. These rooms should be chosen so as to be remote from noisy air vents and cage washers, and should be identical with respect to background noise levels in the frequency range of 50 Hz to 10 kHz. Ambient and experimental noise sound pressure levels can be measured with a calibrated ANSI type 1 sound level meter and octave band filter. It is important that the background noise has a similar amplitude (approx 50 dB) and frequency distribution in both rooms.

The number of times personnel enter and leave the rooms should be mini-mized by only housing those rats participating in this study in the chosen rooms. A noise generator should be placed in one of the rooms and activated for 15 min each day (*see* **Note 2 *[13–15]***). This procedure has been shown to stress rats and cause mast cell degranulation after a period of 3 wk *(16,17)*. The rats in the room without the noise generator form the unstressed control group.

3.1.2. Mesenteric Surgery and Preparation for Microscopy

1. Rats are anesthetized, and when the rat has reached a suitable level of anesthesia (no eye or foot reflex), the abdomen is shaved and a tracheotomy is performed, using PE 240 tubing, so that the animal can be artificially ventilated.
2. A midline incision, from the pubis to the sternum, is made along the linea alba, the intestine is carefully externalized, and a portion of the mesentery is gently spread flat over a Plexiglas platform integrated into the Plexiglas animal surgery tray.
3. The exposed mesentery is kept warm and moist with a constant trickle of HEPES saline (pH 7.4) at 37°C.
4. Next, the HEPES is replaced by a fixative consisting of 3% formaldehyde in HEPES at 4°C, and the animal is sacrificed with an intravenous injection (0.5 mL) of Beuthanasia.
5. After 1 h, the mesenteric tissue is carefully excised and divided into separate "windows," a window being defined as the portion of mesenteric tissue bordered by two adjacent pairs of feeding arterioles and collecting venules, and the attached intestine (**Fig. 2**).
6. The intestine is cut away from the mesenteric window, as is most of the adjacent adipose fat.
7. Each window of the preparation is mounted between two thin glass cover slips using aqueous mounting medium.
8. At this point the specimens may be examined microscopically and photographed or videotaped before staining for mast cells. The subsequent mast cell staining procedure will obscure any fluorescent stains that may have been used to identify other structures earlier in the experiment.

3.1.3. Intestinal Surgery and Preparation for Microscopy

1. The rats are prepared as for the mesentery surgery and a portion of the intestine (ileum) is carefully externalized, wrapped in HEPES-soaked gauze, and positioned on a HEPES-saturated gauze platform that is arranged adjacent to the abdomen.
2. The intestine is kept warm and moist with a constant drip of HEPES at 37°C. The abdominal aorta is exposed, and a cannula is placed retrograde, distal to the superior mesenteric artery.
3. The aorta is clamped just proximal to the superior mesenteric artery, and the circulation is flushed free of blood with approx 5 mL of HEPES.
4. The animal is killed by intravenously injecting Beuthanasia, and the HEPES is replaced by phosphate-buffered Karnovsky's fixative (pH 7.4) for perfusion fixation. Pressure is maintained at 30 mmHg, and the portal vein is clamped. Fixative also is applied to the outside of the intestine.
5. After 1 h, a 4-cm segment of distal ileum is excised and divided into four equal portions; one for light microscopy and three for electron microscopy. These portions are placed in fixative for an additional hour. The tissue segments are then rinsed in 0.2 M sodium cacodylate buffer and incubated overnight in 2% diaminobenzidine (DAB) at room temperature in the dark (*see* **Note 3**).

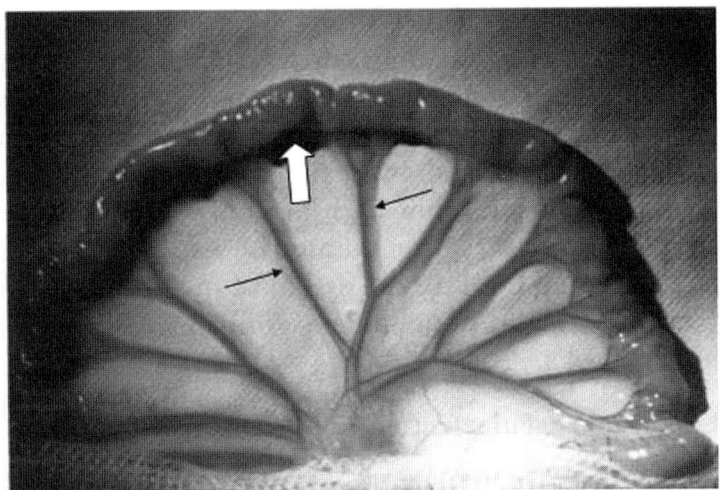

Fig. 2. Intestine and mesentery of rat, showing mesenteric windows between adjacent pairs of feeding arterioles and collecting venules. After 1 h, the mesenteric tissue is carefully excised and divided into separate "windows," a window being defined as the portion of mesenteric tissue bordered by two adjacent pairs of feeding arterioles and collecting venules (**black arrows**), and the attached intestine (**white arrow**).

6. The next day, the segments are re-immersed in DAB solution, containing H_2O_2 to a concentration of 0.2%, for 1 h, rinsed three times in 0.15 M sodium cacodylate buffer, postfixed in osmium tetroxide, dehydrated in increasing concentrations of ethanol, and embedded in Spurr's resin for light and electron microscopy.
7. The pieces of tissue are oriented in the resin so that the blocks can be sectioned longitudinally through the intestinal villi. This orientation allows the whole length of each villus to be visualized and increases the chances of seeing mast cells in the villus interstitium. Thick sections (2 µm) are cut for light microscopy and ultrathin sections for electron microscopy. These latter sections are stained with uranyl acetate and lead citrate.

3.2. Connective Tissue Mast Cells

3.2.1. Mast Cell Staining

1. Slides with mesenteric windows are rehydrated with distilled water and then stained with 0.1% Alcian blue in 0.7 M HCl for 30 min, rinsed in 0.7 M HCl, and subsequently stained with 0.5% Safranin O in 0.125 M HCl for 5 min (*see* **Note 4**).
2. They are then rinsed in distilled water, counterstained with 0.1% eosin for 30 s, and gradually dehydrated in a series of 70%, 80%, 90%, 95%, and 100% ethanol.
3. The slides are cleared in xylene and mounted with mounting medium.
4. This staining procedure is modified from Mayrhofer (*15*). For a faster, less-complicated staining technique (*see* **Note 5**).

3.2.2. Mast Cell Observation

1. Connective tissue mast cells degranulate to release biogenic amine granules, such as histamine granules, which stain blue (**Fig. 3A**). At this stage, the cell body also stains blue. The mast cells are often located near venules.
2. Intact mast cells stain blue but do not show any free granules.
3. Mast cells that are extensively degranulated are almost depleted of histamine and just show a thin rim of blue stain around the outside (**Fig. 3B**). Occasionally, the extensively degranulated mast cells show some red staining, which indicates the presence of the proteoglycan, heparin.
4. Mast cells within small windows, without a well-developed vasculature, show more of the red stain than those within the larger windows.
5. Using this staining technique, the mast cells can be classified as intact, moderately degranulated, or extensively degranulated and the major type of granule constituents can be characterized.
6. A useful way to evaluate the numbers of mast cells in each state of granulation is to examine the tissue under a ×20 power microscopic objective and count the number of cells per field of view, using a ×10 power eyepiece. Rows of fields can be counted systematically from left to right.

3.3. Mucosal Mast Cells

3.3.1. Mast Cell Staining

For light microscopy, thick sections (2-μm thick), cut longitudinally through the intestinal villi, are stained with 1% Toluidine blue (pH 7.0) for 15 min and then washed in distilled water. This technique has been modified from Conroy and Toledo (*18*).

3.3.2. Mast Cell Observation

1. The mast cells can be visualized easily under low-power (×10 objective) light microscopy. At this magnification, degranulated mast cells are easy to identify by the presence of empty vacuoles (**Fig. 4**).
2. Mucosal villi from unstressed animals rarely show vacuolated mast cells. At higher power, water-immersion objectives, such as a 340, 0.75 n/a show greater detail and the intense Toluidine blue-stained granules remaining in the mast cells can be resolved.
3. Intact mast cells show blue-stained granules in the cytoplasm but no vacuoles.
4. The total numbers of degranulated mast cells per each villus cross-section can be counted in a chosen number of villi (i.e., 20–30) per animal. If the tissue also is stained with DAB, eosinophils can be easily differentiated from mast cells because their peroxidase granules stain brown, in contrast to the mast cell granules that stain blue. A photograph of part of a villus cross-section containing eosinophils is shown in **Fig. 5**.
5. Under electron microscopy, mast cells can be identified by their granules, made electron dense by staining the sections with uranyl acetate and lead citrate (**Figs. 6** and **7**).

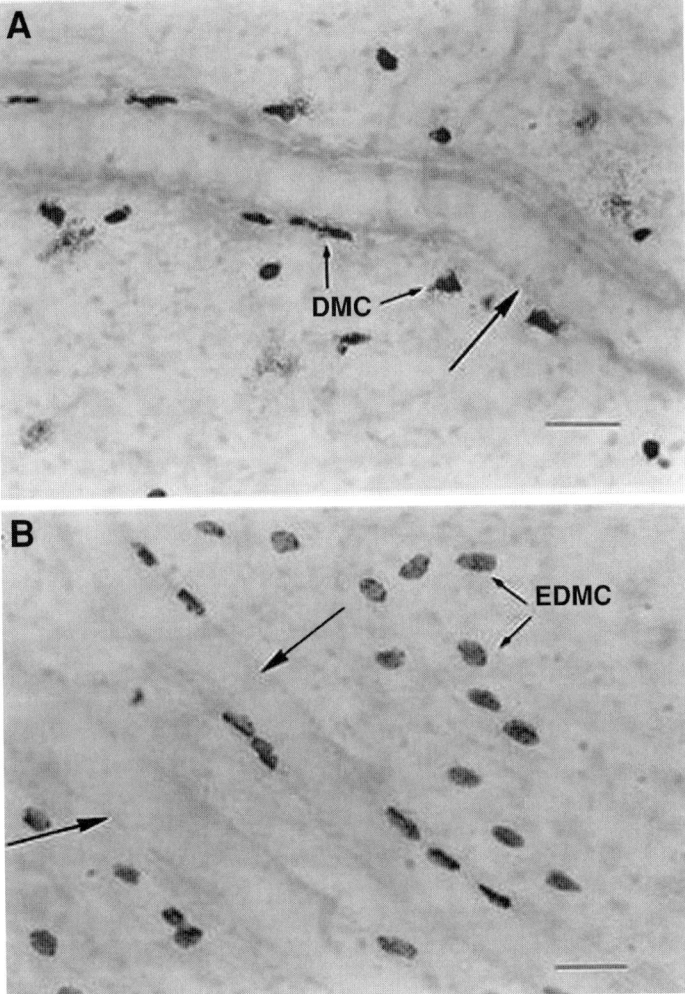

Fig. 3. Photomicrograph of degranulated mesenteric mast cells (DMCs) and extensively degranulated mast cells (EDMCs). Scale bar: 25 µm. The mast cells are often located near venules **(large arrow)**.

6. Vacuoles are seen in degranulating mast cells **(Fig. 6)**, and some areas of cytoplasm appear to be disintegrating, perhaps because a granule has just been released.
7. **Figure 7** also shows an eosinophil characterized by the oval shaped granules bisected by a thin layer of more electron-dense material.
8. Preparing the tissue for both light and electron microscopy gives one the advantage of being able to count cells over a wide area and also to determine the proximity of the mast cells to fine structures, such as peripheral nerves.

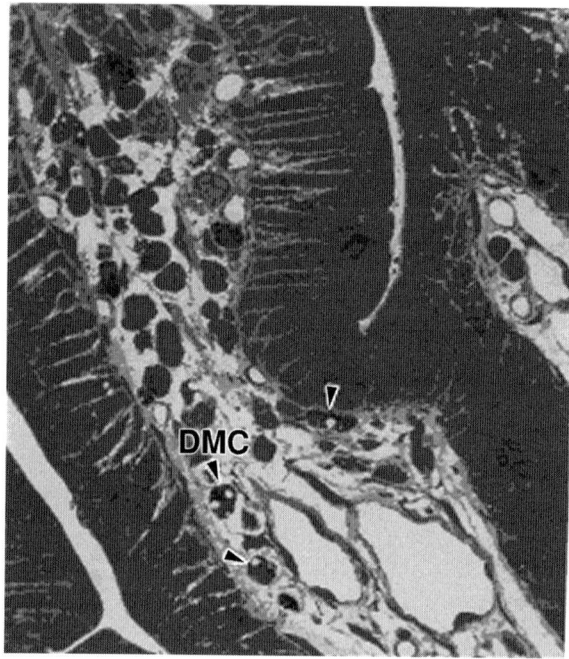

Fig. 4. Photomicrograph of section though intestinal mucosal villus showing degranulated mesenteric mast cells (DMCs). The mast cells can be visualized easily under low-power (×10 objective) light microscopy. At this magnification, degranulated mast cells are easy to identify by the presence of empty vacuoles **(arrowheads)**.

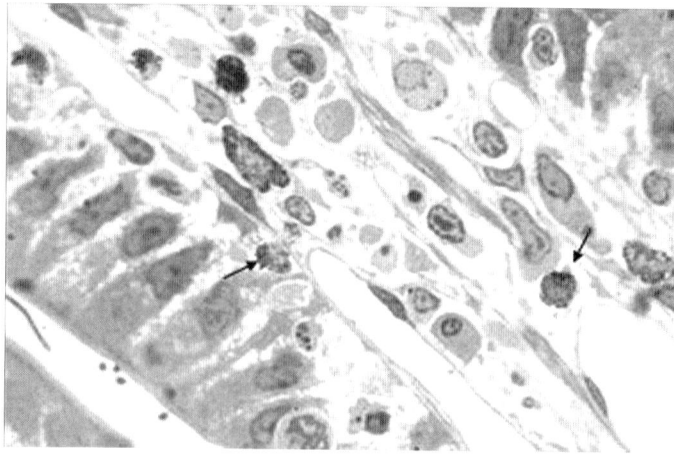

Fig. 5. Photomicrograph of section though intestinal mucosal villus showing eosinophils stained with DAB **(arrows)**.

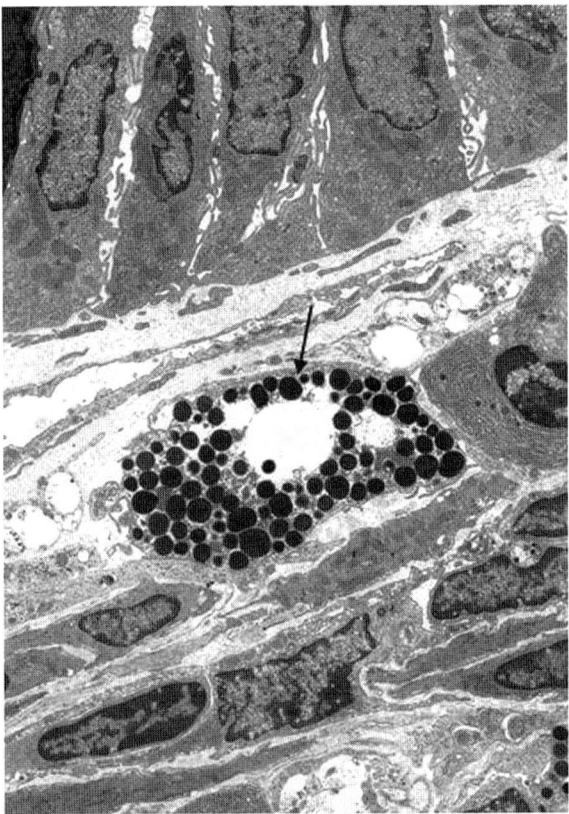

Fig. 6. Electron micrograph of section through intestinal mucosal villus showing degranulated mast cell (**arrow**).

4. Notes

1. To ensure that the animals have a low baseline level of stress, they should be housed in open wire cages (39 cm × 30 cm × 30 cm) such as those sold in pet stores for hamsters. One model that is particularly suitable has two levels linked by a wire mesh slope. In addition, it is advisable to provide each cage with woodchip bedding and one black, PVC tunnel (11 cm diameter × 17 cm length). Such a tunnel is large enough to accommodate both rats when they sleep during the day. When rats are housed in this way they rarely fight at night, unlike rats that are housed in standard, institutional cages (polycarbonate, suspended, solid-bottom cages [40.8 cm × 21.0 cm × 16.8 cm] with woodchip bedding and no other enrichment). In addition, rats housed in enriched cages as described previously, spend more than half of their time either in or on the tunnel, or on the shelf or ramp at night. Rats housed in standard cages fight continually at night and the

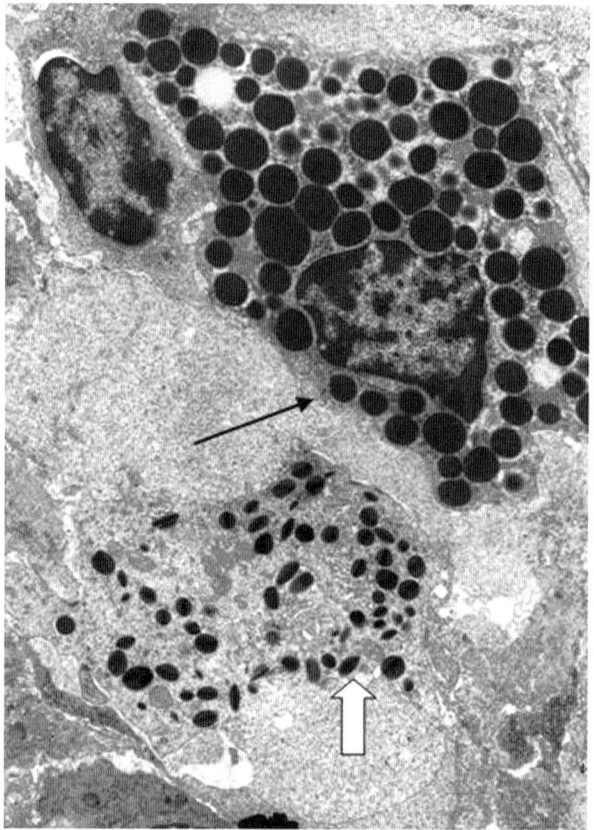

Fig. 7. Electron micrograph of section through intestinal villus showing an intact mast cell (**black arrow**) and eosinophil (**white arrow**).

fights usually involve a single "aggressor" and a single "victim." These rats also squeak frequently and show significantly more rearing than those in enriched cages. Thus rats housed in the standard cages do not provide a good, unstressed control because they are unable to avoid their cagemate if they so desire. In fact, a previous study stated that one third of bladder mast cells were degranulated in control animals, probably as a result of the stress of handling the animals and the mechanical damage during tissue removal (*1*). It is not necessary, or desirable, to accept such a high level of mast cell degranulation in control animals. In experiments in which the animals are housed appropriately, as described previously, mast cell degranulation in control animals varies between 5 and 10%.

2. An effective noise generator consists of an audio CD player with a white noise recording played in a loop mode and set to 90 dB. One speaker is positioned in the room equidistant from the animal cages. A water sprinkler timer is connected

into the circuit so that the noise is automatically activated every day at a selected time and stopped 15 min later. The noise level of 90 dB (averaged over frequencies from 10 to 10,000 Hz) is similar to that produced by cage washers and air conditioners unless adequate care is taken, and is relatively low compared with the 110-dB tolerance level of rats *(13)*. Thus, rats that are housed in many institutional animal facilities are stressed in an uncontrolled manner just by the environmental noise *(14,15)*.

3. DAB is used because it stains peroxidase-containing granules in immune cells, such as eosinophils, and thus makes the cells easier to distinguish from mast cells. The DAB is prepared as follows *(16)*: DAB (0.1 g) is added to 50 mL of 0.1 M monobasic phosphate buffer, and the pH is adjusted to 7.2 very gradually with concentrated NH_4OH. The solution becomes a light tannish-pink color. Next, the tissue squares are rinsed in distilled water. Meanwhile, 25 mL of DAB solution is added to 1.66 mL of 3% H_2O_2 to give a final concentration of 0.2%.

4. There is a wide heterogeneity in the structure and function of mast cells that has been documented both in vitro and in vivo *(19)*. For this reason the Alcian blue–Safranin method for mast cell staining is used in order to differentiate between the mast cells containing proteoglycan heparin (red stain) and those with biogenic amines (blue stain).

5. To stain mesenteric mast cells more quickly, after fixation suffuse the tissue with 1% Toluidine blue for 20 s, rinse with HEPES-buffered saline (pH 7.4), and remount. Degranulated mast cells can be recognized by the presence of intracellular granules released into the surrounding tissue. This technique is fast and simple but it has the disadvantages that the Toluidine blue diffuses from the mast cells into the tissue very quickly (within 20 min), and that only the histamine is visualized, not the heparin.

Acknowledgments

This work was funded by NIH grant R21 AT 1124.

References

1. Spanos, C., Pang, X., Ligris, K., et al. (1997) Stress-induced bladder mast cell activation: implications for interstitial cystitis. *J. Urol.* **157,** 669–672.
2. Kimata, H. (2003) Enhancement of allergic skin wheal responses in patients with atopic eczema/dermatitis syndrome by playing video games or by a frequently ringing mobile phone. *Eur. J. Clin. Invest.* **33,** 513–517.
3. Singh, L. K., Pang, X., Alexacos, N., Letourneau, R., and Theoharides, C. (1999) Acute immobilization stress triggers skin mast cell degranulation via corticotrophin releasing hormone, neurotensin, and substance P: a link to neurogenic skin disorders. *Brain Behav. Immun.* **13,** 225–239.
4. Theoharides, T. C., Singh, L. K., Boucher, W., et al. (1998) Corticotropin-releasing hormone induces skin mast cell degranulation and increased vascular permeability, a possible explanation for its proinflammatory effects. *Endocrinology* **139,** 403–413.

5. Theoharides, T. C., Spanos, C. P., Pang, X., et al. (1995) Stress-induced intracranial mast cell degranulation. A corticotrophin releasing hormone-mediated effect. *Endocrinology* **136,** 5745–5750.

6. Castagliuolo, I., LaMont, J. T., Qiu, B., et al. (1996) Acute stress causes mucin release from rat colon: role of corticotrophin releasing factor and mast cells. *Am. J. Physiol.* **271,** 884–892.

7. Soderholm, J. D., Yang, P. C., Ceponis, P., et al. (2002) Chronic stress induces mast cell-dependent bacterial adherence and initiates mucosal inflammation in rat intestine. *Gastroenterology* **123,** 1099–1108.

8. Skofitsch, G., Savitt, J. M., and Jacobowitz, D. M. (1985) Suggestive evidence for a functional unit between mast cells and substance P fibres in the rat diaphragm and mesentery. *Histochemistry* **82,** 5–8.

9. Fewtrell, C. M. S., Foreman, J. C., Jordan, C. C., Oehme, P., Renner, H., and Stewart, J. M. (1982) The effects of substance P on histamine and 5-hydroxytryptamine release in the rat. *J. Physiol.* **330,** 393–411.

10. Alexacos, N., Pang, X., Boucher, W. Cochrane, D. E., Sant, G. R., and Theoharides, T. C. (1999) Neurotensin mediates rat bladder mast cell degranulation triggered by acute psychological stress. *Urology* **53,** 1035–1040.

11. Imaki, T., Xiao-Quan, W., Shibasaki, T., et al. (1995) Stress-induced activation of neuronal activity and corticotrophin-releasing factor gene expression in the paraventricular nucleus is modulated by glucocorticoids in rats. *J. Clin. Invest.* **96,** 231–238.

12. Playfair, J. H. L. (1996) *Immunology at a Glance, Sixth edition.* Blackwell Science, London, UK.

13. Riley, V. (1981) Psychoneuroendocrine influences on immunocompetence and neoplasia. *Science* **212,** 1100–1109.

14. Milici, A. J. and Bankston, P. W. (1982) Fetal and neonatal rat intestinal capillaries: permeability to carbon, ferritin, hemoglobin and myoglobin. *Am. J. Anat.* **165,** 165–186.

15. Mayrhofer, G. (1980) Fixation and staining of granules in mucosal mast cells and intraepithelial lymphocytes in the rat jejunum, with special reference to the relationship between the acid glycosaminoglycans in the two cell types. *Histochem. J.* **12,** 513–526.

16. Baldwin, A. L. and Wilson, L. M. (1999) Effects of noise on mesenteric permeability in the rat. *FASEB J.* **13,** 1.3, A1.

17. Baldwin, A. L. (2000) Effect of noise on the intestinal exchange barrier. *FASEB J.* **14,** 315, A22.

18. Conroy, J. D. and Toledo, A. B. (1976) Metachromasia and improved histologic detail with toluidine blue-hematoxylin and eosin. *Veterinary Pathol.* **13,** 78–80.

19. Katz, H. R., Stevens, R. L., and Austen, K. F. (1985) Heterogeneity of mammalian mast cells differentiated in vivo and in vitro. *J. Allergy Clin. Immunol.* **76,** 250–259.

VIII

Roles of Mast Cells in Host Defense

27

In Vivo Models for Studying Mast Cell-Dependent Responses to Bacterial Infection

Christopher P. Shelburne, James B. McLachlan, and Soman N. Abraham

Summary

Mast cells are a critical component of host defense against bacterial infections. Activation of these cells during infection induces both innate and adaptive aspects of protective immunity needed for the elimination of the bacteria and survival of the host. These functional roles for the mast cell have been principally characterized using two in vivo models of acute bacterial infection featuring Gram-negative pathogens such as *Escherichia coli*. Here, we present basic protocols for the identification of mast cell-dependent biological functions during bacterial infection. These include the use of mast cell-deficient mice, the identification of mast cells in tissue, the culture of uropathogenic *E. coli*, and the basic analysis of mast cell-dependent functions in the peritoneal cavity and footpad models of bacterial pathogenesis.

Key Words: Mast cell; bacteria; *E. coli*; UPEC; tumor necrosis factor; peritoneal cavity; footpad; draining popliteal lymph node.

1. Introduction

Mast cells are granulated leukocytes present in most vascularized tissues but are especially prominent along host–environmental interfaces, such as the skin, lung, and intestines *(1)*. The activation of these cells is primarily associated with pathogenic inflammatory reactions such as that found in IgE-dependent hypersensitivity reactions *(2,3)*, autoimmune conditions, or fibrosis *(4–7)*. However, recent evidence has suggested that mast cells contribute beneficial functions to both innate and adaptive immunity during infection. For instance, mast cell activation is required for the clearance of bacteria at the sites of infection *(8,9)*, as well as for the sequestration of lymphocytes in distal draining lymph nodes after bacterial infection in tissue *(10)*.

From: *Methods in Molecular Biology, vol. 315: Mast Cells: Methods and Protocols*
Edited by: G. Krishnaswamy and D. S. Chi © Humana Press Inc., Totowa, NJ

Here, we present protocols that this laboratory has used to characterize mast cell-dependent functional responses to infectious challenge by Gram-negative pathogens such as *Escherichia coli*. These protocols characterize the use of genetically mast cell-deficient mice, the detection of mast cells in tissue, the preparation and injection of pathogenic *E. coli*, and the analysis of two separate mast cell dependent biological functions in two in vivo settings, the peritoneal cavity and the footpad.

2. Materials

2.1. Studying the Role of Mast Cells in Bacterial Infection In Vivo and Bone Marrow-Derived Mast Cells

1. Mast cell-deficient WBB6F1-W/W^v mice at 4–6 wk of age (Jackson Laboratories, Bar Harbor, ME).
2. Congenic littermate control WWB6F1-+/+ mice at 4–6 wk of age (Jackson Laboratories).
3. Complete RPMI medium (cRPMI): 10% fetal bovine serum (FBS), 100 U/mL penicillin, 0.1 mg/mL streptomycin, 25 m*M* HEPES, 2 m*M* L-glutamine, 1 m*M* sodium pyruvate, 1 m*M* nonessential amino acids, and 1 m*M* MEM amino acids (Invitrogen, Carlsbad, CA). cRPMI should be filter sterilized and stored at 4°C.
4. Recombinant interleukin-3 (R&D Systems, Minneapolis, MN), reconstituted in cRPMI and stored in 100-µL aliquots at 5 µg/mL at –80°C.
5. Recombinant stem cell factor (R&D Systems) reconstituted in cRPMI and stored in 100-µL aliquots at 5 µg/mL at –80°C (optional).
6. Sterile Tissue Forceps (Roboz Surgical Instrument, Gaitherburg, MD).
7. Sterile Scissors (Roboz Surgical Instrument).
8. 10-mL syringes (Becton Dickinson, San Diego, CA).
9. 22.5 gage 1.5-cm needles (Becton Dickinson).
10. 50-mL polypropylene tubes.
11. Ethanol 70%.
12. 75-cm^3 tissue culture flasks.

2.2. Preparation of E. coli

1. Uropathogenic *E. coli* strain J96.
2. Luria-Bertani medium.
3. MacConkey agar plates.
4. 10% bleach.

2.3. Identification of Mast Cells in Tissue

1. Prepared tissue sections.
2. Blocking buffer: 1% bovine serum albumin, 10% fetal calf serum (FCS) in 1X phosphate-buffered saline (PBS), pH 7.2.
3. Alexa-488 labeled avidin (Molecular Probes, Eugene, OR).

4. ProLong anti-fade reagent (Molecular Probes).
5. Carnoy's Fixative: 60% ethanol, 30% chloroform, and 10% glacial acetic acid. This medium should be prepared fresh each time.
6. Toluidine blue-O (EM Science, Gibbstown, NJ).
7. Toludine blue-O Solution: 0.5 g of toluidine blue-O in 99.5 mL in 0.5 N HCl. It may take a while for the toluidine blue to go into solution. Filter the solution after preparation and store at room temperature.
8. Xylenes.
9. 100%, 95%, 70%, and 50% ethanol (these should be freshly prepared).
10. Eosin Y.
11. Shandon Cytospin, cytoclips, absorbent pads, and cytofunnels.

2.4. Study of Mast Cell-Dependent Functions in the Peritoneal Cavity During Bacterial Infection

1. Commercial mouse restraint system (Plas Labs, Lansing MI).
2. 1-mL syringes (Becton Dickinson).
3. 30 gage 0.5-cm needles (Becton Dickinson).
4. Hank's Balanced Salt Solution (HBSS) without calcium, magnesium, or phenol Red (Invitrogen).
5. Sterile glass pipets.
6. anti-$F_c\gamma$RII/III (Clone 2.4G2; Becton Dickinson BioSciences).
7. FITC-conjugated Rat IgG2b anti-mouse GR-1 antibody (Clone RB6.8C5; Becton Dickinson BioSciences).
8. FITC-conjugated Rat IgG2b isotype-matched control (Clone A95-1; Becton Dickinson BioSciences).
9. PE-conjugated rat IgG2a anti-mouse neutrophil antibody (Clone 7/4; Caltag, Burlingame, CA).
10. PE-conjugated Rat IgG2a isotype matched control (Clone R35-95; Becton Dickinson BioSciences).
11. Tumor Necrosis Factor enzyme-linked immunoassay (ELISA) Kit (R&D Systems).

2.5. Studies of Mast Cell-Dependent Functions in the Footpad

1. Microdissecting scissors (Roboz Surgical Instrument Company).
2. Microdissecting tweezers (Roboz Surgical Instrument Company).
3. Collagenase Type IA (Sigma, St. Louis, MO).
4. 70-μM cell straining filter (Becton Dickinson Biosciences).
5. Ethylene diamine tetraacetic acid (EDTA) solution: prepare a 100 mM solution in 1X PBS and adjust the pH to 7.2.
6. Fluorescein isothiocyanate (FITC)-conjugated hamster anti-mouse $CD3_e$ chain (Clone 17A2; Becton Dickinson Biosciences).
7. FITC-conjugated hamster IgG isotype matched control (Clone A19-3; Becton Dickinson Biosciences).
8. PE-conjugated rat anti-mouse CD4 (Clone L3T4; Becton Dickinson Biosciences).

9. PE-conjugated rat IgG2a isotype matched control (Clone R35-95; Becton Dickinson Biosciences).
10. Biotin-conjugated rat anti-mouse B220 (Clone RA3-6B2; Becton Dickinson Biosciences).
11. Biotin-conjugated rat IgG2a isotype matched control (Clone R35-95; Becton Dickinson Biosciences).
12. Strepavidin-cychrome (Becton Dickinson Biosciences).
13. 4% paraformaldehyde: mix 4 g of paraformaldehyde (Sigma) into 95 mL of 1X PBS. This will require heating of the solution and mixing with a stir-bar. Once the paraformaldehyde has gone into solution, let it cool, and adjust the pH to 7.2. Add 1X PBS to a total volume of 100 mL. This solution should be freshly prepared prior to use each time or stored at $-80°C$.
14. Flow Cytometer (FACscan; Becton Dickinson Biosciences).
15. MPER protein extraction buffer (Pierce, Rockford, IL).
16. Complete protease inhibitor tablets (Roche, Indianapolis, IN).
17. TRIzol buffer (Invitrogen).
18. Maxim Biotech Multi-Cytokine reverse transcription polymerase chain reaction (RT-PCR) Kit (San Francisco, CA).
19. PCR Thermocycler.
20. Agarose and Gel Apparatus Equipment.
21. Ethidum Bromide
22. Eagle Eye II Cabinet (Stratagene, La Jolla, CA) or UV gel box.

3. Methods

3.1. Studying the Role of Mast Cells in Bacterial Infection In Vivo

Characterization of mast cell-dependent processes in vivo has been greatly aided by the use of mice that are genetically deficient in mast cells. Although several genetically mast cell-deficient strains of mice exist, the most widely used is the WBB6F1-Kit^{W}/Kit^{W-v} (W/W^v) strain, which contains less than 0.1% of the total number of mast cells found in their congenic littermates (11). The genetic defect in these mice is intrinsic to the mast cell and does not appear to affect the tissue environment or the expression of proteins required for mast cell viability in vivo. Therefore, W/W^v mice may be selectively or systemically reconstituted with mast cells derived from genetically compatible mice. This very valuable feature permits confirmation that: (1) any observed functional deficiency in W/W^v mice is in fact caused by the absence of mast cells; and (2) that the observed functional deficiency is not to the result of any of the additional system abnormalities present in these mice, which include anemia, a lack of cutaneous melanocytes, germ cells, and interstitial cells of Cajal (11).

Examination of mast cell-dependent biological functions during bacterial infection should follow this general protocol. (1) Determine that a functional deficiency exists between W/W^v mice and wild-type congenic controls after bacterial challenge. (2) Determine that either local or systemic reconstitution

Table 1
Procedure for the Analysis of Mast Cell-Dependent
Biological Responses During Bacterial Challenge In Vivo

1. Establish that a functional deficiency exists in mast cell-deficient W/W^v mice relative to congenic wild-type mast cell-sufficient mice after bacterial challenge.
2. Determine whether the biological response can be repaired by reconstitution of W/W^v mice with mast cells. This repair will determine whether the functional deficiency is truly mast cell dependent and not the result of other defects present in W/W^v mice.
3. Determine the mechanism by which mast cells contribute to the biological response by reconstituting W/W^v mice with mast cells containing gene-specific gene deletions or modifications.

of W/W^v mice with mast cells repairs the observed functional deficiency. (3) Finally, determine the contribution of specific mast cell proteins to the biological response in question by reconstituting W/W^v mice with mast cells deficient in those proteins or containing mutations that alter the function of those proteins (**Table 1**).

3.2. Bone Marrow-Derived Mast Cells

Mast cells are rather difficult to procure from tissue in the large numbers required for the reconstitution of W/W^v mice. This problem is circumvented by the use of mast cells cultured from bone marrow. This procedure involves obtaining bone marrow from murine femurs, and culturing the cells in the presence of interleukin (IL)-3 for 4 wk (*12*). Reintroduction of these cultured mast cells into W/W^v mice will successfully repopulate most tissues, where they will adopt phenotypic characteristics of mast cells found in wild-type littermates (*12*).

IL-3 may be obtained from recombinant sources or from the supernatant of the WEHI-3 monomyelocytic leukemia cell line (*13*). In most cases, mast cells can be successfully generated from bone marrow using this protocol, even when the mice are genetically deficient in select genes (*see* **Note 1**). In cases where genetically deficient mice are not viable, mast cells may alternatively be cultured from fetal liver (*14*), or directly from embryonic stem cells as has been reported (*15*).

3.2.1. Preparation of Mast Cells From Bone Marrow

1. Sacrifice four mice by CO_2 inhalation.
2. Thoroughly soak the mice with 70% ethanol (*see* **Note 2**).
3. Remove the femurs and scrape them free of tissue with your scissors, then place them into a dish containing ice-cold cRPMI.
4. Attach a 10-mL syringe to a 26 gage 1.5 cm needle, and fill it with ice-cold cRPMI.

5. Gently grind the needle into the end of one of the procured femurs.
6. Holding the femur over a tube with forceps, gently push the syringe plunger to force the cRPMI into the femur. The bone marrow within the femur will be flushed into the tube. Repeat this for the remaining femurs.
7. Place the tube on ice and let any particulate fragments of bone settle to the bottom.
8. Remove the cell suspension to a fresh tube and centrifuge the cells at 300 RCF for 10 min at 4°C.
9. Remove the supernatant and slurry the cell pellet.
10. Resuspend the cells in ice cold cRPMI.
11. Count the cells by Trypan blue exclusion. Adjust the cells to 1 million mononuclear cells/mL in cRPMI containing 5 ng/mL IL-3, or 10% WEHI-3 conditioned medium (*see* **Note 3**).
12. Culture the bone marrow cells for 4 wk. Every 2–3 d, the nonadherent fraction should be removed from the adherent fraction and placed into a fresh flask with fresh medium (*see* **Note 4**).
13. After 4 wk, mast cells should comprise nearly 100% of the culture. This should be confirmed by staining cytospin preparations of the mast cell culture with Toluidine Blue.
14. Cultures can be expanded and maintained in bulk for several months in the presence of 5 ng/mL IL-3 with or without 10 ng/mL stem cell factor (SCF; *see* **Note 5**).

3.3. Preparation of E. coli

Infection of host tissues by Gram-negative opportunistic pathogens such as *E. coli* is usually resolved by the host immune response. Therefore, use of these pathogens, as opposed to more sophisticated immunosuppressive bacterial pathogens such as *Salmonella typhimurium*, is an opportunity to study what happens during a successful host immune response to infection. The uropathogenic *E. coli* strain J96 (UPEC) is easily cultured in traditional medium such as Luria Broth (LB). In our studies, we use log phase UPEC. This ensures that the injected bacterial suspension is consistently viable and active from experiment to experiment (*see* **Note 6**).

1. Place 5 mL of sterile LB medium into a 50-mL tube.
2. Obtain a small frozen piece of UPEC stock with a sterile pipet tip, and place it into the sterile LB.
3. Place the culture into a 37°C incubator and culture overnight.
4. The next morning, transfer 100 μL of the static phase UPEC culture to 6 mL of fresh sterile LB.
5. Place the culture into a 37°C incubator and shake the culture for 2 h.
6. Wash the culture free of LB by adding 44 mL of 1X PBS to the UPEC culture and centrifuge the culture at 3000*g* RCF for 10 min.
7. Drain the pellet by decanting the supernatant into 10% bleach.
8. Slurry the pellet, and resuspend the pellet in 5 mL of sterile saline.

9. Determine the number of UPEC present by spectrophotometric analysis at O.D.$_{600}$. A typical O.D. should be between 0.05 and 0.1.
10. UPEC total numbers can be determined by multiplying the optical density (OD)$_{600}$ X 1×10^9 to give you UPEC per milliliter of saline.

3.4. Identification of Mast Cells in Tissue

A requirement for the study of mast cells in vivo is the ability to detect their presence in the tissue of interest. This may be accomplished by any one of several histochemical staining techniques that will allow a determination of the total number of mast cells in a given tissue, the spatial orientation of mast cells relative to other cells or pertinent structures, and a determination that a particular tissue in W/W^v mice has been successfully reconstituted with mast cells.

Another useful feature of mast cells that can be assessed by the same staining techniques used to detect their presence is their granularity. Most mast cell-dependent functional responses feature a rapid exocytic process termed degranulation, whereby mast cells release preformed granules containing mediators, such as histamine, tumor necrosis factor, serotonin, and numerous proteases. Therefore, determination that a mast cell has undergone degranulation is a good indicator that mast cells may participate in a particular biological response (*see* **Note 7**). Most methods used to detect mast cells in tissue rely on techniques that depend on the presence of mast cell granule constituents such as heparin. Therefore, the presence of mast cells in tissue and their activation status can be assessed simultaneously.

3.4.1. Identification of Mast Cells in Frozen Tissue: Avidin

Avidin is a glycoprotein with a specific binding affinity for heparin, a major constituent of mast cell granules *(16)*. The use of avidin coupled to fluorochromes offers several practical advantages to the routine detection of mast cells in tissue: (1) it can be used in conjunction with other fluorochrome coupled antibodies to detect additional cells or epitopes; and (2) it can be used to detect mast cells in tissues that have undergone extreme fixation treatments such as when decalcifying tissue to remove bone. Although there are many avidin–fluorochrome products, we prefer avidin coupled to Alexa-488 from Molecular Probes, Inc. This is a highly stable and very bright fluorochrome relative to other fluorochromes such as FITC. Avidin-Alexa-488 will stain individual granules of mast cells in tissue that can be easily identified as tiny spherical bodies in the main body of the mast cell (*see* **Note 8**). Please note that strepavidin does not bind to mast cell granules.

1. Rehydrate prepared tissue sections in blocking buffer for 1 h at room temperature.
2. Dilute stock avidin-Alexa-488 1:1000 in blocking buffer.

3. Remove blocking solution from tissue sections, and add avidin-Alexa-488 solution to tissue sections for 1 h at room temperature in the dark.
4. Wash the sections three times in room temperature with 1 mL of 1X PBS for 10 min.
5. Cover slip the slide with Molecular Probes anti-fade Pro-long reagent. Be certain to remove all of the air-bubbles. Let the slide dry.
6. Analyze the tissue sections by fluorescent microscopy. Excitation of Alexa-488 can be achieved by a 488-nm laser and detected by optical filter sets that permit visualization of green light, around 515 nm (*see* **Note 9**).
7. View sections with a ×20 objective to count cells.

3.4.2. Identification of Mast Cells by Toluidine Blue Staining

Toluidine blue is an aniline dye that is widely used to identify mast cells and to determine the granular status of mast cells. Interaction of toluidine blue with mast cell granules induces this stain to undergo a metachromatic shift in color from blue to a deep purple. This staining technique can be done on frozen or paraffin embedded tissues, as well as cytospin preparations. It may also be used in conjunction with colorimetric techniques to detect other cells or cell products in tissue (*17,18*).

3.4.2.1. STAINING FROZEN TISSUE SECTIONS WITH TOLUIDINE BLUE

1. Cut thin 5-μm sections and place onto slides.
2. Fix tissue sections for 1 h in Carnoy's fixative.
3. Stain sections for 45 min at room temperature with 0.5% toluidine blue solution.
4. Rinse the slides with distilled water.
5. View sections with a ×20 objective to count mast cells.

3.4.2.2. STAINING OF PARAFFIN-EMBEDDED SECTIONS WITH TOLUIDINE BLUE

1. Fix thinly cut tissue in Carnoy's fixative for at least 1 h. Carnoy's fixative must be present in at least a 10-fold excess volume of the sample. The sample must be cut thin enough to allow penetration of the fixative.
2. Embed samples in paraffin.
3. Cut paraffin embedded sections to 4–6 μm.
4. Dry slides in 60°C oven for 30 min.
5. Deparaffinize sections by serially transferring slides into xylene twice (5 min each), 100% ethanol (two changes for 2 min each), 95% ethanol (two changes), 70% ethanol (two changes), 50% ethanol (two changes), followed by transfer to deionized water.
6. Stain sections in 0.5% toluidine blue solution overnight.
7. Rinse slides three times in deionized water.
8. Counterstain in Eosin Y for 30 s to 1 min.
9. Rinse slides in deionized water.
10. Dehydrate the sections in two changes of 95% and two changes of 100% alcohols.
11. Clear slides in two changes of Xylenes.

12. Cover slip the slide.
13. View sections with a ×20 objective to count mast cells.

3.4.2.3. STAINING CYTOSPIN PREPARATIONS WITH TOLUIDINE BLUE

This approach should be used when staining cultured mast cells or when you want to specifically detect mast cells in peritoneal lavage fluid.

1. Using a Shandon cytospin, cytospin 100 µL of cells or 200 µL of peritoneal exudates onto a clean slide at 600 RPM for 6 min. The volume used will ultimately be dependent upon the cell concentration in the sample. It is important not to cytospin too many cells onto the slide.
2. Air-dry the cytospin slides.
3. Flood the slide with 0.5% toludine blue solution for 5 min.
4. Rinse the slide three times with distilled water.
5. Cover slip the slide with mounting medium and view with a ×20 objective.

3.4.2.4. DETERMINATION OF MAST CELL DEGRANULATION

Mast cell degranulation is determined by comparing an unchallenged control sample with the challenged sample. Typically, the granules in a nondegranulated mast cell are tightly associated with the cellular body with no evidence of discharge. The granules will be purple in color. A degranulated mast cell will exhibit comparatively fewer granules located within the cell body, with evidence of many exuded granules loosely associated with the outside of the cell. These released granules will be purple or blue in color (*see* **Note 10**).

3.5. Study of Mast Cell-Dependent Functions in the Peritoneal Cavity During Bacterial Infection

The peritoneal cavity has been widely used as a model site for the study of mast cell-dependent biological responses during bacterial infection. Infection models include the cecal ligation and puncture technique (*9,19*), as well as the direct injection of bacterial pathogens such as *E. coli* (*8*). We favor the latter approach because the pathogen is defined and the approach is less susceptible to experimental variations that can occur during the cecal ligation and puncture surgical procedure. As a model site to study bacterial infection, the peritoneal cavity is readily accessible to injection and for the extraction of cells or cell products for analysis. The peritoneal cavity of W/W^v mice is also easily reconstituted with mast cells. Here, we will describe the procedures used to study the mast cell recruitment of neutrophils during bacterial infection.

3.5.1. Reconstitution of Mast Cells Into the Peritoneal Cavity of W/W^N Mice

1. Resuspend cultured mast cells in sterile saline at a concentration of 1×10^8 cells/mL.

2. Fill a 1-mL syringe with the mast cell preparation, and attached a 27 gage 0.5-cm needle. Be certain to remove any air bubbles or excess air. Place the syringe to one side.

3. Firmly grip a W/W^v mouse behind the head and secure the tail so that the mouse is prostrate in your hand.

4. Flip the mouse over with the abdomen facing upwards and tilt the head slightly forward towards the ground.

5. Insert the needle of the syringe into the lower right hand quadrant of the abdomen, and inject 100 µL of the cells (1×10^7 cells).

6. Mice should be allowed to recover for a minimum of 5 wk.

7. Before experimentation, some mast cell reconstituted W/W^v mice should be examined after the 5-wk period for the presence of mast cells to demonstrate that the reconstitution was successful.

8. Subsequent experiments should be performed with age matched wild-type congenic controls and nonreconstituted W/W^v mice.

3.5.2. Injection of Bacteria Into the Peritoneal Cavity

1. Resuspend UPEC at 1×10^7 bacteria/mL in sterile saline.

2. Fill a 1-mL syringe with the UPEC preparation and attach a 30 gage 0.5-cm needle. Be certain to remove any bubbles or excess air from the syringe.

3. Firmly grip a mouse behind the head and secure the tail so that the mouse is prostrate in your hand.

4. Flip the mouse over with the abdomen facing upwards, and tilt the head slightly forward towards the ground.

5. Insert the needle of the syringe into the lower right hand quadrant of the abdomen, and inject 100 µL of the cells (1×10^6 UPEC).

6. The viability and concentration of the UPEC inoculum should be confirmed by culturing serial dilutions of the inoculum on LB plates, overnight at 37°C.

3.5.3. Lavage of the Peritoneal Cavity

One of the principal functional responses to UPEC-induced mast cell activation in the peritoneal cavity is the rapid recruitment of neutrophils. Neutrophil recruitment is required to clear the bacterial burden; therefore, determination of total neutrophil numbers and the total number of UPEC in the peritoneal cavity are suitable endpoints for determining that mast cells have reacted to the presence of a pathogen. Determination of the types of cells present in the peritoneal cavity, as well as the determination of bacterial numbers, can be assessed by obtaining the components of the peritoneal cavity with a lavage.

1. Fill a 10-mL syringe with ice-cold HBSS and attach a 22 gage 1.5 cm needle.

2. Sacrifice the mice by CO_2 inhalation (*see* **Note 11**).

3. Turn the mouse over (abdomen side up) and pin the mouse down through the arm pits.

4. Thoroughly wet the mouse with 70% ethanol.

5. Using a pair of tissue forceps, gently grab and lift the skin at the base of the abdomen, and make a midline incision along the abdomen using a pair of sharp scissors. Be certain to cut only the skin and not the underlying peritoneal membrane.
6. Using the tissue forceps, gently pinch and lift a small portion of the exposed peritoneal membrane near the base of the mouse. Insert the needle of the syringe filled with ice-cold HBSS, bevel side up, through the peritoneal membrane held by the forceps.
7. Inject 5 mL of ice-cold HBSS into the peritoneal cavity taking care not to introduce additional puncture holes into the peritoneal membrane or any or the underlying organs. Gently withdraw the needle (*see* **Note 12**).
8. Gently massage the inflated peritoneal cavity to induce peritoneal cells to dislodge into the HBSS.
9. To retrieve the peritoneal exudate (the HBSS with cells), begin by placing a sterile glass pipet into a pipetteman and place to one side within easy reach.
10. Gently grab the peritoneal membrane with forceps and pull slightly upwards. This position will have to be maintained for **steps 11–13**.
11. Weaken the membrane near the point held by the forceps with a pair of sharp scissors. Do not cut through the membrane.
12. Gently work the pipet attached to the pipetteman through the weakened membrane.
13. Once the pipet is through the membrane, gently draw the fluid out and place into a fresh tube on ice. Continue to retrieve the peritoneal exudates until most of the 5-mL volume has been retrieved.
14. Record the total collected volume per mouse.

3.5.4. Detection of Neutrophils in the Peritoneal Cavity

The detection of neutrophils can be performed in several ways, including myeloperoxidase activity assays *(8)*, or by counting the number of neutrophils on cytospin preparations of peritoneal exudates stained with the Wright-Giemsa stain *(20)*. We assess neutrophil numbers by staining peritoneal exudates for two neutrophil markers using the anti-GR-1 and anti-7/4 antibodies, followed by analysis by flow cytometry. Very few neutrophils should be detected in the peritoneal cavities of saline or unchallenged mice.

1. Inject UPEC or saline into the peritoneal cavity as described.
2. At 1, 3, 6, 12, 24, or 48 h, collect the peritoneal lavage fluid and adjust the cell suspension to 1 million cells/mL of cRPMI.
3. Add 10 μg/mL anti-$F_c\gamma$RII/III for 30 min on ice.
4. Add 2.5 μg/mL of FITC-labeled anti-GR-1 and 2.5 μg/mL PE-labeled anti-7/4 antibodies or FITC- and PE-labeled isotype matched controls to the appropriate samples.
5. Incubate samples for 30 min on ice.
6. Wash samples with 10 mL of ice-cold 1X PBS.
7. Decant supernatant, dry the tube, slurry the cells, and add 4% freshly prepared paraformaldehyde.
8. Analyze the samples by flow cytometry.

3.5.5. Determination of UPEC Numbers in the Peritoneal Cavity

Total UPEC numbers can be assessed by plating serial dilutions of the peritoneal lavage fluid on MacConkey agar plates. Plates are incubated at 37°C overnight, and colonies are counted the next day. A differential in total UPEC numbers in the peritoneal lavage fluid derived from W/W^v mice, wild-type mice, and mast cell reconstituted W/W^v mice can be best appreciated several hours after infection.

3.5.6. Detection of Tumor Necrosis Factor in Peritoneal Exudates

Tumor necrosis factor (TNF) is a proinflammatory cytokine made by many types of cells, including mast cells, macrophages, and neutrophils. Mast cells are the only cell type known to presynthesize and store this cytokine in its granules *(21)*. Therefore, mast cells are an important source of this cytokine, especially during the early stages of bacterial infection. Mast cell-derived TNF is absolutely required for the recruitment of neutrophils during bacterial infection *(8,9)*. This protocol also can be used to detect additional mast cell products or additional cytokines.

1. Obtain peritoneal exudates by lavage as described.
2. Centrifuge peritoneal lavage fluid at 300 RCF for 10 min at 4°C to remove cells.
3. Add complete protease inhibitors prepared in HBSS to a final 1X concentration.
4. Perform an ELISA on the samples using an ELISA kit. Typically, TNF levels derived from wild-type or mast cell reconstituted mice can be maximally detected within 1 h.

3.6. Studies of Mast Cell-Dependent Functions in the Footpad

The footpad represents a tissue site long used by immunologists to study the effects of pathogens or adjuvants on the recruitment of different cells types and their organization in the local popliteal draining lymph node *(22)*. We adopted this model to study the effects of footpad mast cells on the recruitment of T- and B-lymphocyte populations into the draining lymph node during bacterial infection. The use of the footpad model is advantageous because the popliteal lymph node is the sole draining lymph node for this tissue. Furthermore, the footpad is very accessible and relatively easy to inject. This site also may be a more relevant model for the study of bacterial infection in that the footpad contains significant tissue barriers not present in the peritoneal cavity.

3.6.1. Reconstitution of Mast Cells Into the Footpad of W/W^v Mice

1. Prepare a 1-mL syringe attached to a 27 gage 0.5-cm needle containing 5 million bone marrow-derived cells per 20 µL volume of sterile saline. The bone marrow derived mast cells should be derived from an autologous donor.
2. Turn the needle so that the bevel side corresponds to the measurement markings on the side of the syringe.
3. To inject the mast cells into the W/W^v footpad, pull a mouse into a restraint with the relevant footpad protruding. Push the restraining bolt onto the snout of the

mouse making certain that the snout is centered in the opening of the bolt. Failure to do this could cause the mouse to suffocate.

4. Remove the cap from the needle of the syringe. Place the syringe to one side.
5. Tightly grab the toes of the extended foot and pull slightly outward. This should expose the whole of the footpad. Keep a firm grip, as the mouse may jerk when the needle is inserted.
6. Gently wipe the footpad with a clean Kimwipe.
7. Subcutaneously insert the needle, bevel side up, into the foot.
8. Gently press the plunger and expel 20 µL of the mast cell suspension into the foot as determined by the measurement markings.
9. Hold the needle in place for 5–10 s and then gently remove.
10. Release the mouse from the restrainer.
11. Mice should be allowed to recover for at least 5 wk.
12. Before experimentation, some of the mast cell reconstituted W/W^v footpads should be examined after the 5-wk period for the presence of mast cells to demonstrate that the reconstitution was successful.
13. Experiments should be carried out with age matched congenic wild-type and non-reconstituted W/W^v mice.

3.6.2. Injection of Bacteria Into Footpad

A key issue to working with the footpad as a model system for bacterial infection is to make certain that the mice have suitable housing with regular cage changes. Second, a major objective for the researcher should be to minimize the degree of collateral damage instigated by the injection. This will significantly reduce background. This can be accomplished with practice and the use of small bore needles.

1. Adjust UPEC concentration to 5 million bacteria/mL in normal saline.
2. Fill a 1-mL syringe with the UPEC solution, and attach a 30 gage 0.5-cm needle. Prepare a similar syringe containing only saline.
3. Turn the needle so that the bevel side corresponds to the measurement markings on the side of the syringe. Remove the cap from the needle, and press the plunger to push some of the bacterial suspension through (once again, into bleach).
4. To inject the bacterial solution into the footpad, pull a mouse into the restrainer with the relevant footpad sticking out. Push the restraining bolt onto the snout of the mouse making certain that the snout is centered in the opening of the bolt.
5. Remove the cap from the needle of the syringe. Place the syringe to one side.
6. Tightly grab the toes of the extended foot and pull slightly outward. This should expose the whole of the footpad. Keep a firm grip, as the mouse may jerk when the needle is inserted.
7. Gently wipe the footpad with a clean Kimwipe.
8. Subcutaneously insert the needle, bevel side up, into the foot (*see* **Note 13**).
9. Gently press the plunger and expel 20 µL of the bacterial suspension into the foot as determined by the measurement markings (*see* **Note 14**).
10. Hold the needle in place for 5–10 s and then gently remove.

11. Release the mouse from the restrainer.
12. Once again, confirm the viability and concentration of the UPEC inoculum by culturing dilutions of the inoculum on LB plates, overnight, at 37°C.

3.6.3. Obtaining Single Cell Suspensions From Draining Lymph Nodes

1. Add 5 mL of cRPMI to each well of a 12-well plate. There should be one well of cRPMI per popliteal lymph node.
2. Collect popliteal lymph nodes, and place them individually into wells containing cRPMI.
3. Cut the popliteal lymphs node into fine pieces using microdissecting scissors and microdissecting tweezers.
4. Add Collagenase A to each well to a final concentration of 100 U/mL.
5. Incubate for 1 h at 37°C.
6. Add EDTA to the solution to a final concentration of 10 mM and mix. Let the mixture stand for 5 min.
7. Transfer the tissue suspensions into a 70-μm cell strainer that has been fitted into a 50-mL test tube. Most of the tissue suspension should pass through the strainer into the test tube. Be certain to rinse out the 12-well plates with 1X PBS and add this to your total cell volume.
8. Work the remaining undigested tissue against the cell strainer with a 1-mL plunger. Very little tissue should remain when you are done. Be sure not to miss any tissue that may have been caught up on the sides of the strainer.
9. Wash the cell strainer with 45 mL of cold 1X PBS. Draw the flow-through up into a 25-mL pipet and use it to extensively wash the strainer. Do this twice. When you arc donc, siphon any remaining fluid in the cell strainer through the mesh from the bottom side and add it to the 50-mL tube.
10. Centrifuge the cells at 300g for 10 min at 4°C. Decant the supernatant and slurry the pellet.
11. Popliteal lymph nodes derived from saline and UPEC treated footpads after 24 h should yield approx 250,000 and 1 million cells, respectively.

3.6.4. Flow Cytometry of Draining Lymph Node Preparations for T and B Lymphocytes

One of the earliest mast cell-dependent functional responses to UPEC challenge in the footpad is the distal sequestration of B and T lymphocytes in the draining popliteal lymph node. This process can be quantitatively measured by flow cytometry of single cell suspensions of isolated popliteal draining lymph nodes for total numbers of B and T lymphocytes.

1. Inject footpads with saline or UPEC as described.
2. Prepare blocking solution containing 1% BSA, 10% FCS with 10 μg/mL of anti-F$_c$γRII/III in 1X PBS. This solution should be ice cold.
3. Isolate draining popliteal lymph nodes at 24 h and prepare single cell suspensions as described.
4. To each sample, add 0.5 mL of blocking solution to each cell suspension for 30 min at 4°C.

5. To each sample, add 0.5 mL of blocking solution containing 2.5 µg/mL each of biotin-conjugated rat anti-mouse B220 (recognizes B-lymphocytes), FITC-conjugated hamster anti-mouse CD3$_e$ chain, and PE-conjugated rat anti-mouse CD4 (both anti-CD3 and anti-CD4 distinguish T-cells).
6. To a control sample, add 2.5 µg/mL each of biotin-conjugated ratIgG2a, FITC-conjugated hamster IgG, and phycoerythrin conjugated rat IgG2a isotype controls.
7. Incubate cells for 30 min on ice.
8. Add 10 mL of ice-cold 1X PBS and centrifuge cells at 300g at 4°C.
9. Add 1 mL of a 1:5000 dilution of strepavidin–cychrome in blocking buffer each sample. Incubate for 30 min on ice.
10. Add 10 mL of ice-cold 1X PBS and centrifuge cells at 300g at 4°C.
11. Decant supernatant, slurry the cells, and add freshly thawed 4% paraformaldehyde. Store the samples at 4°C until analysis.

3.6.5. Detection of TNF Protein in the Draining Popliteal Lymph Node

The principal mechanism by which mast cells affect the distal sequestration of B and Tlymphocytes in draining popliteal lymph nodes is to release TNF. TNF drains from the footpad into the popliteal lymph node, where it induces an increase in the expression of adhesion molecules, such as VCAM-1, which are involved in trapping and attracting lymphocytes into secondary lymphoid tissues *(10)*. TNF derived from mast cells can be detected in the popliteal lymph node within 1 h. Conversely, TNF mRNA cannot be detected in the popliteal lymph node at this time, confirming that the TNF is derived from an extranodal source *(10)*.

1. Inject UPEC or saline into footpads as described.
2. Collect popliteal lymph nodes at times of 1, 3, 6, and 12 h after injection.
3. Place the lymph nodes into sterile, protease free Eppendorf tubes containing 100 µL of MPER extraction buffer containing 1X Complete protease inhibitors on ice.
4. Homogenize the popliteal lymph nodes using microcentrifuge pestles.
5. Clarify the solution by centrifuging at 16,000g at 4°C.
6. Assay the supernatant for the presence of TNF by ELISA.
7. TNF can be detected within 1 h in the DLN, where it maximally peaks by 3 h.

3.6.6. Detection of TNF mRNA in the Draining Popliteal Lymph Node

1. Place extracted popliteal lymph nodes into 100 mL TRIzol buffer.
2. Increase the volume to 1 mL and extract RNA according to the manufacturer's instructions.
3. Reverse transcribe 1 µg total RNA with one cycle of 42°C for 40 min, 99°C for 5 min, followed by 5°C for 5 min.
4. Perform PCR with an inflammatory cytokine kit from Maxim Biotech. Use the entire reverse transcription product. Separate products by electrophoresis using a 2% agarose gel. Visualize the RT-PCR products by staining the gel with 0.5 µg/mL ethidium bromide solution followed by analysis with an Eagle Eye II.

4. Notes

1. Although IL-3 is the cytokine of choice when culturing mast cells from bone marrow, some researchers include SCF to augment their cultures. SCF is not very efficient by itself in generating mast cells from bone marrow. However, it will greatly enhance the overall numbers of mast cells generated in the cultures. In some cases, the inclusion of both IL-3 and SCF is required for the generation of mast cells from bone marrow, as was found in the generation of bone marrow-derived mast cells from Stat5a/b-deficient mice *(23)*.

2. Spraying the mouse down with 70% ethanol helps to minimize animal dander, which may contain mold or bacteria that could adversely affect later cell cultures.

3. WEHI-3 myelomonocytic cell lines are notoriously variable in their production of IL-3. Never assume that a WEHI-3 cell line automatically makes IL-3, and never assume that a WEHI-3 cell line that makes IL-3 will continue to make IL-3. Batches of conditioned medium should be routinely analyzed for their ability to support mast cell cultures in vitro before their use.

4. The separation of the nonadherent cell fraction from the adherent cell fraction every few days is absolutely critical to the generation of a pure culture of mast cells. Separation of these fractions does several things: (1) it prevents the rapid acidification of the cultures, which will adversely affect cell viability; and (2) it helps to ensure that non-mast cells are removed from the culture. The addition of SCF, which promotes the development of all bone marrow-derived lineages, to these cultures will require that this separation procedure be done more frequently and for a longer duration of time.

5. Mast cell cultures can be maintained for 3 mo without significant loss of surface markers, cytokine dependency, or functional phenotypes. However, this is somewhat dependent upon the strain of mice from which the mast cells are derived. For instance, cultured mast cells derived from Balb/c mice appear will lose responsiveness to IL-4 and will acquire factor independent phenotypes after a few weeks more readily than mast cells derived from C57BL/6 or C57BL/6X129 F1 mice. Therefore, we recommend that mast cell cultures maintained for more than one month be routinely assessed for functional differences or factor dependency.

6. The UPEC strain J96 biosafety Level 1 bacteria that can cause serious illness. Therefore, always wear gloves and suitable lab garments when handling this organism, and always wash your hands after handling this organism.

7. Not all bacterial products induce mast cells to degranulate. For instance, LPS does not induce mast cell degranulation, however, LPS will induce mast cells to secrete TNF *(24)*. Therefore, the presence or absence of mast cell degranulation during a biological response should only be used as an indicator that mast cells take part in a particular response.

8. Staining of tissues with avidin-Alexa-488 requires that the appropriate controls be applied. Other cell types present in tissues may bind avidin. Therefore, the initial experiment utilizing this stain should include a sample of mast cell deficient W/W^v tissue. Also, although avidin interacts with heparin, a component of mast cell granules, the stain may be too intense to reliably distinguish between individual mast cells that have undergone degranulation in tissue. We recom-

mend that toluidine blue be used to distinguish degranulated mast cells as well as the extent of degranulation.

9. Alexa-488 is a very bright fluorochrome that will generate spectral overlap with orange fluorescent dyes, such as Cy3 and Alexa546. Therefore, it is critical to use the appropriate controls to prevent accidental misinterpretation of the data, especially when performing dual labeling studies.

10. Distinctions between moderate and extensive mast cell degranulation, based on the number of granules present in the mast cell body, also may be made. This process requires embedding the tissue in EPON *(3)*.

11. It is best to sacrifice mice by CO_2 inhalation, as opposed to cervical dislocation. Cervical dislocation, if performed improperly, can lead to bleeding into the peritoneal cavity. The presence of red blood cells in peritoneal exudates can interfere with subsequent flow cytometric analysis.

12. Fat present in the base of the abdominal cavity will plug the hole and prevent leakage.

13. It is important to ensure that the mouse does not jerk during the injection process, as this can lead to collateral damage and breakage of the major blood vessels. If bleeding is observed, be certain to note it. One can utilize an inhaled anesthetic such as Isofluorane if required to minimize uncontrolled movements by the mouse.

14. Titration of UPEC concentrations has indicated that this concentration (1×10^5 per footpad) elicits a consistent inflammatory response and lymph node hypertrophy.

Acknowledgments

This work was supported by funds from the National Institutes of Health DK50814 and AI50021 and the Sandler Foundation for Asthma Research.

References

1. Galli, S. J. and Hammel, I. (1994) Mast cell and basophil development. *Curr. Opin. Hematol.* **1,** 33–39.
2. Wershil, B. K., Furuta, G. T., Wang, Z. S., and Galli, S. J. (1996) Mast cell-dependent neutrophil and mononuclear cell recruitment in immunoglobulin E-induced gastric reactions in mice. *Gastroenterology* **110,** 1482–1490.
3. Wershil, B. K., Wang, Z. S., Gordon, J. R., and Galli, S. J. (1991) Recruitment of neutrophils during IgE-dependent cutaneous late phase reactions in the mouse is mast cell-dependent. Partial inhibition of the reaction with antiserum against tumor necrosis factor-alpha. *J. Clin. Invest.* **87,** 446–453.
4. Secor, V. H., Secor, W. E., Gutekunst, C. A., and Brown, M. A. (2000) Mast cells are essential for early onset and severe disease in a murine model of multiple sclerosis. *J. Exp. Med.* **191,** 813–822.
5. Lee, D. M., Friend, D. S., Gurish, M. F., Benoist, C., Mathis, D., and Brenner, M. B. (2002) Mast cells: a cellular link between autoantibodies and inflammatory arthritis. *Science* **297,** 1689–1692.

6. Chen, R., Fairley, J. A., Zhao, M. L., et al. (2002) Macrophages, but not T and B lymphocytes, are critical for subepidermal blister formation in experimental bullous pemphigoid: macrophage-mediated neutrophil infiltration depends on mast cell activation. *J. Immunol.* **169,** 3987–3992.

7. Marshall, J. S. and Bienenstock, J. (1994) The role of mast cells in inflammatory reactions of the airways, skin and intestine. *Curr. Opin. Immunol.* **6,** 853–859.

8. Malaviya, R., Ikeda, T., Ross, E., and Abraham, S. N. (1996) Mast cell modulation of neutrophil influx and bacterial clearance at sites of infection through TNF-alpha. *Nature* **381,** 77–80.

9. Echtenacher, B., Mannel, D. N., and Hultner, L. (1996) Critical protective role of mast cells in a model of acute septic peritonitis. *Nature* **381,** 75–77.

10. McLachlan, J. B., Hart, J. P., Pizzo, S. V., et al. (2003) Mast cell-derived tumor necrosis factor induces hypertrophy of draining lymph nodes during infection. *Nat. Immunol.* **4,** 1199–1205.

11. Galli, S. J., Tsai, M., and Wershil, B. K. (1993) The c-kit receptor, stem cell factor, and mast cells. What each is teaching us about the others. *Am. J. Pathol.* **142,** 965–974.

12. Nakano, T., Sonoda, T., Hayashi, C., et al. (1985) Fate of bone marrow-derived cultured mast cells after intracutaneous, intraperitoneal, and intravenous transfer into genetically mast cell-deficient W/Wv mice. Evidence that cultured mast cells can give rise to both connective tissue type and mucosal mast cells. *J. Exp. Med.* **162,** 1025–1043.

13. Ihle, J. N., Keller, J., Oroszlan, S., et al. (1983) Biologic properties of homogeneous interleukin 3. I. Demonstration of WEHI-3 growth factor activity, mast cell growth factor activity, p cell-stimulating factor activity, colony-stimulating factor activity, and histamine-producing cell-stimulating factor activity. *J. Immunol.* **131,** 282–287.

14. Ryan, J. J., DeSimone, S., Klisch, G., et al. (1998) IL-4 inhibits mouse mast cell Fc epsilonRI expression through a STAT6-dependent mechanism. *J. Immunol.* **161,** 6915–6923.

15. Galli, S. J., Wedemeyer, J., and Tsai, M. (2002) Analyzing the roles of mast cells and basophils in host defense and other biological responses. *Int. J. Hematol.* **75,** 363–369.

16. Weidner, N. and Austen, K. F. (1993) Heterogeneity of mast cells at multiple body sites. Fluorescent determination of avidin binding and immunofluorescent determination of chymase, tryptase, and carboxypeptidase content. *Pathol. Res. Pract.* **189,** 156–162.

17. Biedermann, T., Kneilling, M., Mailhammer, R., et al. (2000) Mast cells control neutrophil recruitment during T cell-mediated delayed-type hypersensitivity reactions through tumor necrosis factor and macrophage inflammatory protein 2. *J. Exp. Med.* **192,** 1441–1452.

18. Anderson, W. H., Davidson, T. M., and Broide, D. H. (1996) Mast cell TNF mRNA expression in nasal mucosa demonstrated by in situ hybridization: a comparison of mast cell detection methods. *J. Immunol. Methods* **189,** 145–155.

19. Prodeus, A. P., Zhou, X., Maurer, M., Galli, S. J., and Carroll, M. C. (1997) Impaired mast cell-dependent natural immunity in complement C3-deficient mice. *Nature* **390,** 172–175.

20. Gommerman, J. L., Oh, D. Y., Zhou, X., et al. (2000) A role for CD21/CD35 and CD19 in responses to acute septic peritonitis: a potential mechanism for mast cell activation. *J. Immunol.* **165,** 6915–6921.

21. Gordon, J. R. and Galli, S. J. (1991) Release of both preformed and newly synthesized tumor necrosis factor alpha (TNF-alpha)/cachectin by mouse mast cells stimulated via the Fc epsilon RI. A mechanism for the sustained action of mast cell-derived TNF-alpha during IgE-dependent biological responses. *J. Exp. Med.* **174,** 103–107.

22. Itano, A. A., McSorley, S. J., Reinhardt, R. L., et al. (2003) Distinct dendritic cell populations sequentially present antigen to CD4 T cells and stimulate different aspects of cell-mediated immunity. *Immunity* **19,** 47–57.

23. Shelburne, C. P., McCoy, M. E., Piekorz, R., et al. (2003) Stat5 expression is critical for mast cell development and survival. *Blood* **102,** 1290–1297.

24. Marshall, J. S., King, C. A., and McCurdy, J. D. (2003) Mast cell cytokine and chemokine responses to bacterial and viral infection. *Curr. Pharm. Des.* **9,** 11–24.

28

Bacterial Activation of Mast Cells

David S. Chi, Elaine S. Walker, Fred E. Hossler,
and Guha Krishnaswamy

Summary

Mast cells often are found in a perivascular location but especially in mucosae, where they may response to various stimuli. They typically associate with immediate hypersensitive responses and are likely to play a critical role in host defense. In this chapter, a common airway pathogen, *Moraxella catarrhalis*, and a commensal bacterium, *Neiserria cinerea*, are used to illustrate activation of human mast cells. A human mast cell line (HMC-1) derived from a patient with mast cell leukemia was activated with varying concentrations of heat-killed bacteria. Active aggregation of bacteria over mast cell surfaces was detected by scanning electron microscopy. The activation of mast cells was analyzed by nuclear factor-κB (NF-κB) activation and cytokine production in culture supernatants. Both *M. catarrhalis* and *N. cinerea* induce mast cell activation and the secretion of two key inflammatory cytokines, interleukin-6 and MCP-1. This is accompanied by NF-κB activation. Direct bacterial contact with mast cells appears to be essential for this activation because neither cell-free bacterial supernatants nor bacterial lipopolysaccharide induce cytokine secretion.

Key Words: Mast cells; *Moraxella catarrhalis*; *Neiserria cinerea*; inflammation; cytokines; interleukin 6; monocyte chemotactic protein-1; nuclear factor-κB (NF-κB); signaling mechanisms; Bay 11; scanning electron microscopy; bacterial growth.

1. Introduction

Mast cells are multifunctional, tissue-dwelling cells capable of producing and secreting a wide variety of lipid mediators, histamine, cytokines, and chemokines (*1,2*). Although typically associated with immediate hypersensitive responses (*3–5*), mast cells also are likely to play a critical role in immune surveillance and contribute to host defense (*5*), especially in the lung (*6*). Good evidence exists to suggest that mast cells are capable of the phagocytosis of a large range of bacteria (*1*). Furthermore, it has been shown that in mast cell-deficient mice, pathogenic bacteria survived 10-fold more than in mice with

From: *Methods in Molecular Biology, vol. 315: Mast Cells: Methods and Protocols*
Edited by: G. Krishnaswamy and D. S. Chi © Humana Press Inc., Totowa, NJ

mast cells *(7)*. Hence, mast cells are likely to play a crucial role in the innate immune response to common bacterial pathogens.

In this chapter, an in vitro model for studying the interaction between bacteria and mast cell is presented. A common airway pathogen, *Moraxella catarrhalis*, and a commensal bacterium, *Neiserria cinerea*, are used to illustrate activation of human mast cells (*see* **Note 1**). The procedure of growing bacteria and the method of activating HMC-1 with varying concentrations of heat-killed suspensions of bacteria are presented. A scanning electron microscopy protocol used to demonstrating active aggregation of bacteria over mast cell surfaces also is offered. The activation of mast cells will be analyzed by nuclear factor-κB (NF-κB) translocation and cytokine production in culture supernatants.

2. Materials

2.1. Preparation and Heat Treatment of Bacteria

1. *M. catarrhalis* strain ATCC no. 25238 and *N. cinerea* strain ATCC no. 14685 (American Type Culture Collection; Manassas, VA).
2. Brain Heart Infusion (BHI) Broth (Difco Laboratory; Detroit, MI).
3. BHI Agar (Difco Laboratory).
4. Phosphate-buffered saline (PBS): 150 mM, PH 7.4. Determined to be endotoxin-free PBS by limulus amebocyte assay (Cambrex Biosciences, Walkersville, MD).
5. Murine-clone medium: RPM1 1640 (Gibco BRL, Frederick, MD) supplemented with 11.1% heat-inactivated fetal bovine serum (Atlanta Biologicals, Atlanta, GA), 2 mM HEPES, pKa 7.55 (Gibco BRL), 50 mg/mL gentamicin, 50 mM 2-mercaptoethanol, 0.09% insulin-transferrin-sodium selenite supplement (Sigma, St. Louis, MO), and 1.5% sodium bicarbonate.
6. Gram stain reagents (Difco Laboratory).

2.2. Activation of Mast Cells With Heat-Treated Bacteria

1. HMC-1 culture medium: RPMI 1640 media supplemented with $2 \times 10^{-5} M$ 2-mercaptoethanol (Sigma), 10 mM HEPES, gentamicin 50 μg/mL, 5 mg/mL insulin-transferrin-sodium selenite supplement (Sigma), 2 mM L-glutamine, and 5% heat-inactivated fetal bovine serum.
2. 24-well Costar tissue culture dishes.
3. Phorbol myristate acetate (PMA; 50 ng/mL).
4. Ionomycin (5 μM).
5. An inhibitor of NF-κB activation: Bay-11 (10 μM final concentration; Biomole Chemicals, Plymouth Meeting, PA).
6. Murine clone medium: *see* **Subheading 2.1.**

2.3. Demonstration of Active Aggregation of Bacteria Over Mast Cell Surfaces by Scanning Electron Microscopy

1. DSM 940 scanning electron microscope (Carl Zeiss SMT, Inc., Thornwood , NY).
2. Desk II Sputter Coater and gold foil cathodes (Denton Vacuum, Cherry Hill, NJ).

3. Sorvall GLC-4 Centrifuge (Dupont, Newtown, CT).
4. Scanning electron microscope stubs, conducting graphite paint, and 25% glutaraldehyde in sealed vials (Ladd Research Industries, Burlington, VT).
5. Sodium cacodylate buffer, 0.25 g of crystalline osmium tetroxide in sealed vials, and paraformaldehyde powder (Electron Microscopy Sciences, Fort Washington, PA).
6. Kodak Professional Sheet Film 4127, D19 Developer, and Kodak Fixer (Calumet Photographic, Bensenville, IL).
7. Fixation Solution I: 2.5% glutaraldehyde, 1% paraformaldehyde in 0.1 M cacodylate-HCl buffer, pH 7.3, containing 0.1% $CaCl_2$.
8. Fixation Solution II: 2% osmium tetroxide in 0.1 M cacodylate-HCl buffer, pH 7.3.
9. Washing buffer: 0.2 M cacodylate-HCl buffer (pH 7.3) containing 0.1% $CaCl_2$.
10. Ethanol.

3. Methods

The methods described in **Subheadings 3.1.–3.3.** outline: (1) the preparation and heat treatment of bacteria; (2) activation of mast cells with heat-killed bacteria; and (3) demonstration of active aggregation of bacteria over mast cell surfaces by scanning electron microscopy. For the methods of growth of HMC-1 cells and cytokine measurement, please *see* Chapter 16. For the detection of NF-κB activation, please *see* Chapter 11.

3.1. Preparation and Heat Treatment of Bacteria

1. Inoculate *M. catarrhalis* and *N. cinerea* on BHI agar. Incubate overnight at 37°C (*see* **Note 2**).
2. Inoculate 10 mL of BHI broth in a 50-mL flask or culture tube with several bacterial colonies from fresh overnight growth on agar media. Incubate broth with shaking overnight at 37°C.
3. Remove and set aside a 1-mL aliquot of broth culture to use in Gram stain and dilution series.
4. Wash and concentrate bacterial cells as follows: transfer remaining overnight culture (9 mL) to a sterile disposable centrifuge tube. Centrifuge at 1500g for 5 min. Filter supernatants through 0.2-μm filter and store at –80°C. Resuspend bacterial cells in 5 mL of PBS.
5. Centrifuge at 1500g for 5 min. Discard supernatant. Repeat resuspension in 5 mL of PBS and centrifugation. Resuspend in 1 mL of PBS.
6. Determine wet weight of bacteria *(8)*. Transfer the bacteria suspension to a preweighed microfuge tube. Centrifuge in microfuge for 15 s at 14,000g (*see* **Note 3**). Remove supernatant with sterile micropipet. Weigh microfuge tube containing the bacteria. Subtract the weight of the empty tube from the weight of the tube containing the bacteria and record the wet weight of the cells in mg.
7. Heat-kill bacterial cells *(9)*. Resuspend bacteria in 1 mL of PBS. Use clamp system to keep tube cap sealed. Place at 60°C for 2 h. Gram stain an aliquot of heat-treated cells. The cells should display normal morphology with no evidence of

cell lysis. To verify complete killing, plate 10 μL of the heat-killed cell suspension on the agar plates and incubate at 37°C overnight. If there is no growth of bacteria, it will indicate that bacteria are completely killed (*see* **Note 4**).

8. Centrifuge the heat-treated bacteria in microfuge for 15 s at 14,000g. Remove supernatant with sterile micropipet. Resuspend to 5 mg/mL (refered to as 100X bacterial concentration) in murine clone medium. Store in 5-mL aliquots at –80°C.

9. While bacteria are being heat-killed, Gram stain is performed using bacteria from the reserved overnight culture. If the Gram stain looks like a pure culture (*see* **Note 5**), plate out a 10-fold dilution series of the reserved bacterial broth culture for determination of the bacterial concentration. Determine the colony-forming units/milliliter (cfu/mL) in the bacterial broth culture from the dilution series. Multiply the cfu/mL by nine (the total number of milliliters that were heat-killed) to derive the total cfu. Divide the total cfu by the wet weight of the bacteria to obtain cfu/μg. The number of bacterial cells extrapolated from determinations of cfu/mL to cfu/μg was 3.5×10^4 cfu/μg for *M. catarrhalis* and 4.2×10^4 cfu/μg for *N. cinerea*.

10. The day of the activation assay, thaw one tube of heat-killed bacterial cells. Reserve an undiluted aliquot for the 100X bacterial concentration, and make a 1:10 dilution (for a 10X bacterial concentration,) and a 1:100 dilution (for a 1X bacterial concentration) in murine clone medium (*see* **Note 6**).

3.2. Activation of Mast Cells With Heat-Killed Bacteria

1. HMC-1 cells, established from a patient with mast cell leukemia, were graciously provided by Dr. J. H. Butterfield (Mayo Clinic, Rochester, MN) and are maintained in HMC-1 culture medium at 37°C and in 5% CO_2 mixture *(10)*. The cells are seeded at 2×10^4 cells/mL density and subcultured every 4 d. Mast cells for this study are seeded at 1.5×10^6 cells/mL in 24-well Costar tissue culture dishes. Cells in media alone serve as negative controls. Cells treated with PMA (50 ng/mL) and 5 μ*M* ionomycin served as positive controls reflecting maximal activation.

2. For bacterial activation, mast cells are incubated with varying concentrations of heat-killed suspensions of *M. catarrhalis* or *N. cinerea* (1.75×10^8, 1.75×10^7, and 1.75×10^6 bacteria/mL for *M. catarrhalis*; *see* **Notes 7** and **8**).

3. To determine a role of NF-κB in mast cell activation by bacteria, Bay-11 (10 μ*M* final concentration), an inhibitor of NF-κB activation, is added to mast cell cultures in presence or absence of bacteria (*see* **Note 9**).

4. HMC-1 cells also are activated with lipopolysaccharide (LPS, 10 ng/mL, Biomole) to determine whether LPS is capable of inducing secretion of cytokines in similar magnitudes as bacterial suspensions.

5. In a selected study, filtered supernatants of bacterial suspensions are added to mast cell cultures to determine whether or not soluble factors are capable of mast cell activation *(11)*.

6. After 24 h of incubation, mast cell cultures are centrifuged at 250g for 10 min to remove cell debris, and cell-free supernatants are collected and stored at –70°C until ready for cytokine assay by ELISA (*see* Chapters 16 and 17).

7. The cell pellet is subjected to nuclear protein isolation for NF-κB activation assay (*see* Chapter 11).

8. Some mast cell cultures are directly subjected to fixation for scanning electron microscopy.

9. Heat-killed *M. catarrhalis* and *N. cinerea* induced a significant secretion of both IL-6 and MCP-1 from mast cells with maximal levels seen with a 100X bacteria to HMC-1 ratio (**Figs. 1** and **2**, respectively *[11]*). Because both LPS and filtered cell-free bacterial supernatant did not induced significant secretion of MCP-1 (166 ± 60 and 297 ± 7 pg/mL, respectively, vs 277 ± 18 pg/mL in the media control group), it suggests that physical contact of bacteria with mast cells appears to be essential for the activation. Nuclear proteins were extracted from mast cells activated for 24 h by PMA and ionomycin or heat killed-bacterial suspensions and assayed for NF-κB nuclear binding activity by electrophoretic mobility shift assay (*see* Chapter 11). The results are shown in **Fig. 3**. In summary, weak activity of NF-κB is observed in unstimulated control cells (integrated intensity [II] were 6.9 and 0.2 for p65 and p50, respectively). This may represent the leukemic nature of this cell line. However, a marked increase of NF-κB nuclear binding activity was observed in samples from cells stimulated with either PMA and ionomycin (II was 12.3 and 24.9 for p65 and p50, respectively) or with both heat-killed *M. catarrhalis* (II was 8.1 and 21.5 for p65 and p50, respectively) and *N. cinerea* (II was 26.1 and 50.4 for p65 and p50, respectively). To confirm the functional significance of NF-kB activation, mast cells were incubated with the NF-κB inhibitor, Bay-11. Bay-11 caused a statistically significant inhibition of MCP-1 production induced by *M. catarrhalis* (382 ± 89 pg/mL vs 828 ± 164 pg/mL in the culture without Bay-11).

3.3. Demonstration of Active Aggregation of Bacteria Over Mast Cell Surfaces by Scanning Electron Microscopy

1. Mast cells are fixed by adding an equal volume of Fixation Solution I directly into culture wells containing growing cell suspensions *(12)*. Fixation is the same for control cultures and for those stimulated with *M. catarrhalis*.

2. Fixation is continued overnight under refrigeration at 4°C.

3. The supernatant is carefully drawn off the visibly settled cells with a pipet, and the cells are washed twice by suspension in the washing buffer and gentle centrifugation (208*g* for 5 min) using a Dupont GLC centrifuge.

4. Cells are subsequently post fixed for 3 h at ambient temperature in Fixation Solution II.

5. Cells are washed by resuspension and gentle centrifugation in distilled water, and placed in 50% ethanol overnight at 4°C.

6. Cells are then further dehydrated in a graduated series of ethanol (50, 80, 95, and 100%).

7. A drop of cell suspension is placed on a glass cover slip and allowed to air dry.

8. The cover slips are attached to aluminum stubs with a drop of graphite paint and air dried under cover overnight.

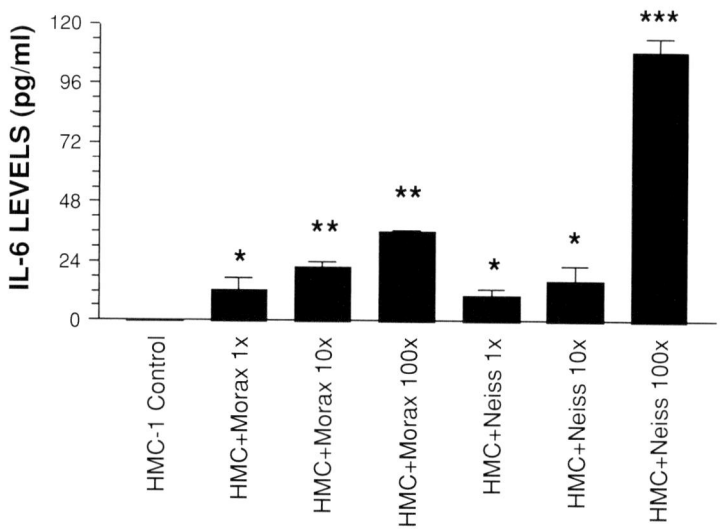

Fig. 1. Activation of mast cells by varying concentrations of *Moraxella catarrhalis* and *Neiserria cinerea* produced a dose-dependent secretion of IL-6, with maximal levels seen with 100X concentrations (1×10^8 bacteria/mL). Cultures with *M. catarrhalis* (Morax) at 1X (* $p < 0.05$), 10X (** $p < 0.005$), and 100X concentrations (** $p < 0.005$), and *N. cinerea* (Neiss) at 1X (* $p < 0.05$), 10X (* $p = 0.05$), and 100X (*** $p = 0.0009$) significantly enhanced IL-6 secretion from HMC-1 cells compared with control cells alone. These experiments were repeated several times and the data shown are representative of a typical experiment. (Reproduced with permission from **ref. *11*.**)

9. The stubs are sputter coated with gold for a total of 3 min (90 s each at 0° and 180° rotation of the stub) in a Desk II Sputter coater.
10. Samples are viewed and photographed in a Zeiss DSM 940 scanning electron microscope at an accelerating voltage of 20 kV.
11. Incubation of heat-killed suspensions of bacteria with mast cells resulted in their aggregation around mast cells. Scanning electron microscopy was performed in resting and heat-killed *M. catarrhalis*-treated HMC-1 cells and the results are shown in **Fig. 4A,B**, respectively. Control mast cells displayed microvilli-like processes on their surfaces (**Fig. 4A**). Treated mast cells had aggregations of *M. catarrhalis* on their surfaces (**Fig. 4B**; *see* **Note 10**).

4. Notes

1. *M. catarrhalis* and *N. cinerea* are Gram-negative, human nasopharyngeal colonists with pathogenic potential. *M. catarrhalis* can cause otitis media, sinusitis, and exacerbation of bronchitis *(13)* and *N. cinerea* is occasionally reported as the causal agent in pediatric ocular infections *(14)*.

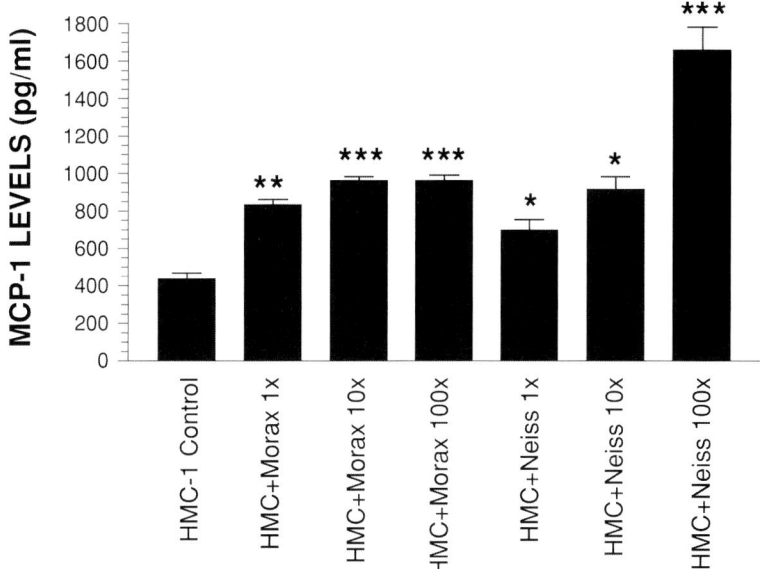

Fig. 2. Activation of mast cells by varying concentrations of *Moraxella catarrhalis* and *Neiserria cinerea* produced a dose-dependent secretion of MCP-1. A dose response curve was again seen with varying concentrations of *M. catarrhalis* and *N. cinerea*, with maximal levels with the 100X concentration (1×10^8 bacteria/mL) of the bacterium. Cultures with *M. catarrhalis* (Morax) at 1X (** $p = 0.007$), 10X (*** $p = 0.001$), and 100X concentrations (*** $p = 0.001$), and *N. cinerea* (Neiss) at 1X (* $p < 0.05$), 10X (* $p < 0.05$), and 100X (*** $p = 0.001$) concentrations significantly enhanced MCP-1 secretion from HMC-1 cells compared with control cells alone. These experiments were repeated several times and the data shown is representative of a typical experiment. (Reproduced with permission from **ref. *11*.)

2. This procedure is suitable for aerobic bacterial species with optimal culture temperature of 37°C. Recommended culture media for specific bacterial species may be found in the *Manual of Clinical Microbiology (15)*.

3. The total centrifugation time should not exceed 15 s. It takes a model 5402 Eppendorf centrifuge approx 9 or 10 s to reach 14,000g, and this time is included in the total run time. Longer centrifugation times will make it difficult to resuspend the cell pellet.

4. If there is any growth of heat-treated bacteria, discard the entire preparation and start the process from **Subheading 3.1., step 2**.

5. Discard the entire preparation if there are any indications of contamination on the Gram stain and start the process from **Subheading 3.1., step 2**.

6. Alternatively, calculate dilutions to fit a desired ratio of bacterial cells:mast cells.

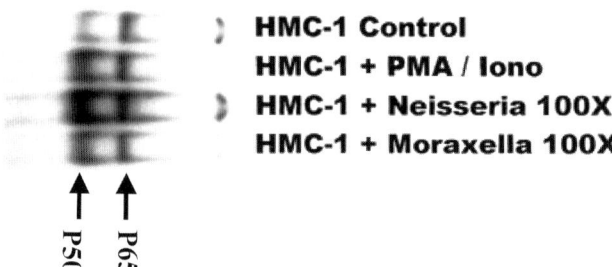

Fig. 3. Representative electrophoretic mobility shift assay showing nuclear factor-κB (NF-κB) binding activity in HMC-1 following stimulation. Weak binding activity of NF-κB is observed in unstimulated cells (Control). However, stimulation with either PMA and ionomycin (Iono) or with bacterial suspensions (both *M. catarrhalis* and *N. cinerea*) increased nuclear binding activity of NF-κB. (Reproduced with permission from **ref. *11***.)

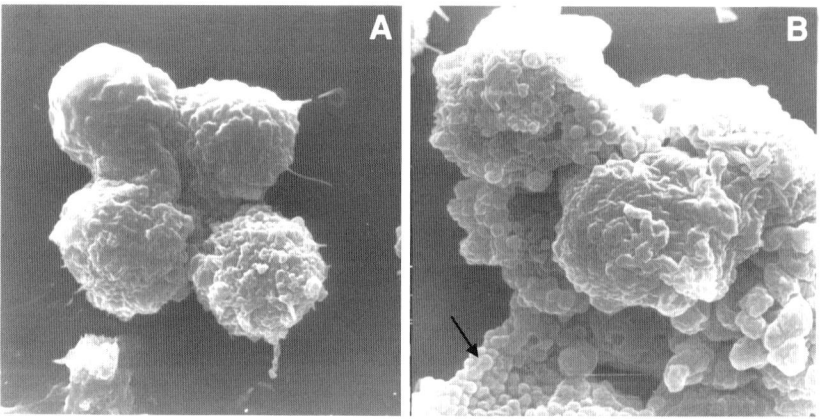

Fig. 4. Scanning electron microscopy of the mast cells. Control mast cells displayed microvilli-like processes on their surfaces (**A**, ×4000). Treated mast cells had aggregations of bacteria (arrow) on their surfaces (**B**, ×5000). These experiments were repeated several times and the data shown is representative of typical experiments. (Reproduced with permission from **ref. *11***.)

7. Equal volumes of bacterial cells (for *M. catarrhalis*, concentrations at 5 mg/mL, 500 µg/mL, and 50 µg/mL are equivalent to 1.75×10^8, 1.75×10^7, and 1.75×10^6 bacteria/mL, respectively) were mixed with murine clone media containing 1.5×10^6 HMC-1 cells/mL.

8. Assay conditions corresponded to 120, 12, or 1.2 *M. catarrhalis* cells/HMC-1 cells, and the bacterial concentration falls within the range reported in sputum from patients with bronchiectasis (*16*).

9. Live bacteria also have been used for this type of experiments. When live bacteria are used, the incubation time usually is shortened to prevent the bacteria taking over the culture. Mast cell responses to live bacteria have been tested at initial ratios of 10 or 100 bacteria to one mast cell, with shortened exposure times (15 min up to 6 h) relative to the time used in this protocol *(1,17)*. Some bacterial species may multiply rapidly in mammalian cell culture media, resulting in a much higher ratio of bacteria to mast cell after several hours.

    Bay-11 has been shown to inhibit cytokine-induced NF-κB-specific inhibitory protein IκBα phosphorylation and NF-κB-dependent expression of adhesion molecules on endothelial cells *(18)*. The concentrations used in studies with BAY-11 inhibitor have varied between 5–20 μ*M* (product data sheet, BIOMOL corporation *[18]*).

10. The attachment of aggregated bacteria onto the surfaces of mast cells appeared to be quite tight, as the mast cells could not be disengaged from the bacteria even by brief vortexing or vigorous pipetting. We have not analyzed actual phagocytosis of bacterial particles by HMC-1 cells because it is beyond the scope of this chapter.

Acknowledgments

This study was supported by USPHS grants AI-43310 and HL-63070, State of Tennessee Grant 20233, RDC grant (ETSU), and Ruth R. Harris Endowment (ETSU).

References

1. Arock, M., Ross, E., Lai-Kuen, R., Averlant, G., Gao, Z., and Abraham, S. N. (1998) Phagocytic and tumor necrosis factor alpha response of human mast cells following exposure to gram-negative and gram-positive bacteria. *Infect. Immun.* **66,** 6030–6034.
2. Abraham, S. N. and Malaviya, R. (1997) Mast cells in infection and immunity. *Infect. Immun.* **65,** 3501–3508.
3. Krishnaswamy, G., Lakshman, T., Miller, A. R., et al. (1997) Multifunctional cytokine expression by human mast cells: regulation by T cell membrane contact and glucocorticoids. *J. Interferon Cytokine Res.* **17,** 167–176.
4. Kelley, J., Chi, D. S., Abou-Auda, W., Smith, J. K., and Krishnaswamy, G. (2000) The molecular role of mast cells in atherosclerotic cardiovascular disease. *Mol. Med. Today* **6,** 304–308.
5. Krishnaswamy, G., Kelley, J., Johnson, D., et al. (2001) The human mast cell: functions in physiology and disease. *Front. Biosci.* **6,** d1109–d1127.
6. Abraham, S. N., Thankavel, K., and Malaviya, R. (1997) Mast cells as modulators of host defense in the lung. *Front. Biosci.* **2,** d78–d87.
7. Malaviya, R., Ikeda, T., Ross, E., and Abraham, S. N. (1996) Mast cell modulation of neutrophil influx and bacterial clearance at sites of infection through TNF-alpha. *Nature* **381,** 77–80.
8. Keller, R., Kiest, R, Joller, P., and Mulsch, A. (1995) Coordinate up- and down-modulation of inducible nitric oxide synthetase, nitric oxide production, and

tumoricidal activity in rat-bone-marrow-derived mononuclear phagocytes by lipopolysacharide and gram-negative bacteria. *Biochem. Biophys. Res. Commun.* **211,** 183–189.

9. Keller, R., Gehri, R., Keist, R., Huf, E., and Kayser, F. H. (1991) The interaction of macrophages and bacteria: a comparative study of the induction of tumoricidal activity and of reactive nitrogen intermediates. *Cell. Immunol.* **134,** 249–256.

10. Butterfield, J. H., Weiler, D., Dewald, G., and Gleich, G. J. (1988) Establishment of an immature mast cell line from a patient with mast cell leukemia. *Leukemia Res.* **12,** 345–355.

11. Krishnaswamy, G., Martin, R., Walker, E., et al. (2003) *Moraxella catarrhalis* induces mast cell activation and nuclear factor kappaB-dependent cytokine synthesis. *Front. Biosci.* **8,** a40–a47.

12. Krishnaswamy, G., Hall, K., Youngberg, G., et al. (2002) Regulation of eosinophil-active cytokine production from human cord blood-derived mast cells. *J. Interferon Cytokine Res.* **22,** 379–388.

13. Catlin, B. W. (1990) *Branhamella catarrhalis*: an organism gaining respect as a pathogen. *Clin. Microbiol. Rev.* **3,** 293–320.

14. Dolter, J., Wong, J., and Janda, J. M. (1998) Association of *Neisseria cinerea* with ocular infections in paediatric patients. *J. Infect.* **36,** 49–52.

15. Murray, P. R., Baron, E. J., Pfaller, M. A., Tenover, F. C., and Yolken, R. H. (1999) *Manual of Clinical Microbiology, Seventh edition.* American Society for Microbiology, Washington, DC.

16. Klingman, K. L., Pye, A., Murphy, T. F., and Hill, S. L. (1995) Dynamics of respiratory tract colonization by *Branhamella catarrhalis* in bronchiectasis. *Am. J. Respir. Crit. Care Med.* **152,** 1072–1078.

17. Munoz, S., Hernanadez-Pando, R., Abraham, S. N., and Enciso, J. A. (2003) Mast cell activation by *Mycobacterium tuberculosis*: mediator release and role of CD48. *J. Immunol.* **170,** 5590–5596.

18. Pierce J. W., Schoenleber, R., Jesmok, G., et al. (1997) Novel inhibitors of cytokine-induced IkappaBalpha phosphorylation and endothelial cell adhesion molecule expression show anti-inflammatory effects in vivo. *J. Biol. Chem.* **272,** 21,096–21,103.

29

Activation of Mast Cells by Streptolysin O and Lipopolysaccharide

Michael Stassen, Angela Valeva, Iwan Walev, and Edgar Schmitt

Summary

This chapter provides protocols to measure the reversible permeabilization of mast cells by streptolysin O (SLO) and to follow SLO-induced activation of mast cells by monitoring degranulation, activation of mitogen-activated protein kinases, and production of tumor necrosis factor-α. A method that uses SLO to deliver molecules into the cytosol of living cells also is described. Furthermore, we outline a procedure to measure the activation of nuclear factor-κB by lipopolysaccharide and ionomycin using transfection of mast cells with reporter genes by electroporation. These protocols should be widely applicable in mast cell research.

Key Words: Murine bone marrow-derived mast cells; streptolysin O; lipopolysaccharide; degranulation; MAP kinases; TNF-α; reversible permeabilization; electroporation; reporter gene.

1. Introduction

A large body of evidence has shed new light on the role of mast cells as critical effectors of innate immune responses, which is attributable to their ability to recognize a variety of microbial constituents (reviewed in **refs.** *1* and *2*). Using murine models, it has been shown that mast cell-derived tumor necrosis factor (TNF)-α plays a crucial role in mediating the influx of neutrophils at the very beginning of the inflammatory response against microbial pathogens *(3,4)*.

Streptolysin O (SLO) is a virulence factor produced by pyogenic streptococci. Upon binding to cholesterol in the membranes of eukaryotic cells, SLO oligomerizes to form transmembrane pores *(5)*. High doses of the toxin are rapidly cytocidal, but low doses are tolerated because a limited number of transmembrane pores can be resealed *(6)*. This process of reversible permeabilization is accompanied by the activation of mast cells as characterized by the activation of mitogen-activated protein (MAP) kinases, degranulation, and the production of TNF-α *(7)*. Expression and purification of recombinant SLO

From: *Methods in Molecular Biology, vol. 315: Mast Cells: Methods and Protocols*
Edited by: G. Krishnaswamy and D. S. Chi © Humana Press Inc., Totowa, NJ

have been described in detail previously (*see* **Note 1** *[8]*). Because slight batch-to-batch variations of different SLO preparations occur, we describe a simple method to determine SLO concentrations that allow the transient permeabilization of murine bone marrow-derived mast cells (BMDMCs) by monitoring cellular adenosine triphosphate (ATP) content. Furthermore, techniques to measure SLO-mediated degranulation and the production of biologically active TNF-α and MAP kinase activation also are given. Finally, we present a method for introducing molecules as large as 100 kDa into cells by reversible permeabilization with SLO.

Lipopolysaccharide (LPS), a cell wall component of Gram-negative bacteria, has been shown to enhance or induce the production of proinflammatory (TNF-α, interleukin [IL]-1, IL-6) and Th2-type cytokines (IL-5, IL-9, IL-10, IL-13) by mast cells *(9–12)*. A distinctive feature of LPS signaling is the activation of nuclear factor-κB (NF-κB) through a Toll-like receptor 4 pathway. Activation of NF-κB can be measured using reporter gene assays, and this example will be used to illustrate the usefulness of introducing plasmids into mast cells via electroporation *(13)*.

2. Materials

1. Minimal essential medium (MEM).
2. Iscove's modified Dulbecco's medium (IMDM) supplemented with 5% heat-inactivated fetal calf serum (FCS), 2 mM L-glutamine, 1 mM pyruvate, 100 U penicillin/mL, and 100 µg/mL streptomycin.
3. 0.55 × 25-mm needles, 1-mL and 5-mL syringes.
4. Gey's lysis buffer: 150 mM NH$_4$Cl, 1 mM KHCO$_3$, 1 mM ethylene diamine tetraacetic acid, pH 7.3.
5. Falcon cell strainer (70-µm nylon, Becton Dickinson, cat. no. 352350).
6. Murine growth factors: IL-3, IL-4, stem cell factor (SCF).
7. SLO.
8. 0.1% and 0.5% Triton X-100 in H$_2$O.
9. ATP Bioluminescence Assay Kit CLS II (Roche).
10. Luminometer.
11. β-hexosaminidase substrate solution: 1.3 mg/mL p-nitrophenyl-N-acetyl-β-D-glucosamine in 0.1 M Na-citrate, pH 4.5.
12. β-hexosaminidase stop solution: 0.2 M glycine, pH 10.7.
13. Actinomycin D.
14. MTT solution: 2.5 mg/mL 3-(4,5-dimethylthiazol-2-yl)-2,5-diphenyl-tetrazolium bromide in phosphate-buffered saline (PBS), pH 7.4.
15. SDS-DMF solution: 20% sodium dodecyl sulfate (SDS), 33% dimethylformamide (DMF) in H$_2$O, pH 4.7.
16. Photometer.
17. TNF-α (murine or human).

18. SDS lysis buffer: 1% SDS, 15% glycerine, 4 M Urea, 50 mM Tris-HCl, pH 6.8.
19. DC protein assay kit (Bio-Rad).
20. Bromophenol blue; β-mercaptoethanol.
21. Protein electrophoresis and blotting equipment.
22. Phospho-MAPK antibody sampler kit (Cell Signaling Technology).
23. ECL chemiluminescence detection kit (Amersham Life Science).
24. Erasure buffer: 2% SDS, 100 mM β-mercaptoethanol, 50 mM Tris-HCl, pH 6.8.
25. Hank's balanced salt solution (HBSS) without Ca^{2+}.
26. Plasmids: NF-κB-dependent luciferase reporter gene; pRL-TK (Promega).
27. Electroporation device: Gene pulser I or II (Bio-Rad).
28. Dual luciferase reporter assay system (Promega).
29. LPS 055:B5 (Sigma).
30. Ionomycin (IO634; Sigma).

3. Methods
3.1. Generation of Murine Bone Marrow-Derived Mast Cells

1. Kill mice (age 5–10 wk) by cervical dislocation and remove intact femurs and tibias from the hind legs.
2. Cut off the tips of the tubular bones with a pair of scissors and put them in MEM. Do not use FCS in the following procedure to avoid foaming.
3. Flush out bone marrow with MEM using a 0.55 × 25-mm needle (24 G × 1 in.) and 5-mL syringe. Thoroughly resuspend the marrow.
4. Centrifuge suspension (10 min, 500g, 4°C), discard supernatant and resuspend pellet in 2 mL (for up to five mice) of Gey's lysis buffer. Incubate 2 min at RT to lyse erythrocytes. Stop reaction by adding 8 mL of MEM.
5. Apply the cell suspension on a BD Falcon cell strainer (70-μm nylon, cat. no. 352350) to remove aggregates.
6. Centrifuge the flow through (10 min, 500g, 4°C) and resuspend cells in an appropiate volume of IMDM/5% FCS as culture medium. After counting, establish bone marrow culture at a density of 2–3 × 10^6 cells/mL IMDM and growth factors (*see* **Note 2**).
7. Every 2–3 d (for a total of 21–28 d), discard half of the medium, carefully resuspend non-adherent cells in the remaining volume, transfer to new culture plates and add fresh medium.

3.2. Determination of Cellular ATP to Monitor Reversible Permeabilization of BMDMCs With SLO

Transient permeabilization of BMDMCs can be followed by monitoring cellular ATP content. At appropriate concentrations of SLO, the ATP levels drop to 30–40% within 30 min and gradually recover, reaching nearly 100% of the original value after 4 h.

1. In a 96-well plate, incubate 10^5 BMDMCs/well with various SLO concentrations (4 μg/mL to 250 ng/mL) in a total volume of 100 μL IMDM/5% FCS. Untreated cells serve as reference. The assay should be performed in triplicates.

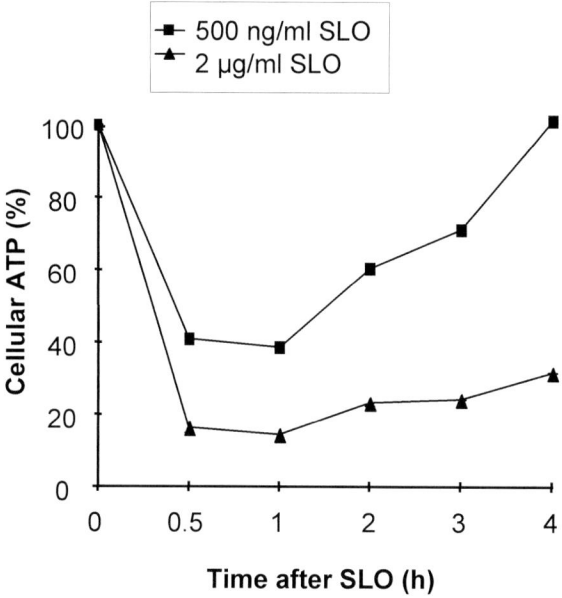

Fig. 1. Reversible permeabilization of bone marrow-derived mast cells (BMDMCs) with streptolysin O (SLO). BMDMCs were treated with SLO as indicated and cellular adenosine triphosphate was measured with luciferase.

2. After $t = 0$, 0.5, 1, 2, 3, and 4 h in an incubator, spin down cells (5 min, 500g), discard supernatant and lyse cell pellet in 100 µL of ice-cold 0.1% Triton X-100 solution.
3. Add 200 µL of luciferase reagent included in the ATP Bioluminescence Assay Kit CLS II (Roche) and measure bioluminescence in a luminometer.
4. Set luminescence of the untreated control as 100% cellular ATP and plot cellular ATP content against time. Optimal reversible permeabilization is characterized by a drop of cellular ATP followed by a gradual recovery, reaching nearly 100% of the initial value after 3–4 h (*see* **Fig. 1**).

3.3. Determination of β-Hexosaminidase Release to Measure SLO-Induced Degranulation

The enzyme β-hexosaminidase is stored in secretory granules and released upon degranulation of BMDMCs.

1. Activate 10^5 cells in a volume of 200 µL (96-well plate) with SLO for 30 min at 37°C.
2. Resuspend cells and transfer to 1.5-mL caps. Spin down cells, carefully remove supernatant, and save it. Lyse cell pellet in 200 µL of 0.5% Triton X-100 by resuspending thoroughly.

3. Transfer 20 µL of supernatant and 20 µL of the corresponding lysate to a fresh 96-well plate seperately and add 50 µL of β-hexosaminidase substrate solution. 20 µL of 0.5% Triton X-100 solution and 20 µL of fresh culture medium should be included as references/blanks. To achieve greatest accuracy, the test should be performed in triplicates. Incubate for 1.5 h at 37°C.

4. Stop enzyme reaction by adding 150 µL of 0.2 M Glycine, pH 10.7, and measure optical density (OD) at 405 nm.

5. Substract the values measured using only 0.5% Triton X-100 and fresh culture medium from the corresponding sample values. Add the background-corrected OD values of cell lysate and supernatant to obtain a measure for the total enzyme activity (100%). Calculate % degranulation = $OD_{supernatant} \times 100\% / (OD_{supernatant} + OD_{lysate})$.

Degranulation in the range of 20–30% can be expected.

3.4. Detection of Biologically Active TNF-α After Treatment of BMDMCs With SLO

This assay is based on the apoptosis-inducing ability of TNF-α on target cells.

1. Incubate mast cells in prewarmed IMDM/5% FCS with SLO at a concentration that allows optimal transient permeabilization (*see* **Figs. 1** and **2A**). Use untreated mast cells as reference. After 0.5, 1, 2, and 4 h (*see* **Fig. 2B**) spin down cells and collect supernatants.

2. Serially dilute (12 steps) culture supernatants in 96-well plates, 50 µL/well. Serial dilutions of TNF-α are used as reference beginning with 10–20 ng/mL.

3. To each well add 40,000 WEHI-164 target cells in 50 µL of IMDM/5% FCS containing 4 µg/mL actinomycin D. Incubate at 37°C for 24 h (*see* **Note 3**).

4. Add 50 µL of MTT solution and incubate at 37°C for 2 h.

5. Add 100 µL of SDS–DMF solution. Mix well and incubate for 3 h at 37°C.

6. Mix well and determine OD at 570 nm; use 690 nm as reference.

7. Plot known TNF-α concentrations of the standard against OD. Determine unknown TNF-α concentrations of samples by using the linear range of the standard curve only.

3.5. Assay of SLO-Induced MAP Kinase Activation

Activation of MAP kinases can be monitored by using antibodies specific for the phosphorylated proteins.

1. To reduce background phosphorylation of MAP kinases, incubate BMDMCs without growth factors in IMDM/5% FCS for 4 h.

2. Stimulate cells with SLO at a concentration that allows optimal reversible permeabilisation for 5, 15, 30, and 60 min. Include an unstimulated control. Use 1.5 to 2×10^6 cells per sample.

3. Harvest cells and spin down briefly. Lyse pellet in 100–150 µL of SDS–lysis buffer and heat samples immediately for 3 min at 100°C.

4. To reduce viscosity, pass solution through a 1-mL syringe six to eight times.

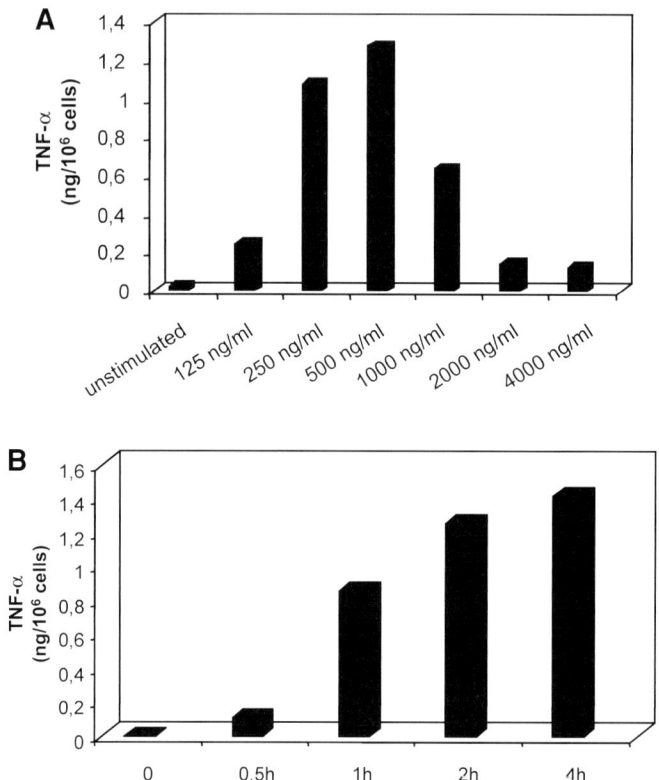

Fig. 2. SLO-induced production of tumor necrosis factor (TNF)-α. **(A)** Bone mar-row-derived mast cells (BMDMCs) were treated for 4 h with variable amounts of SLO and biologically active TNF-α was determined in the supernatants. **(B)** Kinetics of SLO-induced secretion of TNF-α using 500 ng/mL SLO.

5. Determine protein concentration using the DC protein assay kit (Bio-Rad) accord-ing to the instructions of the manufacturer (*see* **Note 4**).
6. Add bromophenol blue and β-mercaptoethanol to final concentrations of 100 ng/ μL and 1%, respectively. Heat samples again at 100°C for 2 min and spin down briefly. Apply 10–15 μg of protein to a 12% SDS polyacrylamide gel electro-phoresis (mini gel). Perform electrophoresis and western blotting according to standard procedures.
7. Use reagents delivered with the Phospho-MAPK Antibody Sampler Kit (Cell Signaling Technology) to assay phosphorylated ERK, JNK and p38 in combina-tion with chemiluminescence detection (ECL, Amersham Life Science).
8. After the first round of detection, blots can be stripped and reused. For this, incubate blots for 2×10 min at 60°C in erasure buffer (2% SDS, 100 m*M* β-mercaptoethanol, 50 m*M* Tris, pH 6.8; *see* **Note 5** and **Fig. 3**).

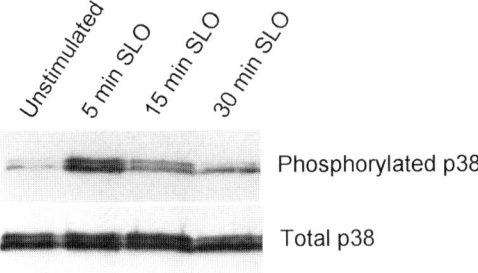

Fig. 3. Streptolysin O- (SLO)-induced phosphorylation of p38 MAP kinase. Bone marrow-derived mast cells (BMDMCs) were treated with 500 ng/mL of SLO and samples were taken at the indicated time points. After detection of phosphorylated p38 using anti phosho-p38 specific antibody, the blot was stripped and probed for total p38.

3.6. Delivery of Molecules Into BMDMCs by Reversible Permeabilization With SLO

It has been shown for several cell lines, that membrane pores formend by SLO allow the entry of molecules up to 100-kDa mass to the cytosol. Because the repair of such pores requires the presence of Ca^{2+}, the agent to be delivered to the cytosol is included at the permeabilization step with SLO in HBSS without Ca^{2+}. Resealing occurs after the addition of medium containing 1–2 mM Ca^{2+} (*see* **Fig. 4** *[6]*).

1. Suspend $1–2 \times 10^6$ cells in 500 µL of HBSS without Ca^{2+} for 15 min.
2. Centrifuge cells (5 min, 500g), discard supernatant and suspend cells in 500 µL of buffer described above. Add SLO and the agent to be delivered into the cytosol at appropriate concentrations (*see* **Note 6**). Incubate at 37°C for 10 min (permeabilization step).
3. Add 1.5 mL of IMDM/5% FCS and incubate for at least 1 h at 37°C (resealing step).

3.7. Transfection of Mast Cells Via Electroporation to Monitor the Activation of NF-κB by LPS

Activation of NF-κB can be measured using a plasmid encoding the luciferase gene whose expression is driven by multiple copies of an NF-κB binding site (GGC CTC TGG AAA GTA CCT TAA ACA TA *[14]*). The promoterless vector pTATALUC+ has been designed for the characterization of *cis*-regulatory elements and can be used for the insertion of NF-κB binding sites by common cloning procedures (*see* **Note 7** *[15]*). As an internal standard for the procedure outlined in **steps 1–6**, a second reporter, pRL-TK (Promega), is used, which contains the constitutively expressed thymidine kinase promoter upstream of the *Renilla reniformis* gene. After cotransfection, activities of both luciferases

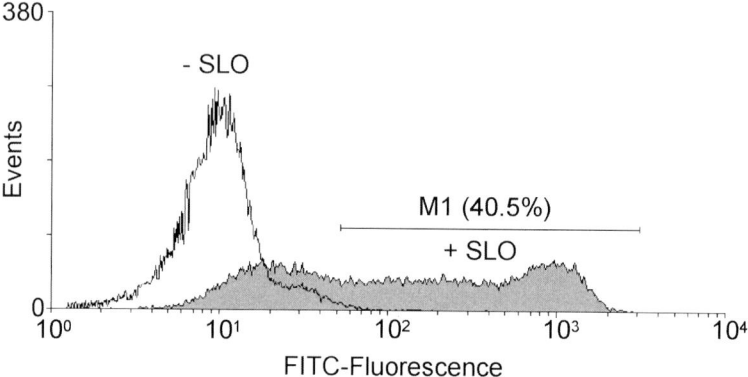

Fig. 4. Flow cytometric determination of FITC–dextran uptake. Bone marrow-derived mast cells (BMDMCs) were permeabilized using 75 ng/mL of streptolysin O (SLO) in the presence of 2.2 µg/mL FITC–dextran (4400 Da; Sigma). After resealing for 1 h in IMDM+5% fetal calf serum (FCS), FACS analysis was performed. Dead cells (25%) were excluded by propidium iodide staining.

can be determined one after the other in the same sample using the dual luciferase reporter assay system (Promega). Parameters for electroporation using two different models of Gene pulser (Bio-Rad) are summarized in **Table 1**.

1. Transfer each $1–2 \times 10^6$ BMDMC in 0.2 mL of IMDM (without FCS) into electroporation cuvets. Perform all of the following steps at RT.
2. Add plasmids in an additional volume of 10 µL to the following final concentrations: NF-κB reporter or empty vector (50 µg/mL); pRL-TK (1–2 µg/mL; to each sample).
3. Pulse cells in electroporation device. Carefully recover cells by adding 0.8 mL of IMDM/5% FCS.
4. Allow cells to recover for 2 h in an incubator.
5. Spin down cells (10 min, 500g).
6. Count viable cells, stimulate cells (1×10^6/mL IMDM/5% FCS) as depicted in **Fig. 5**.
7. Harvest cells after 8–16 h and determine luciferase activity using the dual luciferase reporter assay system (Promega) according to the instructions of the manufacturer (*see* **Fig. 5**).

4. Notes

1. Highly purified SLO can also be obtained from the Institute of Medical Microbiology, Mainz (makowiec@mail.uni-mainz.de). Store SLO in small aliquots at –20°C and thaw only once.
2. For the generation of murine BMDMCs from their bone marrow precursors, it is obligatory to use IL-3 in the culture medium. We use IL-3 purified from WEHI-

Table 1
Parameters for Electroporation of BMDMCs
Using Bio-Rad Devices

	Gene pulser I	Gene pulser II
Cuvets (width)	0.2 cm	0.4 cm
Volume of cells	0.2 mL	0.2 mL
Time constant	app. 30 ms	app. 30 ms
Voltage	350 V	290 V
Capacity	960 μF	600 μF
Resistance	∞	–

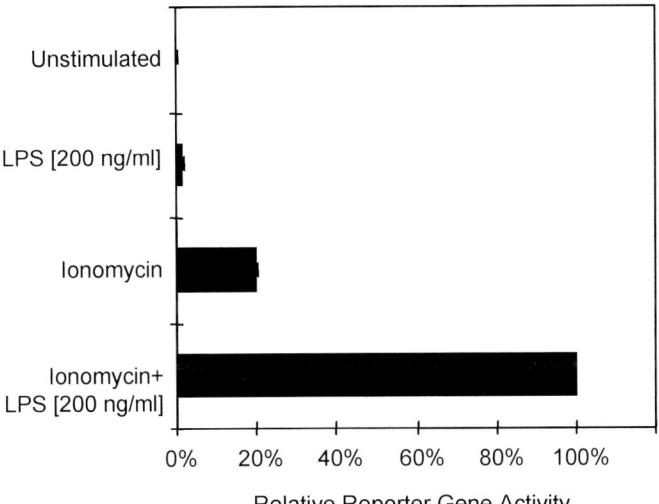

Fig. 5. Expression of an NF-κB-dependent luciferase gene after activation with ionomycin and LPS. Transfected bone marrow-derived mast cells (BMDMCs) were stimulated with ionomycin (0.5 μ*M*) and/or LPS (200 ng/mL). The activity of the pTATALUC+ control vector was substracted from the indicated values, and data were standardized according to the Renilla luciferase activity.

3B supernatant at a concentration of 20 U/mL. 1 U refers to an amount of IL-3, which allows for half-maximum proliferation of the IL-3-dependent cell line DA-1. In addition to IL-3, IL-4, and SCF also can be added.

3. The sensitivity of this assay, if necessary, can be improved by including a final concentration of 20 m*M* LiCl. The cell line L929 can be used instead of WEHI-164 with equal results.

4. Because samples contain high amounts of SDS, coomassie-based procedures cannot be used.

5. After stripping of the antibodies, start with blocking of the membrane before adding the next antibody. For this procedure, it is essential that the blots do not become dry. As a control, chemiluminescence detection can be performed after stripping. Also include an equal loading control (e.g., an antibody directed against total p38 or β-actin). Using this protocol, four rounds of detection can be performed.

6. The required toxin concentration varies depending on the cell type and density and must be determined empirically. Measuring cellular ATP content is a suitable method. Alternatively, resealing is also evidenced by the reduction in numbers of cells staining positive with Trypan blue. Typically, approx 25% of the cells remain nonpermeabilized, 25% are dead, and approx 50% are resealed (*see* **Fig. 4**). In general, permeabilization in HBSS requires less SLO compared with permeabilization in IMDM/5% FCS.

7. Stratagene offers several PathDetect *cis*-reporting systems, including one for NF-κB.

References

1. Stassen, M., Hultner, L., and Schmitt, E. (2002) Classical and alternative pathways of mast cell activation. *Crit. Rev. Immunol.* **22,** 115–140.

2. Stassen, M., Hultner, L., Muller, C., and Schmitt, E. (2002) Mast cells and inflammation. *Arch. Immunol. Ther. Exp. (Warsz.)* **50,** 179–185.

3. Echtenacher, B., Mannel, D. N., and Hultner, L. (1996) Critical protective role of mast cells in a model of acute septic peritonitis. *Nature* **381,** 75–77.

4. Malaviya, R., Ikeda, T., Ross, E., and Abraham, S. N. (1996) Mast cell modulation of neutrophil influx and bacterial clearance at sites of infection through TNF-alpha. *Nature* **381,** 77–80.

5. Bhakdi, S., Bayley, H., Valeva, A., et al. (1996) Staphylococcal alpha-toxin, streptolysin-O, and *Escherichia coli* hemolysin: prototypes of pore-forming bacterial cytolysins. *Arch. Microbiol.* **165,** 73–79.

6. Walev, I., Bhakdi, S. C., Hofmann, F., et al. (2001) Delivery of proteins into living cells by reversible membrane permeabilization with streptolysin-O. *Proc. Natl. Acad. Sci. USA* **98,** 3185–3190.

7. Stassen, M., Muller, C., Richter, C., et al. (2003) The streptococcal exotoxin streptolysin O activates mast cells to produce tumor necrosis factor alpha by p38 mitogen-activated protein kinase- and protein kinase C-dependent pathways. *Infect. Immun.* **71,** 6171–6177.

8. Weller, U., Muller, L., Messner, M., et al. (1996) Expression of active streptolysin O in Escherichia coli as a maltose-binding-protein–streptolysin-O fusion protein. The N-terminal 70 amino acids are not required for hemolytic activity. *Eur. J. Biochem.* **236,** 34–39.

9. Leal-Berumen, I., Conlon, P., and Marshall, J. S. (1994) IL-6 production by rat peritoneal mast cells is not necessarily preceded by histamine release and can be induced by bacterial lipopolysaccharide. *J. Immunol.* **152,** 5468–5476.

10. Stassen, M., Muller, C., Arnold, M., et al. (2001) IL-9 and IL-13 production by activated mast cells is strongly enhanced in the presence of lipopolysaccharide: NF-kappa B is decisively involved in the expression of IL-9. *J. Immunol.* **166,** 4391–4398.

11. Supajatura, V., Ushio, H., Nakao, A., Okumura, K., Ra, C., and Ogawa, H. (2001) Protective roles of mast cells against enterobacterial infection are mediated by toll-like receptor 4. *J. Immunol.* **167,** 2250–2256.

12. Masuda, A., Yoshikai, Y., Aiba, K., and Matsuguchi, T. (2002) Th2 cytokine production from mast cells is directly induced by lipopolysaccharide and distinctly regulated by c-Jun N-terminal kinase and p38 pathways. *J. Immunol.* **169,** 3801–3810.

13. Stassen, M., Arnold, M., Hultner, L., et al. (2000) Murine bone marrow-derived mast cells as potent producers of IL-9: costimulatory function of IL-10 and kit ligand in the presence of IL-1. *J. Immunol.* **164,** 5549–5555.

14. Toth, C. R., Hostutler, R. F., Baldwin, A. S. Jr., and Bender, T. P. (1995) Members of the nuclear factor kappa B family transactivate the murine c-myb gene. *J. Biol. Chem.* **270,** 7661–7671.

15. Altschmied, J. and Duschl, J. (1997) Set of optimized luciferase reporter gene plasmids compatible with widely used CAT vectors. *Biotechniques* **23,** 436–438.

IX

ANALYSIS OF PROGRAMMED CELL DEATH IN MAST CELLS

30

Mast Cell Apoptosis

Alexander Gerbaulet, Karin Hartmann, and Yoseph A. Mekori

Summary

Apoptosis is a physiological form of cell death. Cells undergoing apoptosis execute a genetically controlled program that leads to organized breakdown of cellular structures and ends in phagocytosis of their remains. In mast cells, several mechanisms regulating apoptosis have been identified including growth factors, tumor necrosis factor-α receptors, monomeric IgE, Toll-like receptors, and proteins of the bcl-2 family. Methods used to characterize apoptosis of mast cells are reviewed, with special attention to flow cytometric analysis of annexin V staining, analysis of deoxyribonucleic acid fragmentation by gel electrophoresis and end-labeling techniques, measurement of caspase activity by enzymatic assays, and characterization of pro- and anti-apoptotic proteins by immunoblotting.

Key Words: Annexin V; apoptosis; caspases; DNA fragmentation; flow cytometry; mast cells; mastocytosis; TUNEL; Western blotting.

1. Introduction

There are two major forms of cell death: apoptosis, which is the physiologic form of cell death, and necrosis, an accidental form of cell death. Apoptosis occurs naturally at the end of a cell's life span, during tissue regulation, and in response to events that induce an irreparable damage of cellular structures (*1*). The process of apoptosis is highly complex and resembles a well-organized retreat. Characteristic morphological features of apoptotic cells include cell shrinkage, condensation of chromatin, fragmentation of DNA, and formation of apoptotic bodies (**Fig. 1**). Because of phagocytosis of the apoptotic bodies, there is no inflammation after apoptosis. In contrast, necrosis is provoked by intense stimuli, leading to loss of essential cellular properties, such as the integrity of the cell membrane or maintenance of homeostasis. Necrotic cells show a breakdown of their DNA, destruction of intracellular organelles, and attraction of inflammatory cells. In this technical review, we will focus on char-

From: *Methods in Molecular Biology, vol. 315: Mast Cells: Methods and Protocols*
Edited by: G. Krishnaswamy and D. S. Chi © Humana Press Inc., Totowa, NJ

A

B

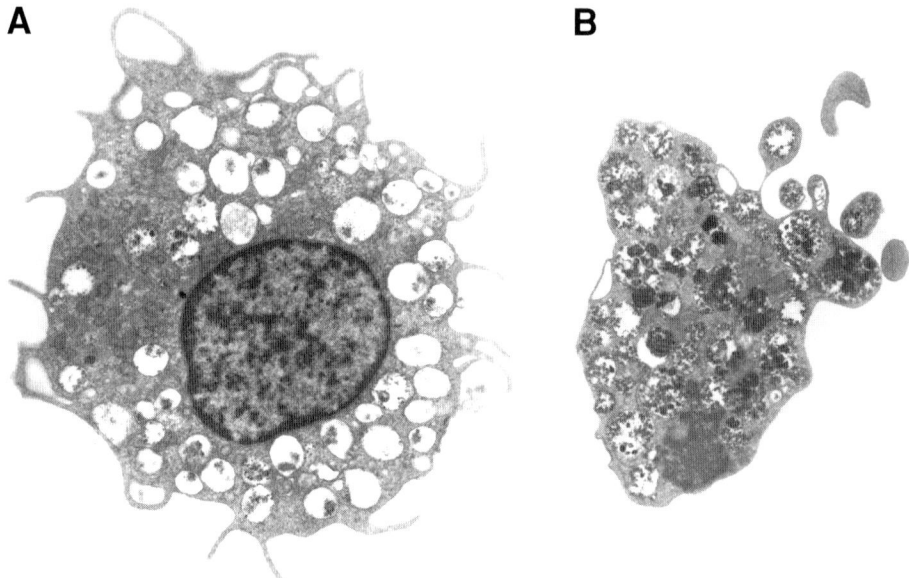

Fig. 1. Ultrastructure of (**A**) an untreated, viable murine bone marrow-cultured mast cell (BMCMC) compared with (**B**) an apoptotic BMCMC. Apoptosis was induced by incubation with anti-CD95 mAb (1 mg/mL) and actinomycin D (40 ng/mL) for 48 h. Control cells (**A**) exhibit a corrugated cell surface and regularly distributed nuclear chromatin. In contrast, apoptotic cells (**B**) show membrane blebbing and formation of apoptotic bodies (electron microscopy, magnification: ×800).

acterization of mast cell apoptosis using biochemical properties of apoptotic cells *(2)*. Apoptosis is induced either by an extrinsic pathway triggered by stimulation of specific surface receptors such as CD95 (Fas, APO-1) and TNF-related apoptosis-inducing ligand (TRAIL) receptors or by an intrinsic pathway mediated through intracellular proteins leading to release of cytochrome c from mitochondria *(3)*. Both signaling pathways share a common end, a cascade of proteases, referred to as caspases *(4)*. Molecules that are referred to by methods reviewed in this chapter include proteins like the bcl-2 family and p53, extracellular expression of phosphatidylserine (PS), and activation of caspases.

1.1. Effect of Growth Factors on Apoptosis of Mast Cells

Mast cells are long-lived cells that derive from CD34-positive hematopoietic progenitor cells *(5,6)*. Growth factors, receptor signaling, antibodies, and lipopolysaccharides tightly regulate their maturation, differentiation, and survival. Stem cell factor (SCF) has been identified as the most important regulator of mast cell maturation and differentiation in vivo and in vitro *(7,8)*. Injection of SCF into mouse skin and spleen induces an increase of mast cells *(9)*. In response to deprivation of SCF, mast cells show signs of apoptosis, and numbers of cells return to baseline *(9,10)*. SCF binds to the receptor KIT, which in turn signals to a series of pathways including phosphatidylinositol 3' kinase, phospholipase C, protein kinase C, the Ras-mitogen activated protein kinase (MAPK) cascade, and Janus tyrosine kinases/signal transducers and activators of transcription (JAK/STAT pathway [11]). Stimulation of mast cells with SCF has been shown to induce upregulation of the antiapoptotic proteins bcl-2 and bcl-x_L *(12,13)*.

In murine mast cells, interleukin (IL)-3 is able to prevent apoptosis in response to deprivation of SCF within one hour of growth factor withdrawal *(10)*. Vice versa, SCF also inhibits apoptosis of murine mast cells following IL-3 deprivation *(9,10,14)*. IL-3 shares with SCF parts of its signaling pathways, mainly phosphatidylinositol 3' kinase, MAPK, and STAT-5, and also exhibits its antiapoptotic effects via upregulation of bcl-2 *(11,14)*. In contrast to murine mast cells, human mature mast cells derived from lung, uterus, kidney, tonsils, and liver fail to express the IL-3 receptor and are not susceptible to an anti-apoptotic effect of IL-3 *(15)*. However, human immature mast cells, cultured cells, and mature intestinal cells have been shown to express the IL-3 receptor *(16)*.

IL-4 has been reported to exhibit proapoptotic as well as antiapoptotic effects depending on maturation of mast cells, tissue subtype, and organism from which mast cells are derived *(17–19)*. In the presence of SCF, IL-4 has been shown to induce apoptosis in human cord blood-derived mast cells (CBMCs), whereas human fetal liver- and lung-derived mast cells are protected from IL-4-induced apoptosis by endogenous production of IL-6 *(17)*. In contrast, skin-derived mast cells are resistant to IL-4-mediated apoptosis, probably as a result of the lack of IL-4 receptors on mast cells of the MC(TC) subtype (mast cells expressing tryptase and chymase [20]). However, coculture with IL-4 and SCF has been found to significantly enhance proliferation and mediator release in mature human intestinal mast cells *(18)*. IL-4 thus suppresses the maturation of progenitor cells but leads to the expansion of certain mature mast cells. It has been speculated that IL-4 exerts its apoptotic effects via downregulation of KIT, whereas its proliferative capabilities are mediated by shifting mature mast cells to the IL-3 receptor-positive MC(T) phenotype (mast cells expressing tryptase only). In murine mast cells, IL-4 has been demonstrated to induce apoptosis through mitochondrial damage and activation of STAT-6 *(19)*.

Transforming growth factor (TGF)-β has been shown to prevent the rescue effect of SCF in murine IL-3-deprived mast cells, probably via downregulation of KIT *(21,22)*. In addition, nerve growth factor has been found to increase mast cell numbers by preventing apoptosis of human CBMC *(23)* and rat peritoneal mast cells *(24)*.

1.2. Regulation of Mast Cell Apoptosis by TNF Receptors

The expression of the surface receptor CD95 (Fas, APO-1), belonging to the family of death or TNF-α receptors, has been reported on different mast cell types, including murine bone marrow-cultured mast cells (BMCMCs); the murine cell lines C57, MCP-5, and P815; and HMC-1 cells *(25,26)*. Stimulation with CD95 ligand (CD95L) or specific anti-CD95 antibodies has been demonstrated to induce apoptosis in C57 and P815 cells, whereas BMCMC and MCP-5 cells are resistant to anti-CD95-induced apoptosis *(25)*. Thus, susceptibility of mast cells to apoptosis mediated by CD95 appears to be associated not only with expression of CD95 but also with intracellular control of signaling pathways. In accordance, the addition of the transcription inhibitor actinomycin D has been shown to render BMCMCs susceptible to anti-CD95-induced apoptosis *(25)*. Murine mast cells have additionally been reported to express CD95L intracellularly; however, a functional expression in mast cells has not been proven *(27)*.

1.3. Effect of Monomeric IgE on Mast Cell Apoptosis

Two independent studies have shown recently that the sensitization of murine mast cells by monomeric IgE, which does not lead to crosslinking of the high-affinity IgE receptor FcεRI, induces prolonged survival *(28,29)*. Kalesnikoff et al. *(28)* showed, in addition to the antiapoptotic effect, marked induction of various proinflammatory cytokines, such as IL-4, IL-6, IL-13, and TNF-α; phosphorylation of MAPK like ERK1/2, JNK; and upregulation of bcl-x_L mRNA upon exposure with monomeric IgE *(28)*. These results suggested that prolonged survival, at least in part, resulted from autocrine stimulation. In contrast, Asai et al. *(29)* failed to detect release of mediators or activation of MAPK in response to monomeric IgE, but also observed inhibition of apoptosis. Kitaura et al. *(30)* were then able to demonstrate that only a subgroup of monomeric IgE antibodies exhibits the cytokinergic effect; however, all monomeric IgEs tested were associated with an antiapoptotic activity *(31)*.

1.4. Regulation of Mast Cell Apoptosis by Toll-Like Receptors

Toll-like receptors (TLRs), which belong to a receptor family sharing homology with the Toll receptor found in *drosophila*, play an important role in the innate recognition of bacterial infections. TLRs recognize lipopolysaccharides (LPS) and peptidoglycans from bacterial walls. Murine mast cells recently have been reported to express TLR-2, TLR-4, and TLR-6 *(32,33)*. Human mast cells showed expression of TLR-1, TLR-2, and TLR-6 *(34)*. Stimulation of TLRs by LPS has been found to inhibit apoptosis of IL-3-deprived murine BMCMC by upregulating bcl-x_L protein *(35)*. Prolonged survival induced by LPS also was enhanced by costimulation with interferon-γ, which leads to an increased expression of TLR-4.

1.5. Altered Expression of Apoptosis Molecules in Mastocytosis

Several studies demonstrated an altered expression of apoptosis molecules in mastocytosis, a rare disease characterized by accumulation of mast cells in tissues *(13,36–39)*. In adults, mastocytosis usually is caused by activating *KIT* mutations *(40)*. Bone marrow mast cells of patients with systemic mastocytosis have been shown to strongly express bcl-xL *(13,37,39)*. In contrast, expression of bcl-2 was absent or low, with the exception of patients with mast cell leukemia that exhibited enhanced levels of bcl-2 in their bone marrow *(13,36,37,39)*. In addition, the cell cycle-regulating protein p21 was overexpressed in bone marrow lesions, whereas the expression of Ki67 and p53 as well as the percentage of apoptotic mast cells was comparable between mastocytosis and controls *(39)*. In contrast to infiltrates of the bone marrow, skin lesions of patients with mastocytosis have been found to be associated with an increased expression of bcl-2 but not bcl-xL *(13,38)*. Thus, an altered rate of apoptosis and cell cycling may also contribute to the pathogenesis of mast cell diseases.

2. Materials

2.1. Flow Cytometric Analysis of Propidium Iodide and Annexin V Staining

1. Phosphate-buffered saline (PBS): 137 m*M* NaCl, pH 7.4, 2.7 m*M* KCl, 8 m*M* Na_2HPO_4, and 1.5 m*M* KH_2PO_4.
2. Binding buffer: 10 m*M* HEPES, 140 m*M* NaCl, 2.5m*M* $CaCl_2$, pH 7.4.
3. Fluorescein isothiocyanate (FITC)-labeled annexin V (BD Pharmingen, San Diego, CA).
4. Propidium iodide (PI), 50 µg/mL in PBS.

2.2. Analysis of DNA Fragmentation by Gel Electrophoresis

1. PBS: 137 m*M* NaCl, pH 7.4, 2.7 m*M* KCl, 8 m*M* Na_2HPO_4, 1.5 m*M* KH_2PO_4.
2. Lysis buffer: 5 m*M* Tris-HCl, pH 8.0, 5 m*M* ethylene diamine tetraacetic acid (EDTA), 0.5% Triton X-100.
3. TE buffer: 10 m*M* Tris-HCl, pH 7.4, 1 m*M* EDTA.
4. Phenol chloroform solution, phenol:chloroform 3:4 (v/v) water-saturated.
5. Proteinase K, 20 mg/mL in PBS.
6. RNase A, 20 mg/mL in PBS (DNase-free).
7. Electrophoresis equipment.

8. TAE buffer: 40 mM Tris, pH 8.0, 20 mM acetic acid, 50 mM EDTA.
9. 10X loading buffer: 30% (v/v) glycerol, 1% (w/v) sodium dodecyl sulfate (SDS), 0.25% (w/v) bromophenol blue.
10. Agarose gel (*see* **Note 1**).

2.3. Analysis of DNA Fragmentation by End-Labeling Techniques

2.3.1. Histochemical Staining

1. PBS: 137 mM NaCl, pH 7.4, 2.7 mM KCl, 8 mM Na$_2$HPO$_4$, 1.5 mM KH$_2$PO$_4$.
2. Formaldehyde solution, 3.7% (w/v) in PBS.
3. Cacodylate buffer: 30 mM Tris-HCl, pH 7.2, 1 mM CoCl$_2$, 10 mM sodium cacodylate.
4. Reaction buffer: cacodylate buffer containing 20 mM dUTP, 4 mM biotin-16-dUTP, 250 U/mL TdT (freshly prepared).
5. Termination buffer: 300 mM NaCl, 30 mM sodium citrate.
6. Acetate buffer: 50 mM CH$_3$COOH-NaOH, pH 5.0.
7. Horseradish peroxidase-labeled streptavidin, 10 mg/mL in PBS.
8. AEC reagent: dissolve 20 mg of 3-amino-9-ethylcarbazole in 2.5 mL of *N,N*-dimethylformamide and add acetate buffer to a final volume of 50 mL. Before use, add 25 mL of 30% (w/w) H$_2$O$_2$.

2.3.2. Flow Cytometry

1. 1% formaldehyde: 1% (w/v) formaldehyde in PBS. Prepare fresh from paraformaldehyde.
2. 70% ethanol.
3. 5X reaction buffer: 1 M sodium cacodylate; 125 mM Tris-HCl, pH 6.6, bovine serum albumin (BSA) 1.25 mg/mL.
4. 10 mM CoCl$_2$ solution in H$_2$O.
5. TdT 25 U/μL.
6. BrdUTP solution: 2 mM BrdUTP, 50 mM Tris-HCl, pH 7.5.
7. FITC-conjugated anti-BrdU monoclonal antibody solution: 0.3 (m/v) % in PBS, 0.3% (v/v) Triton X-100, 5 mg/mL BSA.
8. Rinsing buffer: 0.1% Triton X-100, 5 mg/mL BSA in PBS.
9. PI solution: 5 μg/mL PI, 200 μg/mL DNase-free RNase A in PBS.
10. Flow cytometer.

2.4. Analysis of Caspase Activation

1. Z-DEVD-7-amino-4-methylcoumarin, 10 mM in dimethyl sulfoxide (DMSO).
2. 7-amino-4-methylcoumarin, 10 mM in DMSO as reference standard.
3. Ac-DEVD-CHO, 1 mM in DMSO as specific caspase inhibitor.
4. 20X lysis buffer: 200 mM Tris-HCl, 2 M NaCl, 20 mM EDTA, 0.2% Triton X-100, pH 7.5.
5. 5X reaction buffer: 50 mM PIPES, 10 mM EDTA, 0.5% CHAPS, pH 7.4.
6. Dithiothreitol, 1 M in H$_2$O.
7. PBS: 137 mM NaCl, pH 7.4, 2.7 mM KCl, 8 mM Na$_2$HPO$_4$, 1.5 mM KH$_2$PO$_4$.
8. ELISA microreader (342 nm excitation/441 nm emission).

2.5. Analysis of Protein Expression by Immunoblotting

1. TBS buffer: 50 mM Tris-HCl, pH 7.6, 1% (m/v) BSA, 0.1% (v/v) Tween-20.
2. Blocking solution: 10% (m/v) nonfat dry milk in TBS buffer.
3. Lysis buffer: PBS, pH 7.4; 1% (v/v) nonidet P-40, 0.5% sodium desoxycholate, 0.1% (m/v) SDS, 0.0005% (m/v) aprotinin, 0.0005% (m/v) leupeptin, 0.1% (m/v) phenylmethylsulfonylfluoride.
4. Incubation buffer: 5% (m/v) nonfat dry milk in TBS.
5. 4X loading buffer: 250 mM Tris-HCl, pH 6.8, 40% (v/v) glycerol, 8% (m/v) SDS, 0.001% (m/v) bromophenol blue.
6. Electrophoresis buffer: 25 mM Tris-HCl, pH 8.3, 192 mM glycine, 0.1% SDS.
7. Electrophoresis stacking gel: 4.85% (m/v) acrylamide, 0.15% (m/v) bisacrylamide, 125 mM Tris-HCl, pH 6.8, 0.1% (m/v) SDS, 0.1% (m/v) ammonium persulfate, 0.01% (m/v) TEMED.
8. Electrophoresis separating gel: 14.6% (m/v) acrylamide, 0.4% (m/v) bisacrylamide, 375 mM Tris-HCl, pH 8.8; 0.1% (m/v) SDS, 0.1% (m/v) ammonium persulfate, 0.01% (m/v) TEMED.
9. Electrophoresis equipment.
10. Anode buffer I: 300 mM Tris-HCl, pH 11.0, 20% (v/v) methanol.
11. Anode buffer II: 25 mM Tris-HCl, pH 10.4, 20% (v/v) methanol.
12. Cathode buffer: 40 mM 6-aminocaproic acid, pH 7.6, 20% (v/v) methanol.
13. Nitrocellulose membrane (e.g., Hybond C, Amersham Biosciences, Amersham, UK).
14. Semi-dry blotting equipment.
15. Primary antibody (e.g., anti-bcl-2 mouse monoclonal IgG1, c = 1.5 μg/mL; cat. no. sc-509, Santa Cruz Biotechnology Inc, Santa Cruz, CA); anti-bcl-x$_L$ mouse monoclonal IgG1, c = 1.5 μg/mL (cat. no. sc-8392, Santa Cruz Biotechnology); anti-bax mouse monoclonal IgG1, c = 2 μg/mL (clone YTH-2D2, Trevigen, Gaithersburg, MD); anti-p53 mouse monoclonal IgG2a, c = 0.25 μg/mL (clone DO1, BD Pharmingen, San Diego, CA).
16. Horseradish peroxidase-conjugated secondary antibody.
17. Anti-beta-actin antibody.
18. Strip buffer: 62.5 mM Tris-HCl, pH 6.8, 100 mM β-mercaptoethanol, 2% (m/v) SDS.

3. Methods

The methods described in **Subheadings 3.1.–3.5.** outline analysis of: (1) propidium iodide and annexin V staining by flow cytometry; (2) DNA fragmentation by gel electrophoresis; (3) end-labeling techniques; (4) caspase activation; and (5) protein expression by immunoblotting.

3.1. Flow Cytometric Analysis of Propidium Iodide and Annexin V Staining

Propidium iodide (PI) intercalates (inserts between adjacent bases) the DNA. Together with DNA, PI forms a fluorescent charge transfer complex. Because PI is unable to cross the intact cell membrane, only necrotic and late apoptotic cells with a defective membrane will show an increased fluorescence after incubation with PI *(41)*. Annexin V, a human protein with anticoagulant, antiphospholipase, and antikinase activities, binds to extracellularly exposed PS in the presence of Ca^{2+}. The lipid double-layer membrane of viable cells is characterized by an asymmetric distribution of phospholipid compounds, with phosphatidylcholine and sphingomyelin being expressed on the outer surface and PS on the cytoplasmatic face. Enzymes called flippases control the asymmetric distribution. Loss of asymmetry, while the membrane remains intact, is an early event during apoptosis *(42)*. Combined staining with fluorochrome-labeled Annexin V that only binds to extracellular PS and PI allows to discriminate between viable (Annexin V-negative/PI-negative), apoptotic (Annexin V-positive/PI-negative), and necrotic (Annexin V-positive/PI-positive) cells (*see* **Note 2**, **Fig. 2**).

1. Wash cells twice with cold PBS and resuspend pellet in binding buffer yielding a concentration of 10^6 cells/mL.
2. Transfer 100 µL of the cell suspension to each round-bottom tube, add 5 µL of annexin V-FITC and 2–10 µL of PI (start with 2 µL, optimal amount should be titrated) per tube, and incubate for 15 min in the dark on ice.
3. Add 400 µL of binding buffer per tube without washing. Analyze with flow cytometer within 1 h.
4. For adjustment and compensation, the following controls should be prepared:
   a. Unstained cells.
   b. Cells incubated with PI only.
   c. Cells incubated with annexin V-FITC only.
5. Before analyzing PI- and annexin V-FITC-stained cells, compensate between FL1 (green fluorescence, FITC) and FL2 (red fluorescence, PI). PI can be detected in FL2 and FL3.

3.2. Analysis of DNA Fragmentation by Gel Electrophoresis

A typical feature of apoptotic cells is the occurrence of DNA fragments with a length of 180–200 bp (which is the size of DNA comprising a nucleosome) and multiples. DNA fragments are generated by an endonuclease, called caspase-activated DNase (CAD), which is set free by cleavage of its inhibitor, ICAD, through activated caspase-3 *(43)*. Fragments can be detected by conventional agarose gel electrophoresis, showing a characteristic "DNA ladder" (*see* **Note 3**, **Fig. 3**).

1. Wash apoptotic cells with cold PBS; lyse the cells with 500 µL of lysis buffer for 1 h at 4°C.
2. Centrifuge at 27,000g for 30 min to pellet the high molecular fraction of the lysate.
3. Separate the supernatant and add proteinase K to yield a final concentration of 0.5 mg/mL and incubate for 30 min at 4°C.
4. Protein contaminants are removed by two extractions with phenol chloroform. Phenol is removed by extraction with chloroform; DNA stays in the aqueous phase.

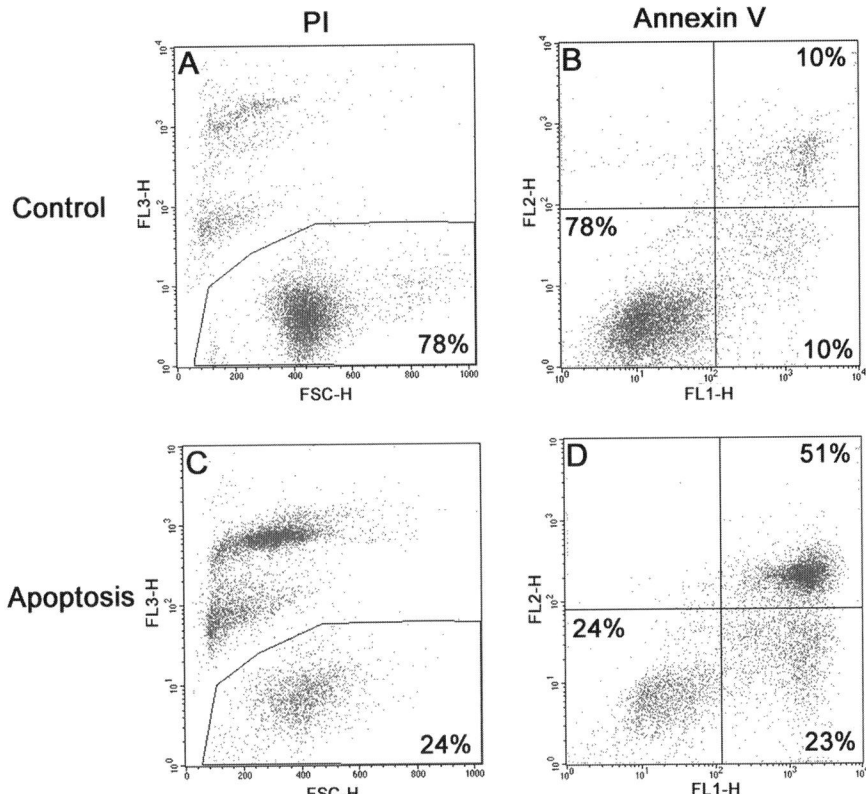

Fig. 2. Flow cytometric staining of apoptotic **(C,D)** and control **(A,B)** HMC-1 cells with PI and FITC-labeled annexin V. Apoptosis **(C,D)** was induced by incubation with rhTRAIL (100 ng/mL) and actinomycin D (20 ng/mL) for 48 h. Cells were either stained with PI only **(A,C)** or double-stained with annexin V and PI **(B,D)**. Dot plots showing FCS (cell size) vs FL-3 **(A,C)** allow to discriminate between two cell populations. Viable, intact cells are shown at low FL-3 fluorescence, whereas necrotic or late apoptotic cells are characterized by high uptake of FL-3. Dot plots analysing FL-1 vs FL-2 **(B,D)** allow to discriminate between viable (FL-1-low/FL-2-low), early apoptotic (FL-1-high/FL-2-low), and late apoptotic or necrotic (FL-1-high/FL-2-high) cells.

5. Precipitate DNA by adding ethanol to 70% (v/v) and NaCl to 0.1 *M* final concentration (*see* **Note 4**).
6. Resuspend DNA in TE buffer yielding approximately 100 ng/µL and digest with RNase A (final concentration: 0.5 mg/mL) for 30 min at 37°C.
7. Subject DNA to gel electrophoresis and stain with ethidium bromide at 0.1 µg/mL (*see* **Note 5**).

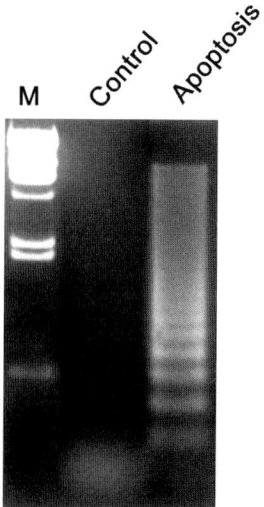

Fig. 3. DNA fragmentation of apoptotic C57 cells demonstrated by gel electrophoresis. M, DNA molecular weight marker; Control, untreated C57 cells; Apoptosis, C57 cells incubated with anti-CD95 MAb (1 mg/mL) and actinomycin D (10 ng/mL) for 12 h.

3.3. Analysis of DNA Fragmentation by End-Labeling Techniques

End-labeling techniques are based on the detection of free 3'-hydroxyl termini, generated by DNA cleavage *(43)*, with marked nucleotides. Examples for marked nucleoside triphosphates (dNTPs) are biotinylated dUTP or 5-bromo-dUTP (BrdUTP). The TUNEL (terminal desoxynucleotidyl transferase dUTP nick end labeling) method uses terminal desoxynucleotidyl transferase (TdT) to append tagged dUTP to free 3'-OH ends of double-stranded DNA fragments *(44)*. Visualization of marked complexes can be performed using FITC-conjugated streptavidin, horseradish peroxidase-conjugated streptavidin, or FITC-labeled anti-BrdU antibodies. Techniques used for the detection and quantification of TUNEL staining include light or fluorescence microscopy and flow cytometry (*see* **Note 6 [41]**).

3.3.1. Histochemical Staining

1. Spin cells on a slide (cytospin). Fix with fresh formaldehyde solution for 10 min; wash three times in PBS for 5 min (*see* **Note 7**).
2. Quench endogenous peroxidase with 3% (v/v) H_2O_2 for 5 min, followed by two 5-min washes in PBS.
3. Equilibrate in cacodylate buffer for 10 min. Once treated with cacodylate buffer do not allow to dry.

4. Immerse slide in reaction buffer and incubate for 1 h in a humidified chamber at 37°C.
5. Stop the labeling reaction by immersion into termination buffer. Wash slide with PBS for 10 min.
6. Add a small volume of peroxidase-labeled streptavidin. Incubate for 30 min in a humidified chamber at 37°C. Afterwards wash several times with PBS.
7. Immerse slide for 10 min in AEC reagent at room temperature. After washing twice for 5 min with PBS and once with water, subject samples to light microscopy.

3.3.2. Flow Cytometry

1. Fix cells (10^6 cells) in 1% formaldehyde for 15 min on ice (*see* **Note 8**).
2. Wash with PBS (centrifuge at $300g$, 5 min, 5 mL PBS), resuspend in PBS, yielding 10^6 cells/0.5 mL.
3. Add 5 mL of ice-cold 70% ethanol (*see* **Note 9**). Centrifuge at $200g$ for 3 min, remove the supernatant, wash with PBS.
4. Resuspend cells in a solution containing 10-μL reaction buffer, 2 μL of BrdUTP, 0.5 μL of (12,5 U) TdT, 5 μL of $CoCl_2$, 33.5 μL H_2O. Incubate for 40 min at 37°C.
5. Add 1.5 mL of rinsing buffer and centrifuge ($300g$, 5 min).
6. Resuspend cells in 100 μL of FITC-conjugated anti-BrdU MAb solution and incubate for 1 h at room temperature.
7. Add 2 mL of rinsing buffer and centrifuge ($300g$, 5 min).
8. Resuspend cell pellet in 1 mL of PI solution. Incubate for 15 min in the dark.
9. Analyze cells by flow cytometry. The following samples should be prepared for compensation, positive and negative control:
   a. Unstained cells.
   b. Cells stained with FITC-anti-BrdU MAb only.
   c. Cells stained with PI only.
   d. Negative control: cells treated according to the protocol, but with exclusion of TdT in the BrdUTP/TdT incubation step.
   e. Positive control: cells that are known to be apoptotic treated according to the protocol.
10. Compensate between FL1 (green fluorescence, FITC) and FL2 (red fluorescence, PI). PI can be detected in FL2 and FL3.

3.4. Analysis of Caspase Activation

The protease family of caspases (aspartate-specific cysteine proteases) plays a central role in the initiation and execution of apoptosis *(4)*. Both, the extrinsic and intrinsic apoptotic pathways lead to activation of a cascade of caspases. Initiator caspases (caspase-2, -8, -9, and -10) autocatalytically initiate the cascade and transmit the apoptotic signal by cleavage and activation of effector caspases (caspase-3, -6, and -7) that in turn mediate DNA fragmentation, chromatin condensation, and membrane blebbing. Caspase-3 appears to be the key effector, which cleaves different other intracellular substrates such as inhibitor of caspase-activated DNase (ICAD), poly-ADP-ribosepolymerase, actin, fodrin, and lamin. Therefore, caspase-3 is the main target for the assessment of apoptosis. Methods to detect activation of caspases include immunoblotting of activated caspases or caspase substrates, enzymatic assays (cleavage of synthetic substrates, specific caspase inhibitors), and measurement of fluorogenic caspase substrates by flow cytometry *(45)*. An enzymatic assay uses a fluorochrome-conjugated tetrapeptide bearing the consensus sequence Asp-Glu-Val-Asp (DEVD) that is recognized by effector caspases. Upon cleavage of the tetrapeptide, fluorescence is enhanced. The enzymatic assay described below is available as a commercial kit from Molecular Probes (Leiden, The Netherlands; *see* **Note 10**).

1. Induce apoptosis in cells, also prepare a control of untreated cells (10^6 cells/sample).
2. Harvest cells and wash with PBS.
3. Dilute the 20X lysis buffer to a 1X working solution (1 mL is sufficient for 20 assays). Resuspend cells in 50 μL of 1X lysis buffer, lyse by subjecting cells to a freeze-thaw cycle (freeze cells in a dry ice/ethanol bath for 5 min, then thaw).
4. Prepare a solution of 2X reaction buffer: Add 400 μL of 5X reaction buffer and 10 μL of 1 *M* dithiothreitol to 590 μL of H_2O. Mix well, precipitation and coalescence of the reagents may be observed (1 mL is sufficient for 20 samples).
5. Centrifuge the lysate at 1000*g* to spin down cellular debris. Transfer 50 μL of the supernatant to individual microplate wells. Use 50 μL of 1X lysis buffer as negative control to determine background fluorescence. As an additional control, the inhibitor Ac-DEVD-CHO can be incubated with caspase-containing samples. Add 1 μL of 1 m*M* Ac-DEVD-CHO and keep for 10 min at room temperature, while the other samples are stored on ice. 1 μL of DMSO can be added to the remaining no-inhibitor samples as a control for DMSO.
6. Prepare a 2X substrate working solution by adding 20 μL of 10 m*M* Z-DEVD-AMC to 980 μL of 2X reaction buffer (*see* **Note 11**).
7. Add 50 μL of 2X substrate working solution to each sample and control wells. Cover the microplate and incubate at room temperature for 30 min.
8. Measure the plate using 342 nm for excitation and 441 nm for emission. Measurements can be performed at several time points.

3.5. Analysis of Protein Expression by Immunoblotting

Immunoblotting is an immunochemical technique based on separating proteins by polyacrylamide gel electrophoresis according to size. Proteins are then immobilized by transferring them to a membrane and finally probing them with a specific antibody. The expression rate of a protein is measured by the optical density of its band compared to beta-actin or other reference proteins *(2)*.

1. Lyse cells using 200 μL of lysis buffer. For cultured human mast cell line-1 (HMC-1) cells, we use 10^7 cells, yielding an average of 1 mg total protein. Total protein can be measured using a Bradford assay.
2. Add 4X loading buffer to the lysate containing 50 μg of protein.

3. Samples are subjected to SDS discontinuous polyacrylamide gel electrophoresis according to Laemmli using electrophoresis buffer and a 15% (m/v) polyacrylamide separating gel.

4. Cut nitrocellulose membrane to the size of the gel. Equilibrate gel in cathode buffer, the membrane in anode buffer II. Cut 10 pieces of filter paper to the size of the gel. Soak four papers in cathode buffer, four papers in anode buffer I, and two papers in anode buffer II. Starting from the anode of the semi-dry blotting chamber, pile four anode buffer I papers, followed by two papers of anode buffer II, the membrane, the PA gel, four cathode buffer papers, and finish with the cathode of the blotting chamber.

5. Apply a current of 1 mA/cm^2 for 1 h. When desired, membrane can be stained with Ponceaux red, gel with Coomassie blue.

6. Wash membrane in dematerialized water.

7. Wash membrane in TBS.

8. Block with blocking solution for 1 h.

9. Incubate with primary antibody in incubation buffer at 4°C overnight.

10. Wash three times for 10 min with TBS.

11. Block with blocking solution for 1 h.

12. Incubate with secondary antibody for 1 h and develop.

13. Shake blot in strip buffer for half an hour at 50°C. Wash twice with TBS buffer. Reblock with blocking solution and reprobe with anti-beta-actin antibody (or other reference antibody) and develop.

14. Expression of the protein is quantified by its optical density using beta-actin as an internal standard.

4. Notes

1. Agarose concentration can vary between 1% and 2% (w/v), according to the separation properties needed. A total of 1.2% (w/v) agarose in TAE buffer is recommended for the start.

2. The major advantage of flow cytometric methods is that they allow to rapidly analyzing large quantities of cells. Because of the large cell numbers measured, quantification of apoptotic cells by flow cytometry is highly reproducible. Combining annexin V staining with other markers also allows calculating the rate of apoptosis of a certain subpopulation of cells.

3. The occurrence of a "DNA ladder" is a characteristic sign of late stages of apoptosis, making it a robust, but not very sensitive (requires an apoptotic rate of at least 20%) method.

4. If samples are lysed in a small volume (e.g., 20 μL per 10^6 cells), precipitation is not obligatory.

5. A standard protocol for agarose gel electrophoresis can be applied: add 1 μL of 10X loading buffer to 9 μL of sample DNA (100 ng/μL). Load samples, positive control, and molecular weight marker into gel pockets; cover gel with TAE buffer; and set voltage to 5 V/cm. Turn off when bromophenol blue has almost reached the anode.

6. Histochemical methods allow localization and morphological evaluation of apoptotic cells. By using TdT, the sensitivity for detection of DNA fragments is increased compared to the analysis using gel electrophoresis. Apoptosis is detected at an earlier stage, because 3'-OH strand breaks occur before complete DNA fragmentation. For flow cytometry, above discussed advantages apply (*see* **Note 2**). False-positive results have been reported, probably due to the occurrence of free 3'-OH ends that are not related to apoptosis.

7. Paraffin-embedded tissue sections are deparaffinized by washing with xylene, ethanol 100%, 95%, 70% (for each step, wash 5 min twice), followed by two 10-min PBS washing steps, treated with proteinase K (20 mg/mL), and finally washed twice with PBS for 5 min.

8. Proper fixation is mandatory to avoid depletion of DNA fragments. Use methanol-free formaldehyde derived from paraformaldehyde.

9. Cells can be stored in ethanol at −20°C for several weeks.

10. Caspase activity is a specific sign of apoptosis. During necrosis, activation of caspases has not been detected so far. However, there are also caspase-independent pathways of apoptosis like the perforin/granzyme pathway. Because different apoptotic pathways are associated with activation of specific caspase subfamilies, analysis of caspase activity allows to differentiate between in- and extrinsic apoptotic pathways.

11. An AMC standard reference curve can be created by diluting the 10 mM AMC with 1X reaction buffer (made from 5X) to solutions ranging from 0 to 100 µM AMC. Apply 100 µL of each standard per well before measuring the plate.

Acknowledgments

We thank C. Berns, Department of Dermatology, University of Cologne, Germany, for excellent technical assistance. This work was supported by a grant from the Wilhelm Sander Foundation (99.049.2) to K. Hartmann.

References

1. Lawen, A. (2003) Apoptosis—an introduction. *Bioessays* **25,** 888–896.
2. Otsuki, Y., Li, Z., and Shibata, M. A. (2003) Apoptotic detection methods—from morphology to gene. *Prog. Histochem. Cytochem.* **38,** 273–339.
3. Danial, N. N. and Korsmeyer, S. J. (2004) Cell death: critical control points. *Cell* **116,** 205–219.
4. Degterev, A., Boyce, M., and Yuan, J. (2003) A decade of caspases. *Oncogene* **22,** 8543–8567.
5. Kirshenbaum, A. S., Kessler, S. W., Goff, J. P., and Metcalfe, D.D. (1991) Demonstration of the origin of human mast cells from CD34+ bone marrow progenitor cells. *J. Immunol.* **146,** 1410–1415.
6. Foedinger, M., Fritsch, G., Winkler, K., et al. (1994) Origin of human mast cells: development from transplanted hematopoetic stem cells after allogenic bone marrow transplantation. *Blood* **84,** 2954–2959.

7. Flanagan, J. G. and Leder, P. (1990) The *c-kit* ligand: a cell surface molecule altered in steel mutant fibroblasts. *Cell* **63,** 185–194.

8. Martin, F.H., Suggs, S. V., and Langely, K. E. (1990) Primary structure and functional expression of rat and human stem cell factor DNAs. *Cell* **63,** 203–211.

9. Iemura, A., Tsai, M., Ando, A., Wershil, B. K., and Galli, S. J. (1994) The c-kit ligand, stem cell factor, promotes mast cell survival by suppressing apoptosis. *Am. J. Pathol.* **144,** 321–328.

10. Mekori, Y. A., Oh, C. K., and Metcalfe, D. D. (1993) IL-3-dependent murine mast cells undergo apoptosis on removal of IL-3. Prevention of apoptosis by c-kit ligand. *J. Immunol.* **151,** 3775–3784.

11. Shelburne, C. P., McCoy, M. E., Piekorz, R., et al. (2003) Stat5 expression is critical for mast cell development and survival. *Blood* **102,** 1290–1297.

12. Mekori, Y. A., Gilfillian, A. M., Akin, C., Hartmann, K., and Metcalfe, D. D. (2001) Human mast cell apoptosis is regulated through Bcl-2 and Bcl-X_L. *J. Clin. Immunol.* **21,** 171–174.

13. Hartmann, K., Artuc, M., Baldus, S. E., et al. (2003) Expression of Bcl-2 and Bcl-X_L in cutaneous and bone marrow lesions of mastocytosis. *Am. J. Pathol.* **163,** 819–826.

14. Yee, N. S., Paek, I., and Besmer, P. (1994) Role of kit-ligand in proliferation and suppression of apoptosis in mast cells: basis for radiosensitivity of white spotting and steel mutant mice. *J. Exp. Med.* **179,** 1777–1787.

15. Valent, P., Besemer, J., Sillaber, C., et al. (1990) Failure to detect IL-3 binding sites on human mast cells. *J. Immunol.* **145,** 3432–3437.

16. Gebhardt, T., Sellge, G., Lorentz, A., Raab, R., Manns, M. P., and Bischoff, S. C. (2002) Cultured human intestinal mast cells express functional IL-3 receptors and respond to IL-3 by enhancing growth and IgE receptor-dependent mediator release. *Eur. J. Immunol.* **32,** 2308–2316.

17. Oskeritzian, C. A., Wang, Z., Kochan, J. P., et al. (1999) Recombinant human (rh) IL-4 –mediated apoptosis and recombinant human IL-6-mediated protection of recombinant human stem cell factor-dependent human mast cells derived from cord blood mononuclear cell progenitors. *J. Immunol.* **163,** 5105–5115.

18. Bischoff, S. C., Sellge, G., Lorentz, A., Sebald, W., Raab, R., and Manns, M. P. (1999) IL-4 enhances proliferation and mediator release in mature human mast cells. *Proc. Natl. Acad. Sci. USA* **96,** 8080–8085.

19. Bailey, D. P., Kashyap, M., Mirmonsef, P., et al. (2004) Interleukin-4 elicits apoptosis of developing mast cells via a Stat6-dependent mitochondrial pathway. *Exp. Hematol.* **32,** 52–59.

20. Oskeritzian, C. A., Zhao, W., Pozez, A. L., Cohen, N. M., Grimes, M., and Schwartz, L. B. (2004) Neutralizing endogenous IL-6 renders mast cells of the MCT type from lung, but not the MCTC type from skin and lung, susceptible to human recombinant IL-4-induced apoptosis. *J. Immunol.* **172,** 593–600.

21. Mekori, Y. A. and Metcalfe, D. D. (1994) Transforming growth factor-beta prevents stem cell factor-mediated rescue of mast cells from apoptosis after IL-3 deprivation. *J. Immunol.* **153,** 2194–2203.

22. Dubois, C. M., Ruscetti, F. W., Stankova, J., and Keller, J. R. (1994) Transforming growth factor-beta regulates *c-kit* message stability and cell-surface protein expression in hematopoetic progenitors. *Blood* **83,** 3138–3145.

23. Kanbe, N., Kurosawa, M., Miyachi, Y., Kanbe, M., Saitoh, H., and Matsuda, H. (2000) Nerve growth factor prevents apoptosis of cord blood-derived human cultured mast cells synergistically with stem cell factor. *Clin. Exp. Allergy* **30,** 1113–1120.

24. Horigome, K., Bullock, E. D., and Johnson, E. M. (1994) Effects of nerve growth factor on rat peritoneal mast cells. Survival promotion and immediate-early gene induction. *J. Biol. Chem.* **269,** 2695–2702.

25. Hartmann, K., Wagelie-Steffen, A. L., von Stebut, E., and Metcalfe, D. D. (1997) Fas (CD95, APO-1) antigen expression and function in murine mast cells. *J. Immunol.* **159,** 4006–4014.

26. Hartmann, K., Worobec, A. S., Bianchine, P. J., Mekori, Y. A., and Metcalfe, D. D. (1996) Expression of Fas antigen on human and on murine mast cell lines: antibody to Fas antigen induces mast cell apoptosis (abstract). *J. Allergy Clin. Immunol.* **97,** 261.

27. Wagelie-Steffen, A. L., Hartmann, K., Vliagoftis, H., and Metcalfe, D. D. (1998) Fas ligand (FasL, C95L, APO-1L) expression in murine mast cells. *Immunology* **94,** 569–574.

28. Kalesnikoff, J., Huber, M., Lam, V., et al. (2001) Monomeric IgE stimulates signaling pathways in mast cells that lead to cytokine production and cell survival. *Immunity* **14,** 801–811.

29. Asai, K., Kitaura, J., Kawakami, Y., et al. (2001) Regulation of mast cell survival by IgE. *Immunity* **14,** 791–800.

30. Kitaura, J., Song, J., Tsai M., et al. (2003) Evidence that IgE molecules mediate a spectrum of effects on mast cell survival and activation via aggregation of FcepsilonRI. *Proc. Natl. Acad. Sci. USA* **100,** 12,911–12,916.

31. Kawakami, T. and Galli, S. J., (2002), Regulation of mast-cell and basophil function and survival by IgE. *Nat. Rev. Immunol.* **2,** 773–786.

32. Supajatura, V. Ushio, H., Nakao, A., Okumura, K., Ra, C., and Ogawa, H. (2001) Protective roles of mast cells against enterobacterial infection are mediated by Toll-like receptor 4. *J. Immunol.* **167,** 2250–2256.

33. McCurdy, J. D., Lin, T. J., and Marshall, J. S. (2001) Toll-like receptor 4-mediated activation of murine mast cells. *J. Leukoc. Biol.* **70,** 977–984.

34. McCurdy, J. D., Olynych, T. J., Maher, L. H., and Marshall, J. S. (2003) Disting Toll-like receptor 2 activators selectively induce different classes of mediator production from human mast cells. *J. Immunol.* **170,** 1625–1629.

35. Yoshikawa, H. and Tasaka, K. (2003) Caspase-dependent and -independent apoptosis of mast cells induced by withdrawal of IL-3 is prevented by Toll-like receptor 4-mediated lipopolysaccharide stimulation. *Eur. J. Immunol.* **33,** 2149–2159.

36. Cervero, C., Escribano, L., San Miguel, J. F., et al. (1999) Expression of Bcl-2 by human bone marrow mast cells and its overexpression in mast cell leukemia. *Am. J. Hematol.* **60,** 191–195.

37. Jordan, J. H., Walchshofer, S., Jurecka, W., et al. (2001) Immunohistochemical properties of bone marrow mast cells in systemic mastocytosis: evidence for expression of CD2, CD117/Kit, and bcl-x(L). *Hum. Pathol.* **32,** 545–552.
38. Hartmann, K., Hermes, B., Rappersberger, K., Sepp, N., Mekori, Y. A., and Henz, B. M. (2003) Evidence for altered mast cell proliferation and apoptosis in cutaneous mastocytosis. *Br. J. Dermatol.* **149,** 554–559.
39. Baldus, S. E., Zirbes, T. K., Thiele, J., Eming, S. A., Henz, B. M., and Hartmann, K. (2004) Altered apoptosis and cell cycling of mast cells in bone marrow lesions of patients with systemic mastocytosis. *Haematologica* **89,** 1525–1527.
40. Nagata, H., Worobec, A. S., Oh, C. K., et al. (1995) Identification of a point mutation in the catalytic domain of the protooncogene c-kit in peripheral blood mononuclear cells of patients who have mastocytosis with an associated hematologic disorder. *Proc. Natl. Acad. Sci. USA* **92,** 10,560–10,564.
41. Vermes, I., Haanen, C., and Reutelingsperger, C. (2000) Flow cytometry of apoptotic cell death. *J. Immunol. Methods* **243,** 167–190.
42. Van Engeland, M., Nieland, L. J. W., Ramaekers, F. C. S., Schutte, B., and Reutelingsperger, C. P. M. (1998) Annexin V-affinity assay: a review on an apoptosis detection system based on phosphatidylserine exposure. *Cytometry* **31,** 1–9.
43. Nagata, S., Nagase, H., Kawane, K., Mukae, N., and Fukuyama, H. (2003) Degradation of chromosomal DNA during apoptosis. *Cell Death Differ.* **10,** 108–116.
44. Willingham, M. C. (1999) Cytochemical methods for the detection of apoptosis. *J. Histochem. Cytochem.* **47,** 1101–1109.
45. Köhler, C., Orrenius, S., and Zhivotovsky, B. (2002) Evaluation of caspase activity in apoptotic cells. *J. Immunol. Methods* **265,** 97–110.

Index